ADVANCED DIGESTIVE ENDOSCOPY:
PRACTICE AND SAFETY

ADVANCED DIGESTIVE ENDOSCOPY: PRACTICE AND SAFETY

EDITED BY

PETER B. COTTON

Blackwell
Publishing

© 2008 by Blackwell Publishing
Blackwell Publishing, Inc., 350 Main Street, Malden, Massachusetts 02148-5020, USA
Blackwell Publishing Ltd, 9600 Garsington Road, Oxford OX4 2DQ, UK
Blackwell Publishing Asia Pty Ltd, 550 Swanston Street, Carlton, Victoria 3053, Australia

The right of the Author to be identified as the Author of this Work has been asserted in accordance with the
Copyright, Designs and Patents Act 1988.

First published 2008
1   2008

Library of Congress Cataloging-in-Publication Data

Advanced digestive endoscopy : practice and safety / edited by Peter B. Cotton.
      p. ; cm. – (Advanced digestive endoscopy)
   Includes bibliographical references and index.
   ISBN 978-1-4051-5858-9 (alk. paper)
   1. Endoscopy.   2. Digestive organs–Diseases–Diagnosis.   I. Cotton, Peter B.   II. Series.
   [DNLM: 1. Endoscopy, Digestive System–methods.   2. Digestive System Diseases–diagnosis.
3. Endoscopy, Digestive System–standards.   WI 141 A244 2008]
   RC804.E6A38 2008
   616.3'07545–dc22

                                                                               2007050630

ISBN: 978-1-4051-5858-9

A catalogue record for this title is available from the British Library

Set in 10/13.5 Sabon by Graphicraft Limited, Hong Kong
Printed and bound in Singapore by COS Printers Pte Ltd

For further information on Blackwell Publishing, visit our website:
http://www.blackwellpublishing.com

The publisher's policy is to use permanent paper from mills that operate a sustainable forestry policy, and
which has been manufactured from pulp processed using acid-free and elementary chlorine-free practices.
Furthermore, the publisher ensures that the text paper and cover board used have met acceptable
environmental accreditation standards.

Contents

List of contributors

AABAKKEN, LARS *Department of Medicine, Rikshospitalet, N-0027 Oslo, Norway*

COHEN, JONATHAN *524 East 72nd Street, Apt 30DE, New York, NY 10021, USA*

COTTON, PETER B. *Medical University of South Carolina, PO Box 250327, Ste 210 CSB, 96 Jonathan Lucas Street, Charleston, SC 29425, USA*

COWEN, ALISTAIR *Emeritus Consultant Gastroenterologist, Royal Brisbane Hospital, Brisbane, Australia*

EVANS, JONATHAN S. *Nemours Childrens Clinic, Division of Pediatric GI & Nutrition, 807Nira Street, Jacksonville, FL 32207, USA*

FARIN, GUENTER *Kapellenweg 9, D-72070 Tuebingen, Germany*

GINSBERG, GREGORY G. *Gastroenterology Division, Hospital of the University of Pennsylvania, 3 Ravdin Building, 3400 Spruce Street, Philadelphia, PA 19104, USA*

GRUND, KARL E. *Professor of Surgery, Department of Surgical Endoscopy, Center for Medical Research, Eberhard-Karls University, University Hospital Tuebingen, Germany*

JONES, DIANNE *Logan Hospital, Queensland, Australia*

LEWIN, DAVID N. *Associate Professor of Pathology, Medical University of South Carolina, Pathology and Laboratory Medicine Services, Charleston, SC 29425, USA*

MAHAJAN, LORI *Fellowship Director, Department of Pediatric. Gastroenterology and Nutrition, Cleveland Clinic Children's Hospital, Cleveland, Ohio, USA*

OTT, BEVERLY *Endoscopy Systems Coordinator, Mayo Clinic, Rochester, MN 55905, USA*

PETERSEN, BRET T. *Mayo Clinic, Division of GI/Hepatology, 200 First Street SW, West 19-A, Rochester, MN 55905, USA*

VALORI, ROLAND *National Clinical Lead for Endoscopy in England, Gloucestershire Royal Hospital, Gloucester, UK*

VARGO, JOHN J. *Cleveland Clinic Foundation, Department of GI, Desk S40, 9500 Euclid Avenue, Cleveland, OH 44195, USA*

CHAPTER 1

Overview

PETER B. COTTON

Flexible endoscopy is now a major diagnostic and therapeutic tool in the management of patients with digestive disorders. It was not always so. The discovery of X-rays just over 100 years ago led quickly to the development of the 'barium meal'. This, and the barium enema, rapidly became the workhorses for the diagnosis of luminal disease. Proctoscopy gave visual access to the anus and rectum, and rigid esophagoscopes were used by a few intrepid surgeons, at some risk. The preoccupation of the Japanese with gastric cancer (and their well-known engineering talents) led to the development of gastro-cameras in the 1950s and 1960s, which were used (along with barium radiology) in massive screening programs. 'Semi-flexible' gastroscopes were developed in the mid-part of the century, but did not achieve widespread use, because they were cumbersome and the views were incomplete.

The key modern landmark was the harnessing of fiberoptics in the 1960s. Pioneering work in Britain and USA allowed the development of truly flexible endoscopes, which greatly facilitated esophagoscopy and gastroscopy, and allowed further exploration of the small intestine and the whole colon. Video-endoscopy added an important new dimension, since the images could be widely shared. The ability to take target biopsies added scientific respectability to procedures which were initially ignored, even ridiculed, by the academic establishment. The development and dissemination of a large variety of therapeutic procedures catapulted endoscopy into the mainstream of gastroenterology (and surgery).

The endoscopy success story brought growing pains and increasing responsibilities. What started for many of us 30 or more years ago as an amusing sideline has now become a huge and complex business. We started with one endoscope in a side-room, sometimes with the assistance of a passing nurse, understanding little about the complexities of the tools we were testing, or the diseases we were exploring. We had a naïve belief that only good could come from our activities, with little concept of infection control, the complexities of safe sedation, or how to run an efficient unit.

Now it is universally accepted that high-quality endoscopy demands a sophisticated organization. Patients expect their procedures to be successful and comfortable, and with minimal risk. Fully trained and accredited endoscopists work with expert professional staff, using optimal equipment, in purpose-designed endoscopy units. We need to understand many things outside gastroenterology, such as electrosurgery, lasers, computers, image management, pathology, radiology, and ultrasound, as well as infection control and sedation. Endoscopy unit managers have to be skilled in leadership, business principles, efficiency, and quality improvement.

This book is intended to provide practical guidance for all those attempting to offer (and to teach) quality endoscopy services. This complements and builds on our popular basic book *Practical Gastrointestinal Endoscopy – the fundamentals*, now in it's 6th edition. The material in this Advanced Endoscopy series will be updated regularly, and comments are always welcome. I am delighted that so many distinguished colleagues have kindly agreed to share their wisdom on these important topics, to help us in our goal of delivering optimal endoscopic care.

CHAPTER 2

Design and management of gastrointestinal endoscopy units

BRET T. PETERSEN AND BEVERLY OTT

Synopsis

The specialty of gastrointestinal endoscopy has evolved to the point where it requires specific attention to many aspects of facility design and unit management. Important design elements that require consideration include regulatory mandates, space planning, and infrastructure for health-care facilities, with specific attention to water supplies, forced air, vacuum capability, and waste disposal. Experience has generated numerous specific recommendations for design of the individual portions of the endoscopy suite to enhance both quality and efficiency. Administrative oversight is required for issues specific to physician, nursing, and business concerns. Besides those tasks common to most of health care (such as licensure, competency, and personnel issues) administrative arenas include scheduling of procedures and staff; purchasing of endoscopes, therapeutic devices, and endoscopic databases; reprocessing of endoscopes and related infection control issues; accreditation; efficiency and quality improvement efforts.

Introduction

The growth of gastrointestinal endoscopy as a specialized activity within health care has increased the need for specialization in both facility design and management skills. Historically, endoscopic facilities grew within hospital environments, often using existing patient rooms or wards and the existing skills of generic hospital personnel. Administration was commonly assumed by hospital-based departments responsible for surgical suites or emergency departments, with academic attachments to departments of medicine or surgery. The increasing demand for greater volume and complexity of services commonly strained these original arrangements. This led to the design of purpose-specific facilities and greater specialization by staff and administrators. The subsequent evolution from specialized hospital-based units to office endoscopy and accredited ambulatory surgical centers led to further complexity in the planning and administration of endoscopy units. This chapter will review the broad elements of facility design and unit administration that are important for successful development of a gastrointestinal endoscopy unit today.

Some elements particular to ambulatory surgical centers (ASCs) will be mentioned or referenced. Ambulatory endoscopy centers (AECs) are ASCs specific to one specialty, but they share essentially the same regulatory and design issues. There are extensive published and commercial guides regarding development of such units and professional consultation is typically useful during their planning [1]. This outline should not be considered definitive guidance on issues pertinent to their establishment or administration.

Unit design

A variety of external standards dictate the design of facilities for endoscopic services [2]. Architectural guidelines pertaining to construction of health-care facilities, including ambulatory centers, come from local and state building and fire codes, medicare mandates, accrediting organizations, and the industry standards espoused by the American Institute of Architecture [3]. They vary in specificity, but are generally coherent and well-known to architects working in the health-care field. Facility licensure and medicare certification require strict attention to the details of design [4]. Inquiry about requirements and guidance regarding details should be sought from state agencies that will be providing licensure. In many states there is a requirement to obtain a certificate of need (CON) prior to construction. This approval process confirms the regional or local need for an additional new facility.

Important elements requiring close attention pertain to infrastructure, people, equipment, supplies, and services. Table 2.1 delineates many of the various elements that fall into these categories. Most of them are generic to health care, while some are highly peculiar to sedation-based endoscopy practices, training environments, etc. Each should be considered both separately and as part of the whole. While not all are pertinent in every endoscopy unit, their consideration will ensure that major needs are not overlooked.

Space planning

Architectural form has a major influence on the function of a facility. Considerations given to the space allocated to specific activities, and their adjacency or proximity, greatly affect the resulting efficiency, and even safety, of the services delivered in the environment.

When considering development of a new or remodeled facility, two of the most important considerations pertain to the space available for the project and

Table 2.1 Design and space considerations

Consideration and planning is required for the following elements pertaining to the infrastructure, people, equipment, supplies, and services during design and planning of an endoscopy facility. Many elements require specifically designated locations and space.

Space
- Space: to efficiently accommodate people, current activities, growth (see Table 2.2)
- Adjacency, proximity
- Flow: of patients, staff, equipment, biologic samples, waste, etc.
- Entries and exits for patients and staff

Infrastructure
- Utilities: electrical, HVAC, wet and dry (clean/soiled) vacuum; oxygen, compressed air, anesthesia gases
- Communications: internet, intranet, phone, dictation, call systems for emergency or assistance, visual systems (lights) for monitoring current room use, endoscope or patient status, alarm systems

People
- Patients and family: arrival, waiting rooms, restrooms
  - Specific accommodation may be required for patients with various disabilities, paralysis, overweight, etc.
  - Secure, tamper-evident storage for patient belongings
- Staff: nursing, physicians, receptionists, administrative, housekeeping, transcription
  - Private phone/work space: nursing, physicians, fellows
  - Lockers, changing, coat/personal item storage
  - Break area
  - Conferences/training
- Professional/academic visitors
- Vendors

Equipment
- Endoscopes, light sources, image processors
  - Accommodation for equipment care and upkeep
  - Specialized storage, closets, etc.
  - Space for repair or shipping and receiving
- Image recording/printing devices vs. infrastructure
- Reprocessing machines for endoscopes/devices
- Disposable vs. reusable endoscopic devices
- Stretchers: in use and spare
- Wheelchairs, lifts
- Fluoroscopy equipment
- Anesthesia equipment: in use, storage
- Resuscitation equipment: code cart

Supplies
- Linens: clean, dirty, hamper space per room
- Biological samples, containers: prep, storage, and transport
- Reprocessing fluids
- Disposables: i.e. personal protective ware, etc.
- Medications: controlled and non-controlled substances

Continued p. 6

Table 2.1 (*cont'd*)

Services
- IV starts, lab drawing
- Colon preparation
- Documentation of care
- Consultation
- Conferences/education
- Emergency care/resuscitation
- Fluoroscopy
- Procedural components
  - Check-in, procedure, recovery
  - Changing area
  - Patient lockers or tamper-evident bags to secure clothing storage
  - Procedure waiting: ambulatory or inpatient; chairs vs. stretchers
  - Sedation and analgesia; anesthesia services
- GI endoscopy vs. mixed services/specialties
  - Colonoscopy/EGD
  - ERCP; other fluoro based
  - EUS
  - Capsule endoscopy
  - Esophageal/other manometry
  - Breath testing
  - Pancreatic function testing
  - Bronchoscopy/other non-GI testing

the spectrum and volume of services that must be provided by the facility. Space projections should include the likelihood for growth in volume and potential expansion of services over 5–8 years, allowing for construction of a facility that can either accommodate growth or expand into adjacent space. Considerations of space are among the most difficult and carry the greatest implications for overall construction costs.

Anticipated procedure volumes provide useful space estimates based on planned procedure-room utilization rates and ratios of procedure rooms to waiting spaces and recovery beds [2]. Facilities intended for modest numbers of procedures can utilize space more flexibly than those with significant requirements for patient throughput and efficiency of personnel (Fig. 2.1). Small units often share public and clinical space with other departments that require similar accommodations for waiting, reception, pre- and postprocedure patient care, and administrative services. Examples include small emergency departments, outpatient surgery services, cardiology, pulmonary, or urological procedural areas. Note that ASC guidelines strictly detail which spaces can be shared, with which type of service, and which must be distinct. For instance waiting rooms, entries, and patient care areas must be distinct and separate from contiguous office space, but some staff facilities/break rooms, etc. can be shared [2].

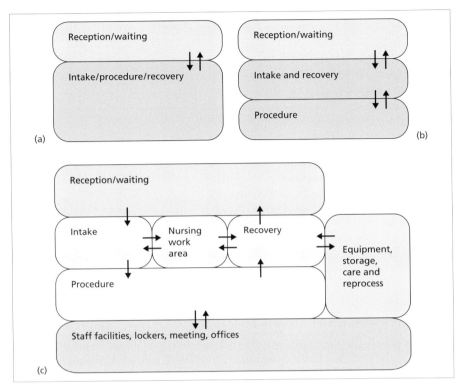

Fig. 2.1 Generic proximity considerations for (a) small, (b) medium, and (c) large units.

Hospital endoscopy is typically less efficient and more space consuming than practice in ambulatory settings due to the mix of inpatients and outpatients and the greater intensity of services required. A variety of ratios pertaining to ancillary activities (such as waiting room capacity per procedure room, recovery capacity per procedure room, etc.) have been used to assist with estimating space needs (Table 2.2) [5].

Daily room volumes

Daily procedure volumes per room vary greatly by type of procedure, patient characteristics, ancillary staffing levels, and process issues such as whether an individual endoscopist works out of one room or two. For high-volume general gastrointestinal endoscopy, daily volumes *per room* can vary from 6 to 10 when physicians use dual rooms and up to 12 or more when they work out of a single room. This equates to 1500–3000 procedures per room, annually [6]. Detailed analysis of procedure types and their mean durations are helpful for estimating

Table 2.2 Ratios for estimating space needs of ancillary functions

Ancillary function	Ratio
Waiting room chairs per procedure room	4–5
Intake beds or stretcher bays per procedure room	1–2
Recovery beds per procedure room based on standard moderate sedation with narcotic and benzodiazepine	1.5–2
Procedure rooms per endoscopist	1–2 colons
	1–3 EGD
	1 ERCP, EUS
Annual volume per procedure room	≥1000+
Space per procedure room: EGD, colonoscopy	220 sq. ft (20 m^2)
Space per procedure room: miscellaneous complex	350+ sq. ft (33+ m^2)
Space per procedure room: ERCP, fluoroscopy	400+ sq. ft (37+ m^2)
Space per recovery bed	60–80 sq. ft (5.6–7.4 m^2)
Space per waiting room chair	15 sq. ft (1.4 m^2)
Space per office	90–120 sq. ft (8.4–11.1 m^2)
Space per examination/consultation room	100–120 sq. ft (9.3–11.1 m^2)

realistic capacities per procedure room and, globally, per unit [5]. For AECs this is straightforward due to the narrow spectrum of procedures performed on relatively well patients. In the hospital setting considerations for both basic and complex procedures in frail and ill patients make estimating more challenging. Procedure and room turnover times specific to the facility and physician mix should be used if available.

Procedure room size

Similarly, space requirements per procedure room vary based upon the antici-pated activity it will need to accommodate [7]. General procedures employing standard moderate sedation without the need for anesthesia monitoring are efficiently accomplished in about 220 square feet (20 m^2). Complex procedures require more equipment and room for more personnel, and are best planned for rooms of 300–350 square feet (28–33 m^2). Fluoroscopy-based procedures can be accommodated in 400 square feet (37 m^2) but often benefit from even larger rooms due to the need for extra rolling equipment, storage for devices, and accommodation for anesthesia. Further comments on individual room design are provided below.

Preparation and recovery ratios

Higher-volume units employing traditional sedation and analgesia work efficiently with one intake space per endoscopist and 1.5–2 recovery beds per procedure room. Adoption of sedation practices utilizing rapidly metabolized sedation agents (propofol, and others) can reduce the need for recovery space but may require larger procedure rooms, depending on the involvement of anesthesia personnel and their equipment requirements in the given facility. Larger-volume units with need for greater efficiency require relatively greater space to accommodate thoroughfares for optimal patient and staff flow. Ideally, alert preprocedure and sedated postprocedure patients are separated in waiting, recovery, and transport areas. The benefit of dual hallways for this purpose is rarely realized due to space constraints.

Separate entrances

Separate entrances for staff access to and from patient-occupied areas help achieve staging for patient care while avoiding unnecessary staff traffic in view of waiting patients and families. In addition, should a problem occur, the separate staff paths for entry and exiting the suite can be utilized for emergency personnel entering the unit or to transport patients from the unit.

Common space problems

Space-planning inefficiencies that are sometimes foisted on staff in endoscopic procedure facilities include:

1 overconsumption of space for very routine procedure rooms, with lost and inefficient square footage between walls and equipment;

2 inadequate space in rooms designed for complex procedures, especially those employing fluoroscopy or other varieties of portable devices or carts;

3 inadequate storage for bulky spare or intermittently utilized equipment (patient lifts, extra monitors, portable recording equipment, argon plasma devices, lasers, etc.);

4 inadequate space for anesthesia staff and equipment at the head of the bed and for storage of anesthesia equipment;

5 inadequate allowance for dictating, conferencing, and downtime of staff and professional visitors.

Physical infrastructure

Most of the infrastructure required for an endoscopy unit, such as electrical, plumbing, and HVAC services, is standard for health-care facilities or ASCs. Infrastructure for communication systems and networking for electronic medical records, image documentation, intranet, etc. is becoming standard.

Particular enhancements must be provided for adequacy of ventilation in reprocessing areas and of vacuum suction in the procedure rooms. Ventilation air exchange rates must maintain ambient levels of reprocessing agent fumes below rigidly defined levels. Vacuum capacity may need local boosters or auxiliary units to accommodate the number and spectrum of active rooms in a unit at any one time. Most facilities use standard 'medical' or 'clean' in-wall vacuum suction attached to disposable waste traps in the room. A useful alternative that may reduce supply expenses, room clutter, and nursing tasks is use of a wet vacuum system which evacuates fluid waste directly into the sewage system. These systems eliminate the need for suction canisters and the infection control issues related to their emptying or disposal. Periodic flushing of lines (1–3 times per week) with a cleaning agent is recommended. Systems can be purchased for a single room or for a suite, floor, or building.

Most endoscope reprocessors are equipped with relatively expensive micron pore filters for removal of bacteria from rinse water. The useful life of these filters can be lengthened with the installation of one or two inexpensive sediment filters in the water supply line to remove larger particles before the water reaches the micron filter. Financial savings can be achieved by having the sediment filters installed on water lines coming to the suite as opposed to lines feeding each endoscope reprocessor.

Intake and recovery areas

The design of facilities for patient intake and recovery varies greatly, based on available space and whether or not the patients are ambulatory. In many units these two activities are combined in one area to allow mobility of space and staff between them. This approach yields maximal flexibility in limited space. We have long maintained separate areas for these activities in order to maintain simplicity and specificity of design, patient confidentiality, and space conservation in the intake area.

Intake areas

Like all hospital-based units, many ambulatory facilities also perform their intake activities while patients are recumbent on a stretcher in hospital attire. This relegates the individual to an unfamiliar and less comfortable patient status early in his or her visit. In contrast we believe it is both efficient and respectful to have patients check-in while still clothed. Subsequently, they change to hospital attire and await their procedure separated by gender in a typically chairbased lounge. They are then escorted to the procedure room where identification is again confirmed before they assume a recumbent position. This approach facilitates family participation in the preprocedure interview and saves on space in the preprocedure area, utilizing about 15 square feet (1.4 m^2) per chair as opposed to 60–80 square feet (5.6–7.4 m^2) per stretcher.

Check-in cubicles can be relatively small (30–40 square feet (2.8–3.7 m^2)) and clustered in close proximity to the entry and changing areas. Their design is analogous to other stations in our institution for performance of phlebotomy or check-in at blood banking areas. They must be designed to preserve confidentiality and to accommodate wheelchairs and an accompanying individual. Requirements include a partial desk or counter for writing and sit-down access to a computer terminal and two chairs. Partial enclosure with three solid walls for improved sound proofing plus one curtain wall can suffice. Full four-walled rooms with doors are generally unnecessary and inefficient.

Managing clothes and valuables

To minimize the space requirement for lockers in the changing area and the need for a patient and nurse escort to return to the check-in changing area prior to departure, patients retain their clothing and accompanying valuables in a tamper-evident plastic bag throughout their visit. In the procedure room the bag is placed in a lockable pouch attached to each stretcher (PHS West, Hanover, MN) where it remains until they redress in the recovery area.

Recovery facilities

Recovery areas can utilize reclining chairs, stretcher bays, or hospital beds. For many years our recovery practice was primarily chair-based due to space constraints, but with the increasing depth of sedation, the frailty of some patients, and enhanced space in new units we have changed to predominantly stretcher-based recovery. Further evolution to propofol sedation could stimulate a return to brief observation intervals in reclining chairs. Facilities serving ambulatory patients with relatively fast turnaround do well with narrow stretcher bays separated by curtains, in which accompanying family members are not well accommodated. Each bay must have monitoring capabilities, emergency call systems and full electronic access to databases and the electronic medical record. Confidential conversations are not pursued in this environment, so a neighboring room for consultation with patients and family is necessary. One bathroom for approximately six recovery bays should be available for changing to street clothes.

In our practice patients undergoing ERCPs and liver biopsy recover in a shared 'short-stay' or 'ambulatory' surgery recovery facility, where family members can easily join the patient for up to several hours of observation. Similar space accommodations can be made in dedicated GI units for those patients in whom observation will be prolonged.

Procedure room reprocessing and storage

The design of individual procedure rooms should be based on careful considerations of their intended use, the tasks of each of the staff members working in the room, need for proximity of equipment and staff to the patient, need for maintenance of relatively clean vs. soiled areas, and patient considerations for safety and ambience. Space requirements are discussed above.

Standard procedure rooms

Generic upper and lower gastrointestinal endoscopy is efficiently performed in relatively smaller rooms with most equipment and storage positioned against the walls [5]. Physician/endoscopist and nurse/assistant areas of activity can be delineated around the patient, who is located in the center of the room. These regions overlap but are largely distinct (Fig. 2.2). Requisite equipment for each individual's activities should be positioned within or accessible to their regions of work. Both endoscopist and nursing areas encompass soiled and clean areas. Separate computer terminals should be provided for the nursing and physician functions. The endoscopist's terminal can be within or just outside of the room,

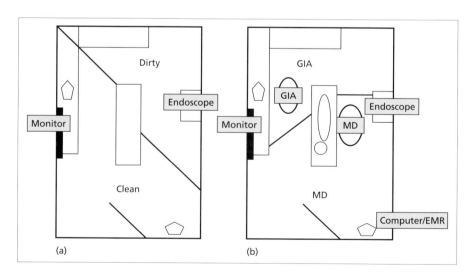

Fig. 2.2 Room design considerations. (a) Clean and dirty regions of the endoscopy room. (b) Functional physician and nursing areas. Note dual computer terminals for electronic medical record and endoscopy database.

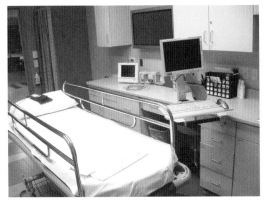

(a)

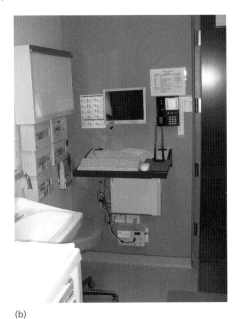

Fig. 2.3 Room pictures of nursing and physician workstations. Note proximity of the nurse's terminal to the patient for ongoing documentation of clinical details of patient monitoring and procedural elements.

(b)

but a nurse's terminal should be in close proximity to the patient and should not require turning away from the patient to access patient medical records or to complete documentation required in the course of the exam (Fig. 2.3). Phones and hand-washing sinks should be accessible to both staff.

Scope reprocessing and storage

Decisions regarding the desired flow of patients and endoscopes influence the design and space requirements. Current architectural standards dictate that endoscope reprocessing areas be located outside of the procedure room. Many units locate endoscope cleaning and reprocessing in nearby anterooms serving only 1–3 procedure rooms (Fig. 2.4), while others employ single dedicated cleaning rooms for the entire suite. The lapsed time from extubation to scope reprocessing will be affected by the location and distance to the reprocessing area as well as by staffing patterns. When the reprocessing room is distant from the procedure room, sinks and space for initial rinsing of soiled equipment

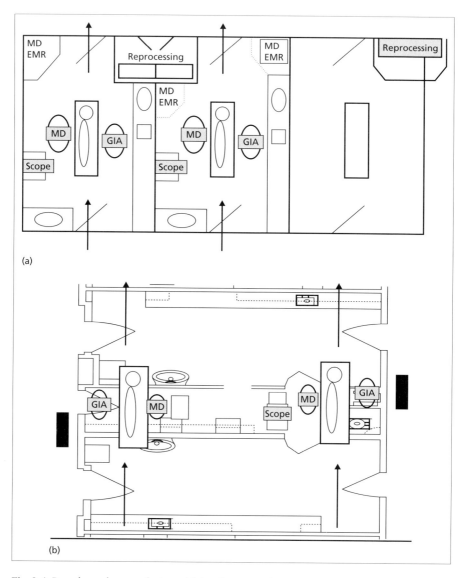

Fig. 2.4 Pass through room design with local reprocessing anterooms. (a) Design options. (b, c) Final design and photo of our reprocessing corridors, which are located between every two general procedure rooms. (d, e, f) Other reprocessing anterooms employed in our units.

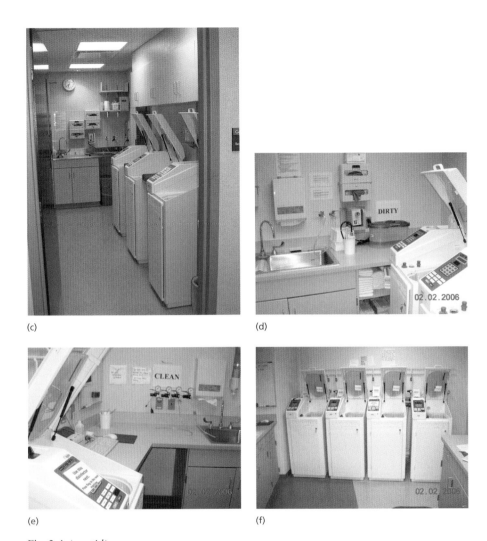

(c)

(d)

(e)

(f)

Fig. 2.4 (cont'd)

(precleaning) should be available in the procedure room. A 'dirty-to-clean' flow of endoscopes and equipment should be maintained in the reprocessing and equipment areas to avoid cross-contamination between soiled and newly cleaned instruments. Adequate counter space on both sides of cleaning areas must be available to accommodate one or more instruments. Counter space with compressed air for drying should be nearby.

Endoscope storage requires a location where instruments can be hung freely without coiling or risk of entrapment by drawers or doors. This does not require significant space. Proprietary cabinets incorporating ventilation and temperature control are available. We employ shallow cabinets lined with brackets that are embedded in the walls of hallways for greater accessibility to all staff. In-room storage is only used for specialty procedure rooms (ERCP and EUS) and storage of prototype and study instruments (Fig. 2.5).

Patient flow issues

Patient flow within the procedure room is largely dictated by door and equipment location. Large units seeking to separate pre- and postprocedure patients employ separate doors at each end of the room for arrival of alert ambulatory patients and departure of wheeled sedated patients on gurneys (Fig. 2.4). This requires additional space for dual hallways. Similarly, larger rooms for complex or fluoroscopic procedures should have an entry at each end for arrival and departure of staff or equipment during the procedures.

Complex procedure rooms

Complex and fluoroscopy-based procedures generally employ greater varieties and numbers of additional devices, often each with their own mobile console. The ability to move additional systems near or far requires adequate space to accommodate movement of ancillary staff around the outside of the equipment near the perimeter of the room (Fig. 2.6). The placement of utilities serving the equipment becomes problematic in larger rooms, as the presence of electrical cords and suction devices on the floor or spanning throughways generates risks to the staff. Options for provision of the utilities to the bedside include mid-floor and ceiling-based utility pillars serving mobile endoscopy carts or semi-mobile hanging bays for stacks of equipment, as has become standard in modern surgical suite. The latter approach keeps the floor clear but requires an even greater space allowance. Anesthesia utilities may be supplied via ceiling attachments for flexible hoses when their use will be relatively intermittent, or via the semimobile hanging bays typical in the operating room. The latter requires greater accommodation for space.

Storage of supplies and medications

Several options are available for in-room storage of linens, commonly used disposables, and other supplies. Adequate quantities of the generic moderate- to high-volume items should be kept in the room to serve only 1–2 days of practice, with daily restocking. This practice can minimize the potential for over-stocking and ordering. It will also minimize the potential waste of accessories by an improved rotation of stock, with the ability to check expiration dates in the primary storage area. Rarely used non-emergency items that may be required

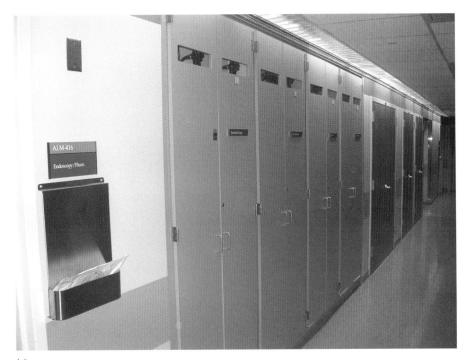

(a)

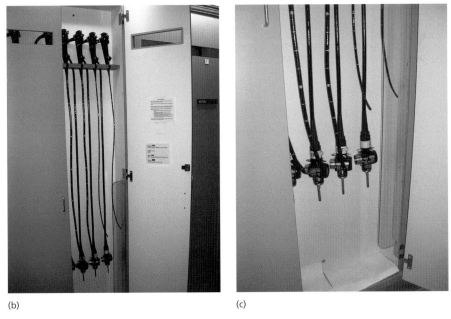

(b)   (c)

Fig. 2.5 (a, b) Endoscope storage in-wall option. (c) Detail demonstrating protective barrier for endoscope tips and placement of paper towels for daily assessment of overnight water dripping. Any evidence of water stains prompts repeated reprocessing in the morning before use.

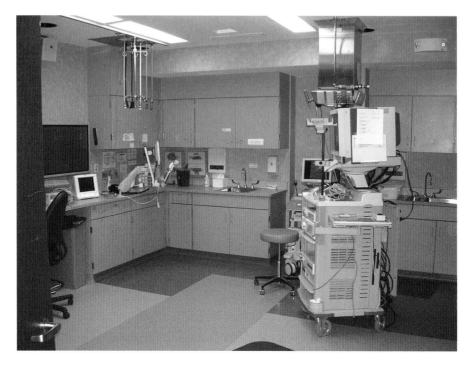

Fig. 2.6 Large complex room design.

in any of several rooms should be kept in a common storage area for the entire suite. Both low- and high-volume specialty items used in only a single room (as with ERCP or EUS equipment) should be efficiently accessible within or very near that specific room. Fluoroscopy rooms dedicated to ERCP practice have the greatest need for organized accessible storage of innumerable devices. Organization can be accomplished with bins, peg-board hanging storage, slotted cupboards, and drawers (Fig. 2.7), or proprietary inventory management systems analogous to pharmaceutical systems noted below. Labeling and lighting should accommodate identification of equipment in dim rooms employing fluoroscopy.

Locked storage and access to pharmaceuticals for both regular and infrequent use should be carefully considered. Options include in-room locked drawers or cabinets with supplies checked out to each nurse for each shift and in-room or unit-wide computerized dispensers (Pyxis Products, Cardinal Health, Inc., San Diego, CA) that are commonly networked to hospital-wide pharmacy systems. Non-controlled medications and intravenous fluid supplies should be kept locked either in the room or in a central storage area, depending upon the frequency and urgency of use.

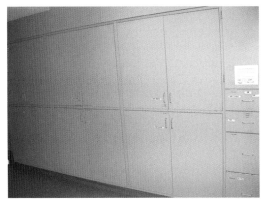

(a)

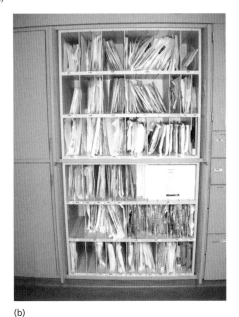

Fig. 2.7 (a, b) Storage for ERCP devices, employing slotted cabinets with recessed doors and labeling for daily 'par' stock control using electronic wands.

(b)

Travel carts for emergencies

Mobile carts are available for transporting the essential elements of the procedure suite to the bedside in the emergency room or intensive care unit. We utilize a self-powered (motorized) design that allows a single nurse to safely drive all equipment to distant locations of the hospital (PHS West, Hanover, MN) (Fig. 2.8). A larger primary cart carries the light source, endoscopes, devices, drugs, and most accessories. A smaller non-powered cart for the monitor and disposable protective equipment links to the larger cart during transportation and separates for positioning across the bed from the endoscopist during the procedure. Vacuum capabilities are generally available in all patient

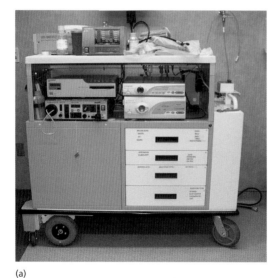

(a)

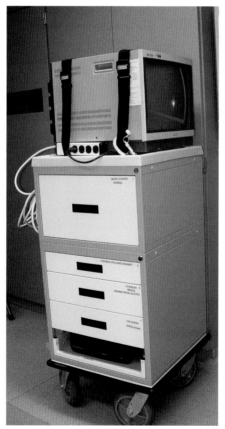

(b)

Fig. 2.8 Mobile cart used for transport of endoscopic services to distant areas throughout the hospital. (a) The main self-powered module containing most equipment. (b) Smaller non-powered module that is linked to the larger unit during travel and unlinked for procedure performance.

areas served. Databases can be linked to the central servers via wireless systems or via hospital-wide intranet jacks.

Unit management

With the trend toward specialization of procedure units there has been a corollary specialization of the administrative tasks for optimal function of such units. Administrative structures will vary greatly depending upon the business model, ownership, and setting of the unit. A variety of structures can function well, as long as the major areas of responsibility are adequately addressed and sufficient communication occurs between the respective roles. Most administrative structures incorporate significant overlap in responsibilities and rely on collaboration in the administration of medical/physician, nursing, and business arenas.

Major areas of responsibility

The major responsibilities of the administrative team are delineated in Table 2.3. Specific comments pertaining to several of these areas of responsibility are

Table 2.3 Major administrative responsibilities for a gastrointestinal endoscopy unit

Medical administration
- Physician credentialing, privileging, calendars
- Definition and maintenance of professional standards
- Sentinel events; complication/outcome tracking; proctoring

Nursing and allied health staff administration
- Hiring, credentialing, training of staff
- Maintenance/demonstration of competency
- Staffing
- Nursing care planning
- Policies and procedures

Other responsibilities variably assigned between physician, nursing, and business administrators
- Purchasing
  - Capital equipment (endoscopes, computers, communications, fluoroscopy, etc.)
  - Software (databases, image management)
  - Devices
- Schedules/calendars
- Medication control
- Equipment maintenance, repair
- Infection control/instrument reprocessing
- Coding and billing
- Accounting
- Accreditation
- Quality Improvement

provided below. Those commonly delegated to the medical administrator include credentialing, privileging, and maintenance/oversight of professional standards for the physician or other professional endoscopists. Many of these issues are managed by a central medical staff office of physician affairs for hospital-based units, while freestanding ambulatory facilities need to attend to them individually.

Responsibilities commonly delegated to the nursing administrator include development and maintenance of nursing care plans, hiring, credentialing, privileging, training, staffing, and maintenance of competencies for nurses and other allied health staff. This individual or their assistant will have significant responsibility for personnel management of the nursing staff. In a hospital setting this is often shared with professionals from the human resources department. Smaller units often place both overall unit management and nursing administration in the hands of the same individual, whereas this would exceed the capacity of one individual in larger units. Reprocessing and repair of equipment is commonly overseen by this member of the team or another staff member with focused expertise.

Administrative tasks that may fall to the medical administrator, head nurse, or a trained business administrator are numerous. They include purchasing (of capital equipment, reusable or disposable devices, and consumables), coding, billing, accounting, image management and electronic medical record databases, and general unit function. Management of non-nursing personnel may fall to this individual as well.

Staffing design

Major staffing issues that influence both efficiency and costs pertain to the level of caregivers employed for varying tasks and the number of staff assigned per room, per physician, or per volume of procedures. Many units staff all procedure rooms with a full-time registered nurse (RN) to administer sedation and monitor the patient and a full-time licensed practical nurse (LPN) or technician as a gastrointestinal assistant (GIA) for assisting with endoscopic interventions. Nursing functions must be in line with state 'scope-of-practice' laws relative to patient monitoring vs. assessment and medication administration. Such rules may vary between settings and states. We staff 1.5 LPNs per general procedure (EGD and colonoscopy) suite, where one staff member monitors patient comfort, vitals, response to medication, and procedural interventions; one joins in to assist with endoscopic interventions; and an RN is available to respond at a moment's notice via a call system in each room. The physician retains global responsibility for assessment, medication management, and initial medication administration. In our advanced procedure suites (ERCP, EUS, miscellaneous complex procedures) and for general procedures in high-risk patients, an RN performs both the monitoring and assessment tasks, an LPN serves as the technical GIA, and the physician retains the responsibility for medication management but not administration.

Nursing staff are also required for the preprocedure assessment and the recovery/dismissal tasks. Other personnel commonly employed in larger units include technical assistants for endoscope reprocessing, skilled technicians for endoscope and other equipment servicing and minor repairs, patient scheduler, and reception and secretarial staff.

Overall staffing levels for endoscopy units can be managed based on indices of productivity, such as procedure unit volume per employee, average total employee hours per procedure [8] or procedure relative value units (RVUs) per non-physician employee. Many varied staff schedules can be used to cover shift responsibilities. Flexibility in staffing for the extremes of high and low demand is useful for the unit manager.

Staffing emergencies

Plans should be made for staffing emergency procedures, both during the workday and during off hours of nights and weekends. If unscheduled procedures are infrequent this activity may be easily absorbed into the existing workday calendar. Many units leave the after-hours technical role of set-up, reprocessing, and procedural assisting to the endoscopist or trainee plus available float staff; however, this diminishes both quality and safety of the procedure and potentially the efficacy of reprocessing. Some units schedule a part time late shift that routinely covers those scheduled procedures that run late plus all emergencies until the morning. We schedule one LPN/GIA to cover emergencies at all times of the day and night for 3–4 day stretches (two per week). They are responsible for transporting the mobile endoscopy cart when necessary, and for the usual elements of procedure set-up, cleaning, and reprocessing. A maximum of 12 individuals rotate through this assignment for after-hour and daytime coverage in order to maintain monthly exposure. They are joined by an RN from the local area being served (emergency room, surgical suite, ICU, floor unit) or from the hospital float pool. During the workday the on-call GIA is available to staff in an unscheduled room or to float as an assistant in the scheduled rooms. During the evenings and on weekends they are available by page for initiation of procedures within 30–45 min.

Weekend ERCP coverage may require specially trained nurses. Historically we required all on-call nurses to have ERCP skills, but the frequency of bleeding and the relative infrequency of weekend ERCPs (~30–40 per year) have prompted us to restrict ERCP call to a smaller group.

Procedure schedules

Attention to the design and completion of daily procedure calendars is critical for unit efficiency and profitability. The major considerations for calendar design include the number of rooms per endoscopist, the time scheduled per procedure of a given type, and the time required for turnover between procedures. When the number of procedure rooms is the predominant constraint for a given unit, efficiency is maximized by utilizing one room per endoscopist while tightly managing room turnover time. In contrast, a surplus of space and procedural demand requires maximizing efficiency of the professional staff by minimizing their between-procedure downtime—usually by provision of multiple rooms per endoscopist. Efficient calendars are more easily designed using block scheduling of endoscopists performing basically similar or uniform procedures. Serial performance of brief EGDs, for instance, allows calculation of average procedure time, average reprocessing and room turnover times, and therefore, the ideal number of rooms per endoscopist—usually two or three depending upon their personal efficiency and the need to intermix other clinical activities or consultative tasks. Outpatient colonoscopies entail longer procedure times but similar turnover times, with two rooms adequate for maximal endoscopist efficiency.

Relative time requirements

We assign a relative time requirement of 1.0 to average risk EGDs in a non-teaching assignment, which we schedule every 15 min—but could just as well list for 10, 12, 18, or 20 min, depending upon the desired pace, documentation requirements, and patient care duties between procedures. In the same system, non-teaching colonoscopies are weighted for a time value of 2.0 (30 min each), and ERCP and EUS procedures, which are always teaching assignments, are assigned a value of ~5 (75–80 min each), including room turnaround. Other complex therapeutic procedures are weighted anywhere between two and five. Thus mixed procedure calendars can be scheduled with some anticipation of workload and appropriate staffing.

Barriers to efficiency

Despite excellent processes, efficiencies can be affected by procedures that go over the time allotted, patients that do not show for appointments, procedures that are cancelled due to inadequate preparation or current health risks, unfilled appointment slots, open blocks in the schedule, or late arriving endoscopists.

Purchasing

Endoscopes

The major purchasing decisions pertain to capital equipment (endoscopes, fluoroscopy units, electrosurgical generators, patient gurneys, databases, etc.). Of these, endoscopes, light sources, and image management systems (endoscopy 'set-ups') are most central to the function of the endoscopy suite. While there are only limited numbers of endoscope vendors in the marketplace and the basic functional aspects of their products are quite similar, endoscopists often develop strong and divergent opinions regarding ergonomics and functionality of each line of equipment. Hence both physician preferences and contractual stipulations are important in the selection of endoscopy equipment. The major options for acquisition of endoscopes are outright purchase of new, refurbished, or used equipment and leasing, typically for terms of 3 or 4 years. The latter approach is often quoted on a price-per-procedure (PPP) basis. Units that purchase endoscopes may do so on a rolling basis, replacing 20–25% of their stock every year, or in bulk fashion every 4–6 years, with amortization/depreciation schedules then spread out over that interval. Purchase with extended use beyond 3–4 years is typically more cost effective than leasing. This approach risks undesirable delays in acquiring new technology and may yield increasingly worn instruments and rising repair costs toward the end of their term. Price-per-procedure leases tend to be more expensive, but they are potentially desirable and cost effective if equipment exchange is planned after shorter time frames of 3 years or so. As with auto leasing, a direct comparison of costs requires quotations for per procedure costs, estimated (contractual) procedure volumes, specific delineation of types and numbers of endoscopes, and contractual residual values at the termination of the contract. Some vendors will not specify all of these elements at the outset, particularly a residual buyout value. Buy-out options for some of the instruments should be considered and negotiated at the time of the lease as they may be useful for subsequent back-up use.

How many endoscopes? For both the purchase and lease options, accurate planning of endoscope requirements contributes to cost constraint, as efficiently reusing fewer instruments is far less costly than having extra instruments hanging largely unused in closets. Appropriate estimates must accommodate instrument breakdowns, repairs, dual procedures, etc. We have successfully utilized the following ratios during equipment planning for several large and small units. One colonoscope, gastroscope, and sigmoidoscope for every 350 procedures per year; one duodenoscope and EUS scope for each 150 procedures per year; one light source and processor per endoscopic procedure room; and one scope reprocessor for each 1000 procedures per year. Some specialty endo-scopes, such as pediatric and therapeutic instruments, may be needed to provide complete basic services. Others may not be economically wise if they require a skill set or instrument that would be infrequently used.

Endoscope repair costs. Endoscope repair costs are a major element of unit finances. Repairs can be purchased on a piecemeal basis, with or without vol-ume discounts, or on a prospective contract basis. Like endoscope leases, pro-spective repair contracts may be negotiated on a per-procedure basis, whether the equipment is purchased or leased. For cash flow purposes this provides useful averaging of expenses over an anticipated range of costs. One typical contract design covers cumulative costs for the department over a range of 90–120% of the face value of the contract. Cumulative actual costs below 90% of the contract value yield a rebate to the unit while costs exceeding 120% yield a liability to the unit. Such contracts typically don't stipulate the cost schedule for various repairs, such that the unit may be unaware they are actually purchasing top-drawer services but paying for them over time. It is useful to have right of acceptance and decline for individually advised repairs, much like that afforded to customers by the service department of a reputable auto dealer. The accept-ance or decline option should be delegated to an individual with knowledge of instrument use and design. This allows staff to learn of instrument frailties and mistreatments that lead to repairs, and provides an avenue for negotiating the price and purpose of some repairs.

Databases. Modern databases for reporting of gastrointestinal endoscopic procedures are available from several vendors as well as via collaboration with the national endoscopy database (CORI System) developed by the University of Oregon and the American Society of Gastrointestinal Endoscopy (ASGE) and funded by the National Institutes of Health. Several major institutions, like ours, employ databases of their own design for meeting documentation require-ments, [9] reporting, and unit management. With the growing emphasis on quality improvement and the coming utilization of pay for performance reim-bursement, computerized databases are becoming inevitable necessities for the endoscopy unit.

Most databases employ, or map to, some version of the internationally developed minimum standard terminology (MST) for endoscopy [10,11]. Most are used for basic scheduling, reporting, billing, and correspondence. Some also provide means of documenting all clinical and nursing care. In our department, the endoscopic database, coupled with interfaces to the institutional electronic medical record and several other systems, provides a completely paperless environment for all aspects of clinical practice, business management, quality assurance, and research. The sophistication and complexity of interfaces needed will be a function of the practice setting and the independence of the unit from a larger institution. Adequate interactivity should negate the need for dual entry of names, numbers, or any variety of data in more than one record or system.

Devices. Next to the cost of personnel, devices are becoming a dominant expense within many endoscopy units, particularly those that deliver complex therapeutic procedures and ERCP and EUS services. The major device decisions any unit faces are: (1) whether to predominantly use reprocessable and reusable devices or single use disposable devices [12,13], and (2) if any devices are reprocessed and reused, whether to do this internally or via a reprocessing vendor.

A variety of considerations may influence these decisions. Single-use devices are typically high quality and sometimes unique in their capabilities. They simplify infection control considerations while generally risking higher costs than reusable devices. Many commonly used devices such as biopsy forceps and single-channel sphincterotomes have reached a commodity status, in that their function and design by different manufacturers are all similar and adequate. This has driven unit costs for single-use designs down to the point where they are cost competitive with the reusable alternatives. Reusable devices typically reduce costs, but require ongoing administration of reprocessing capabilities, including training, quality assurance, risk, etc.

Device costs can be constrained by:

1 the willingness of endoscopists to designate which items are commodities and which are not;
2 willingness to use the lowest cost commodity items;
3 use of an open bid process for competing vendors to propose their best offers based on projections of both uniform large-volume purchasing and single-unit purchasing;
4 purchasing through one of several purchasing collaboratives, which many hospitals participate in across multiple specialties and types of equipment and supplies;
5 concerted effort by physicians and nurses to avoid intraprocedural wastage of expensive items.

Endoscope reprocessing

Endoscope cleaning and reprocessing is perhaps the Achilles heel of the endoscopy suite, as its reliable performance following every procedure is critical for patient safety, yet it is typically performed by the least educated and lowest paid members of the unit team in a fast paced and demanding environment. Lapses in endoscope reprocessing can jeopardize both individual patients and the entire practice, as those incidents that culminate in serious sequelae are often widely publicized.

Cleaning standards are promulgated by the Society of Gastrointestinal Nurses and Associates (SGNA) [14] as well as by many national and international endoscopy societies [15,16]. A number of guidelines are available. All emphasize 'adequate' initial manual cleaning employing soap and enzymatic solutions, rinsing, disinfection in an approved agent for the appropriate duration stipulated in the labeling for the given agent, rinsing, and drying. Most units employ automated reprocessing machines that accomplish reliable flushing of high-level disinfectants, contact times, rinsing, and final alcohol flushes for drying [17].

Written unit standards and processes must be in place for several aspects of the reprocessing task, including:

1   the training of personnel responsible for cleaning and reprocessing equipment;

2   the frequency of strength testing for the disinfectant solutions (usually daily);

3   testing and maintenance of the reprocessing machines;

4   ideally, intermittent and random culture testing for confirmation of the reprocessing outcome.

An individual with a sophisticated understanding of the intricacies of endoscope design and channels is helpful in maintaining optimal cleaning and reprocessing practices in a unit.

Unit design and staffing patterns both influence the efficiency, and hence the safety, of endoscope reprocessing. In our experience, the lapsed time from extubation to placement of the washed instrument in a reprocessing machine is about 8 min when instruments travel directly into a reprocessing room without entering a corridor. When taken to a central reprocessing room the average time is 18 min and when procedures are performed outside of the endoscopy unit, as in an ICU or emergency room, the time to reprocessing can approach a full hour. In the setting of the contiguous reprocessing anteroom, individuals assigned to scope reprocessing can be given visual clues as to when a scope is in need of reprocessing; prompting their proactive retrieval of the soiled instruments. In the alternative scenarios, the endoscope is precleaned locally, but may not be transported for reprocessing until numerous other tasks related to the patient, specimens, or medications are completed.

Coding and billing

Accurate identification of services is the responsibility of the endoscopist. However, endoscopy unit staff, the business manager, and the physician support staff are generally responsible for transfer of the information to the responsible coding and billing personnel [18]. While final coding review and/or billing services may be provided by a department serving a larger institution, expertise in the coding and billing issues specific to the specialty should reside within the endoscopy group. National specialty societies, such as the ASGE [19], and many vendors have useful coding hotlines and/or websites [20,21]. Most endoscopy units utilize a relatively narrow spectrum of billing codes; however, there are nuances and intricacies involved in their selection or combination for some patients and some environments, the details of which are beyond the scope of this review.

Accreditation

Accreditation is the sine qua non for presumed base-level quality and safety of a health care facility. It is also a prerequisite for medicare and some third party reimbursement of both ambulatory and inpatient services. Accreditation for AECs can be obtained through either the Joint Commission for Accreditation of Healthcare Organizations (JCAHO) (Oakbrook Terrace, IL) [22] or the Accreditation Association for Ambulatory Healthcare (AAAHC) (Wilmette, IL) [23,24]. In addition to accreditation, AECs require medicare certification, which may be presumptively granted in so-called 'Deemed Status' when accreditation is received by one of these two organizations. Most hospital and inpatient facilities are accredited as part of their institutional accreditation process with the JCAHO. Elements of an accreditation survey are spread across the spectrum of all administrative and practice functions of a facility. Accreditation therefore requires active attention from all administrative partners in the endoscopy suite, including the medical director, the nursing director, and the business manager. Preparation for an accreditation visit may require 6–12 months of effort. The survey visit itself generally takes 1–2 days, depending on the size and complexity of the unit. For a large institution this may extend over 1–2 weeks. In the past accreditation was typically granted for 3-year intervals; however, the current practice is to require accreditation readiness at all times and to anticipate unannounced accreditation survey activities at any time of the year without advance notice.

Outstanding issues and future trends

The practice of gastrointestinal endoscopy will undoubtedly continue to evolve. Several potential trends can now be anticipated that may influence the size, use, and staffing of our endoscopy units. Many of these trends risk such major change that our current space and capital-heavy investment in existing units will become a liability. Anticipation and planning for how they interact with traditional endoscopy should lessen these risks.

Capsule endoscopy

Capsule endoscopy is now established in the investigation of the small intestine. While this practice does not require an endoscopy environment, the needs for focused nursing skills, billing mechanisms, and a location for computer equipment is prompting its placement in many endoscopy suites. For the most part this has added to the tasks of the suite. Similarly, esophageal capsule exams can be performed almost anywhere, but will end up in many endoscopy suites by convenience. Adoption of the esophageal capsule, however, risks incurring significant erosion of standard upper endoscopy volumes if it proves adequately efficacious and cost-saving. Both remain to be seen at this time. Wireless colon capsule devices for cancer and polyp screening are currently under development.

Colon screening technologies

Colon screening technologies (CT colonography or virtual colonoscopy, stool gene testing, and wireless capsule endoscopes), may significantly erode current screening volumes, while adding lesser numbers of planned therapeutic procedures based on their identification of polyps or other uncertain findings. CT colonography and stool gene testing are both currently available, but remain less adequate than standard colonoscopy. It is likely only a matter of time and almost certain technical advances before they assume a significant role in primary screening. Some gastroenterology practices are investing in their own on-site CT machines to retain the screening practice. Undoubtedly this will lead to difficult interspecialty issues pertaining to quality and competence-based reimbursement.

Endoscopy by non-specialists

Endoscopy by non-specialists is an additional trend that risks eroding volumes and/or reimbursement for high-volume general endoscopy. Both general physicians (GPs, FPs) and licensed non-physicians (RNs, nurse practitioners, and physician assistants) are entering the practice. Arguments about inadequate training of non-specialist physicians are hard to sustain when specialists are training licensed assistants for the same tasks in some practices.

Growth of advanced endoscopy

Growth of advanced endoscopy on the other end of the spectrum encompasses more highly specialized and invasive procedures, including endoscopic mucosal resection (EMR), endoscopic submucosal dissection (ESD), and transgastric intra-abdominal procedures. The latter are becoming known as natural orifice transenteric surgery (NOTES) procedures. At the present time, basic EMR is growing in the form of saline-assisted polypectomy; however, more advanced EMR of very large lesions and ESD of superficially malignant lesions requires lengthy procedures that are not easily adapted to existing Western practices and will likely remain in the hands of tertiary endoscopists. Transgastric NOTES procedures remain highly investigational and many anticipate they will be adopted by general laparoscopic surgeons more readily than by gastroenterologists. For the foreseeable future advanced EMR, ESD, and NOTES procedures are unlikely to greatly influence general endoscopy unit needs. Tertiary centers may need expanded capacity for complex procedures. The NOTES procedures will mostly likely require facilities analogous to operating room suites.

Lastly, two trends of greater immediacy for the general endoscopist, those entering training, and unit personnel are the adoption of simulators for training and of alternative approaches to sedation. Both are beyond the scope of this discussion, but will require some accommodation for space and/or nursing skills.

Summary

Gastrointestinal endoscopy has become a specialty endeavor for physicians and nurses, a primary screening modality for public health purposes, an essential diagnostic and therapeutic service for outpatient and intensive hospital settings, and a big business. Optimal design of facilities and services and professional administration for safety, quality, and efficiency are important to its success on each of these levels.

References

1 http://www.asge.org/pages/practice/sigs/aec.cfm
2 Marasco RF, Marasco JA. Designing the ambulatory endoscopy center. *Gastrointest Endosc Clin N Am* 2002; 12: 185–204.
3 Anonymous (2001). *Guidelines for the design and construction of hospitals and health care facilities.* American Institute of Architecture, Washington, DC.
4 Ganz RA. Regulation certification issues. *Gastrointest Endosc Clin N Am* 2002; 12: 205–14.
5 Burton D, Ott BJ, Gostout CJ, DiMagno EP. Approach to designing a gastrointestinal endoscopy unit. *Gastrointest Endosc Clin N Am* 1993; 3: 525–40.
6 Mulder CJJ. Guidelines for designing an endoscopy unit: Report of the Dutch Society of Gastroenterologists. *Endoscopy* 1997; 29: 1–6.
7 Gostout CJ, Ott BJ, Burton DB, DiMagno EP. Design of the endoscopy procedure room. *Gastrointest Endosc Clin N Am* 1993; 3: 509–24.
8 Ott BJ, Igo M, Shields N. Staffing levels in endoscopy units. *Gastroenterol Nurs* 1994; 13: 224–30.
9 Society of Gastrointestinal Nurses and Associates. Guidelines for documentation in the gastrointestinal endoscopy setting. *Gastroenterol Nurs* 1999; 22: 69–97.
10 Weinstein ML, Korman LY. Information management. *Gastrointest Endosc Clin N Am* 2002; 12: 324.

11 Korman LY. Standardization in endoscopic reporting: implications for clinical practice and research. *J Clin Gastroenterol* 1999; 28: 217–23.

12 Croffie J, Carpenter S, Chuttani R *et al.* ASGE Technology Status Evaluation Report: disposable endoscopic accessories. *Gastrointest Endosc* 2005; 62: 477–9.

13 Petersen BT. Advantages of disposable endoscopic accessories. *Gastrointest Endosc Clin N Am* 2000; 10: 341–8.

14 Walter VA, DiMarino AJ. American Society for Gastrointestinal Endoscopy — Society of Gastroenterology Nurses and Associates endoscope reprocessing guidelines. *Gastrointest Endosc Clin N Am* 2000; 10: 265–74.

15 Nelson DB, Chair, Multisociety Consensus Panel. Multisociety guideline for reprocessing of flexible gastrointestinal endoscopes. *Gastrointest Endosc* 2003; 58: 1–8.

16 http://www.worldgastroenterology.org/?endoscopedisinfection

17 Muscarella LF. Automatic flexible endoscope reprocessors. *Gastrointest Endosc Clin N Am* 2000; 10: 245–58.

18 Stout PL. Coding and billing for gastrointestinal endoscopy. *Gastrointest Endosc Clin N Am* 2002; 12: 335–49.

19 http://www.asge.org/pages/practice/management/nelson.cfm

20 http://www.bostonscientific.com/common_templates/listPages

21 http://www.givenimaging.com/Cultures/en-US/Given/English/Professionals/Reimbursement/

22 http://www.jcaho.org/index.htm

23 http://www.aaahc.org/eweb/StartPage.aspx

24 http://www.asge.org/pages/practice/management/accreditation.

CHAPTER 3

Sedation, analgesia, and monitoring for endoscopy

JOHN J. VARGO

'Sedation and analgesia' represents a continuum ranging from minimal sedation or anxiolysis through general anesthesia. In this era of open access endoscopy, candidacy for sedation and analgesia still must take into account a thorough pre-procedure assessment including a history of present illness, past medical history and a physical examination [1,2]. New practice guidelines put forth by the American Society of Anesthesiologists Committee for Sedation and Analgesia by Non-Anesthesiologists, have classified both moderate and deep sedation and analgesia to the continuum of sedation (Table 3.1) [2]. In most endoscopic cases, moderate sedation is the goal, which is defined as a purposeful response after verbal or tactile (not painful) stimulus, and no compromise of the patient's airway, ventilation or cardiovascular function. In comparison, deep sedation/analgesia may require the use of painful stimuli to elicit responsiveness. Additionally, the patient's airway and spontaneous ventilation may become compromised, and hence, personnel must be designated for the complete and uninterrupted observation of the patient's respiratory and cardiovascular status.

An important component of these guidelines is that the endoscopy team must have the ability to rescue the patient from deeper than expected levels of sedation/analgesia.

We consider that the careful titration of a combination of an opioid and benzodiazepine will result in a predictable targeting of moderate sedation and analgesia, but is this always the case? A balanced cohort of 80 ASA class I and II patients undergoing upper endoscopy, colonoscopy, ERCP and EUS received meperidine and midazolam according to a standardized protocol [3]. Hemodynamic parameters and levels of sedation were determined at 3-minute intervals utilizing the Modified Observer's Assessment of Alertness and Sedation. Deep sedation occurred in 68% of the patients. The procedures with the highest percentage of deep sedation assessments were EUS (29%) and ERCP (35%). Multivariate analysis showed that only ERCP and EUS were independent risk factors for deep sedation and not Body Mass Index, sedation dose or procedure duration.

Table 3.1 Continuum of the depth of sedation

	Minimal sedation (anxiolysis)	Moderate sedation/analgesia (conscious sedation)	Deep sedation/analgesia	General anesthesia
Responsiveness	Normal response to verbal stimulation	Purposeful response to verbal or tactile stimulation	Purposeful response after repeated/painful stimulation	No repsonse, event with painful stimulation
Airway	Unaffected	Unaffected	Intervention may be required	Intervention often required
Spontaneous Respiration	Unaffected	Unaffected	May be inadequate	Intervention often required
Cardiovascular Function	Unaffected	Usually maintained	Usually maintained	May require intervention

Adapted from Gross JB, Bailey PL, Caplan RA *et al.* Practice guidelines for sedation and analgesia by non-anesthesiologists. *Anesthesiology* 2002; 96: 1004–17.

Advances in monitoring during sedation

Cardiorespiratory complications are a leading cause of morbidity and mortality associated with gastrointestinal endoscopy. Both ventilatory depression and oxygen desaturation stemming from the medications used to achieve sedation and analgesia are thought to be important risk components. Pulse oximetry has become the *de facto* standard of care, owing to the evidence that clinical observation alone is inaccurate in the detection of hypoxemia and that supplemental oxygen can minimize the degree of desaturation, and hopefully its deleterious effects. However, to date, neither pulse oximetry nor supplemental oxygen has been shown to decrease the incidence or severity of cardiopulmonary complications.

It is important to point out that pulse oximetry does not detect alveolar hypoventilation, which is measured by hypercapnea or a rise in arterial carbon dioxide pressure [4–6]. Although oxygen administration may prevent hypoxemia and its deleterious effects, it will not detect the development of hypercapnea. Deleterious consequences of alveolar hypoventilation include myocardial depression, acidosis, intracranial hypertension, narcosis, and arterial hypertension or hypotension.

Extended monitoring

Capnography

Capnography is based on the principle that carbon dioxide absorbs light in the infrared region of the electromagnetic spectrum. Quantification of the absorption leads to the generation of a curve, which represents a real-time display of the patient's respiratory activity [5,6]. Randomized trials and case series utilizing capnography have found it to be more sensitive than pulse oximetry or visual assessment in the detection of apneic episodes.

In a series of 80 colonoscopy patients who were randomized to undergo the procedure with and without supplemental oxygen, extended monitoring with capnography was employed [7]. The endoscopist and nursing personnel were blinded to the capnography data. Though the number of apneic events was similar between the two groups, significantly more episodes of apnea were not clinically detected in the group receiving oxygen (7% vs. 42%, $p < 0.001$). Moreover, significantly more patients receiving supplemental oxygen received sedation following an apneic episode. Capnography has also been utilized to allow the safe titration of propofol by a qualified gastroenterologist during ERCP and EUS [6].

A randomized controlled trial of capnography was performed in a group of pediatric patients undergoing elective EGD, colonoscopy or the combination thereof [8]. The primary outcome of this study was to determine whether intervention based on capnographic evidence of alveolar hypoventilation reduced the incidence of hypoxemia undergoing moderate sedation with fentanyl and midazolam. Hypoventilation was defined as a pulse oximetry value <95% for greater than 5 seconds. All procedural personnel were blinded to the capnographic data. Trained observers were utilized to alert the staff of alveolar hypoventilation. In the intervention arm, personnel were alerted if the capnographs indicated alveolar hypoventilation for >15 seconds. In the control arm, the personnel were alerted if alveolar hypoventilation was noted for >60 seconds. In both arms, once the personnel were alerted to the occurrence of alveolar hypoventilation, the subjects were stimulated. A total of 163 patients were randomized. Patients in the intervention arm were significantly less likely to experience hypoxemia when compared to controls (11% vs. 24 %; p < 0.03). The majority of hypoxemic episodes were preceded by alveolar hypoventilation for a median interval of 3.4 minutes. Alveolar hypoventilation occurred in 58% of patients and in 56% of the procedures. Similar data in adults has yet to be published.

BIS monitoring

Bispectral index (BIS) monitoring represents a complex mathematical evaluation of electroencephalographic parameters of frontal cortex activity, corresponding to varying levels of sedation. The BIS scale varies from 0 to 100 (0, no cortical activity or coma; 40–60, unconscious; 70–90, varying levels of conscious sedation, 100, fully awake). Theoretically this index should reflect the same level of sedation regardless of the medications used, except for ketamine. In a preliminary observational study involving 50 patients undergoing ERCP, colonoscopy, and upper endoscopy, BIS levels were found to correlate with a commonly used score for the degree of sedation [9]. A BIS range of 75–85 demonstrated a probability of ≥96% that the patient would have an acceptable sedation score. However, there was increasing variability of the BIS score with deeper levels of sedation. Additionally, there was no correlation between the BIS score and standard physiologic parameters such as pulse oximetry, blood pressure or heart rate.

Further refinements in the BIS algorithm has spawned renewed interest in this technology. Chen and Rex recently employed an updated BIS algorithm that is designed to be more sensitive to variations in lighter levels of procedural sedation for colonoscopy [10]. They found a substantial lag time between the depth of sedation with nurse-administered propofol that was evident clinically via the OAA/S score and the BIS score, for both the induction and recovery phases of the procedure. Moreover, substantial variability in the BIS score (22–88) was seen during the maintenance phase of sedation.

Topical anesthetics: are they worth the effort?

A systematic review was conducted involving five randomized controlled studies comparing topical anesthesia to placebo or no treatment. The primary endpoints of the study were to evaluate the effectiveness of topical anesthetic agents in improving patient tolerance and procedural ease during sedated upper endoscopy [11]. Patients who rated their discomfort as none or minimal were more likely to have received topical anesthesia (OR 1.18, 95% CI: 1.13, 3.12). Endoscopists were more likely to rate the procedure as 'not difficult' for patients who received pharyngeal anesthesia (OR 2.60; 95%: 1.63, 4.17). Drawbacks of the analysis included the heterogeneity of sedation regimens and the lack of standardized outcomes.

Propofol

Propofol (2–6 diisopropylphenol) is classified as an ultra short acting sedative hypnotic agent that provides amnesia, but minimal levels of analgesia. It is very popular with anesthesiologists, and there have been many recent reports of its use by endoscopists. The cumulative experience with non-anesthetist-administered propofol now exceeds more than 300 000 patients [12–21]. Over the course of this experience, there has been an evolution from propofol 'monotherapy' to a 'mixed' approach wherein propofol is used in concert with a narcotic and benzodiazepine [22].

The bulk of the literature focuses on nurse-administered propofol sedation (NAPS). Rex *et al.* reported on 36 743 endoscopic procedures undergoing NAPS from three high volume centers [12]. It is crucial to emphasize that they first established a training program with the assistance of anesthesiologists. The primary outcome of interest in their study was the occurrence of apnea, or other airway compromise (i.e. laryngospasm) that would require would require assisted ventilation. Forty-nine patients required temporary bag mask ventilation: no endotracheal intubation was necessary. The center-specific event rate ranged from 9 per 10 000 to 19 per 10 000. Multivariate analysis did not identify age, gender, or ASA class as risk factors for assisted ventilation at two of the sites. Higher event rates were seen for upper endoscopy at two of the sites. There were no cases of endotracheal intubation, death, neurologic sequelae or other permanent injury

Given the short half-life of propofol, some investigators have combined bolus and infusion administrations. Yusoff *et al.* employed this type of propofol administration in 500 ASA I and II patients undergoing elective upper gastrointestinal EUS [13]. In all cases, the propofol was administered by the gastroenterologist. There were no instances of hypotension, bradycardia or tachycardia.

Minor hypoxemia, defined as a pulse oximetry value <95% but >90%, occurred in 12 (2.4%) patients. Moderate hypoxemia (defined as less than 90% but >85%) occurred in 4 (0.8%) of patients. Nine of these 12 patients responded to an increase in the supplemental oxygen flow rate. One patient required a jaw lift in addition.

Numerous randomized controlled trials have compared propofol to the traditional combination of a narcotic and benzodiazepine, mainly for elective colonoscopy [14–20]. Most showed that propofol resulted in a more rapid attainment of an appropriate level of sedation, and a more rapid recovery to baseline. Interestingly, the patient satisfaction outcomes were mixed. The studies were not powered to detect significant differences in adverse events.

The bulk of the propofol data relies on intermittent boluses which can be labor intensive, and can lead to fluctuating levels of sedation. Target-controlled infusion of propofol should result in a rapid induction to the desired level of sedation and maintenance of the sedation level by achieving a steady state, plasma concentration. Fanti *et al.* utilized anesthesiologist-administered target-controlled infusion in 205 adult inpatients undergoing ERCP [21]. Each patient received premedication with midazolam, and a rescue dose of 50–100 µg of fentanyl was frequently required to provide analgesia. Severe hypoxemia ($S_A O2 < 85\%$) occurred in 4 patients (1.9%) all of whom were ASA physical status III or higher. In three of the cases, hypoxemia resolved with turning the patient to the supine position and 'improving airway patency.' The fourth required manual ventilation for a few minutes.

Though deep sedation is not uncommon during standard sedation and analgesia with an opioid and benzodiazepine, there is a concern that the probability of losing protective airway reflexes and maintaining cardiovascular stability is higher with propofol. The use of triple-agent or 'mixed' sedation with propofol, opioid and benzodiazepine would intuitively be dismissed because of the theoretical risk of pharmacologic synergy and an amplification of sedation-induced untoward events. However, quite the opposite has been found. Cohen *et al.* have employed a mixed sedation protocol for ambulatory upper endoscopy and colonoscopy [22]. The opioid and midazolam were administered by bolus at the beginning of the procedure, and propofol then was administered in intravenous boluses as determined by patient comfort level and physiologic parameters. A total of 100 subjects undergoing either EGD or colonoscopy received the mixed sedation regimen. Of the 729 assessments of the level of sedation, 77% were minimal sedation, 21% were moderate sedation and only 2% were in the deep sedation range. Patient satisfaction with the mixed sedation was quite high (98%) and 71% returned to usual activities within two hours of discharge. In a prospective study comparing propofol 'monotherapy' to the 'mixed' regimens, VanNatta and Rex enrolled 200 ASA Class 1 and 2 subjects undergoing elective outpatient colonoscopy to one of four sedation arms:

1 propofol alone titrated to deep sedation (the classic NAPS protocol);
2 fentanyl plus propofol;
3 midazolam plus propofol; and
4 the combination of fentanyl, midazolam and propofol [23].

It is important to emphasize that the latter three 'mixed' propofol arms were targeted to moderate sedation. Patients receiving propofol alone exhibited deeper sedation scores and longer recovery intervals than the mixed regimens. There were no differences among the study arms in terms of patient satisfaction, changes in vital sings or oxygen desaturation.

As previously pointed out, the current data in randomized controlled trials are insufficient to establish whether propofol or standard sedation/analgesia is safer. Qadeer *et al.* performed a meta-analysis of 12 randomized controlled trials comparing propofol to traditional sedation. Of the 1162 patients, 634 received propofol and 527 received midazolam, meperidine and/or fentanyl [24]. Hypoxemia and hypotension were used as endpoints. The pooled odds ratio with the use of propofol for developing hypoxemia or hypotension during colonoscopy was 0.4 (95% CI: 0.2, 0.79). For upper endoscopy the pooled odds ratio was 0.74 (95% CI: 0.44, 1.44) and for ERCP/EUS 1.07 (95% CI: 0.38, 3.01). This indicates that, for parameters analyzed, propofol mediated sedation is as safe as traditional sedation for EGD, ERCP and EUS and appears to be safer for colonoscopy.

A water soluble prodrug of propofol (fospropofol sodium) has been studied in humans [25]. The pro-drug is activated to propofol after removal of the water-soluble moiety by endothelial alkaline phosphatase. Such a medication would theoretically allow a weight-based bolus frequency similar to traditional agents used for procedural sedation. A potential drawback is that the increased plasma half-life may translate into prolonged recovery. The safety and efficacy of this agent is currently under study.

Droperidol

Droperidol, a narcoleptic of the butyrophenone class, produces a dissociative state while enhancing the effects of other sedative medications. It is routinely used in some centers as a premedication for patients undergoing ERCP. Other indications include: a history of alcohol use or withdrawal, narcotic use, and a history of paradoxical agitation during conventional sedation. In a retrospective study involving 1102 procedures, droperidol was found to be a safe adjunct to the combination of narcotics and benzodiazepines [26]. Complications attributable to droperidol occurred in 1.5% of procedures; this mainly comprised hypotension, responsive to IV fluids. In a prospective, double blind, placebo controlled trial, in 140 patients undergoing elective upper endoscopy, droperidol led to a 10% reduction in procedure time and significantly reduced meperidine and midazolam requirements [27]. However, four patients in the droperidol group received naloxone for excessive drowsiness. Rizzo *et al.* addressed the use of different doses of droperidol in patients undergoing EUS [28]. When compared to placebo, 5 mg of droperidol led to significantly less medication costs, while at the same time, not affecting the mean recovery time. The US Food and Drug Administration required a 'black box warning' for droperidol due to the concern of possible QT interval prolongation leading to fatal arrhythmias [29]. However, a retrospective review of the use of this agent in 3113 ERCPs found that 233 patients (7.48%) developed QT interval prolongation [30]. Only 15 (0.48%) had marked prolongation of the QT interval, but no serious arrhythmias occurred.

Summary

The importance of preprocedural assessment and appropriate monitoring cannot be overemphasized. The endoscopist must have a thorough knowledge of the pharmacology of the agents used for sedation and the training necessary to recognize and manage oversedation. Numerous regulatory groups are carefully scrutinizing the practice of sedation and analgesia. It appears that ventilatory monitoring will be required for at least a subset of our patients. Although both hypercapnea and apnea can be reliably measured, the most important questions to be answered are: will such monitoring affect patient outcomes, and which patients are at risk for apnea and alveolar hypoventilation.

The use of propofol for gastrointestinal endoscopy has been shown to be safe in experienced hands. Its narrow therapeutic window demands that it is administered by specially trained personnel who are not directly involved in the endoscopic procedure. Extended monitoring with capnography appears to offer an advantage over conventional monitoring in that it can detect early phases of respiratory depression, which can allow for a timely adjustment in the propofol infusion and thus prevent significant respiratory depression. Emerging cost effectiveness data suggests that propofol is superior to conventional sedation and analgesia, even with the use of added personnel.

References

1 Waring JP, Baron TH, Hirota WK *et al.* Guidelines for conscious sedation and monitoring during gastrointestinal endoscopy. *Gastrointest Endosc* 2003; 8: 317–22.
2 Gross JB, Bailey PL, Caplan RA, Connis RT *et al.* American Society of Anesthesiologists Task Force on Sedation and Analgesia by Non-Anesthesiologists. Practice guidelines for sedation and analgesia by non-anesthesiologists. *Anesthesiology* 2002; 96: 1004–17.
3 Patel S, Vargo JJ, Khandwala F *et al.* Deep sedation occurs frequently during elective endoscopy with meperidine and midazolam. *Am J Gastroenerol* 2005; 100: 2689–95.

4 Nelson DB, Freeman ML, Silvis SE *et al*. A randomized, controlled trial of transcutaneous carbon dioxide monitoring during ERCP. *Gastrointest Endosc* 2000; 51: 288–95.

5 Vargo JJ, Zuccaro G, Dumot JA, Conwell DL, Morrow JB, Shay SS. Automated assessment of respiratory activity is superior to pulse oximetry and visual assessment for the detection of early respiratory depression during therapeutic upper endoscopy. *Gastrointest Endosc* 2002; 55: 826–31.

6 Vargo JJ, Zuccaro G, Dumot JA *et al*. A prospective, randomized trial of gastroenterologist-administered propofol versus meperidine and midazolam for complex upper endoscopic procedures. *Gastrointest Endosc* 2001; 53: AB79.

7 Zuccaro G, Radaelli F, Vargo J *et al*. Routine use of supplemental oxygen prevents recognition of prolonged apnea during endoscopy. *Gastrointest Endosc* 2000; 51: AB141.

8 Lightdale JR, Goldman DA, Feldman HA, Newburg AR, DiNardo JA, Fox VL. Microstream capnography improves patient monitoring during moderate sedation: a randomized, controlled trial. *Pediatrics* 2006; 117: 1170–8.

9 Bower AL, Ripepi A, Dilger J, Bopari N, Brody FJ, Ponsky JL. Bispectral index monitoring of sedation during endoscopy. *Gastrointest Endosc* 2000; 52: 192–6.

10 Chen SC, Rex DK. An initial investigation of bispectral index monitoring as an adjunct to nurse-administered propofol sedation for colonoscopy. *Am J Gastroenterol* 2004; 99: 1081–86.

11 Evans LT, Saberi S, Kim HM, Elta G, Schoenfeld P. Pharyngeal anesthesia during sedated EGDs: is the 'spray' beneficial? A meta-analysis and systematic review. *Gastrointest Endosc* 2006; 63: 761–6.

12 Rex DK, Heuss LT, Walker JA, Qi R. Trained registered nurses/endoscopy teams can administer propofol safely for endoscopy. *Gastroenterology* 2005; 129: 1384–91.

13 Yusoff IF, Raymond G, Sahai AV. Endoscopist administered propofol for upper-GI EUS is safe and effective: a prospective study in 500 patients. *Gastrointest Endosc* 2004; 60: 356–60.

14 Riphaus A, Stergiou N, Wehrmann T. Sedation with propofol for routine ERCP in high-risk octogenarians: a randomized controlled study. *Am J Gastroenterol* 2005; 100: 1957–63.

15 Wehrmann T, Kokapick S, Lembcke B *et al*. Efficacy and safety of intravenous propofol sedation for routine ERCP: a prospective, controlled study. *Gastrointest Endosc* 1999; 49: 677–83.

16 Ulmer BJ, Hansen JJ, Overly CA *et al*. Propofol versus midazolam/fentanyl for outpatient colonoscopy: administration by nurses supervised by endoscopists. *Clin Gastroenterol Hepatol* 2003; 1: 425–3.

17 Vargo JJ, Zuccaro G, Dumot J *et al*. Gastroenterologist-administered propofol versus meperidine and midazolam for ERCP and EUS: A randomized, controlled trial with cost effectiveness analysis. *Gastroenterology* 2002; 123: 8–16.

18 Sipe BW, Rex DK, Latinovich D, Overly C, Kisner K, Bratcher L, Kareken D. Propofol versus midazolam/meperidine for outpatient colonoscopy: administration by nurses supervised by endoscopists. *Gastrointest Endosc* 2002; 55: 815–25.

19 Wehrmann T, Grotkamp J, Stergiou N, Riphaus A, Kluge A, Lembcke B, Schultz A. Electroencephalogram monitoring facilitates sedation with propofol for routine ERCP: a randomized, controlled trial. *Gastrointest Endosc* 2002; 56: 817–24.

20 Weston BR, Chadalawada V, Chalasani N *et al*. Nurse-administered propofol versus midazolam and meperidine for upper endoscopy in cirrhotic patients. *Am J Gastroenterol* 2003; 98: 2440–7.

21 Fanti L, Agostoni M, Casati A, Guslandi M, Giollo P, Torri G, Testoni A. Target-controlled propofol infusion during monitored anesthesia in patients undergoing ERCP. *Gastrointest Endosc* 2004; 60: 361–6.

22 Cohen LB, Hightower CD, Wood DA, Miller KM, Aisenberg J. Moderate level sedation during endoscopy: a prospective study using low-dose propofol, meperidine/fentanyl, and midazolam. *Gastrointest Endosc* 2004; 59: 795–802.

23 VanNetta M, Rex DK. Propofol alone titrated to deep sedation versus propofol in combination with opioids and/or benzodiazepines and titrated to moderate sedation for colonoscopy. *Am J Gastroenterol* 2006; 101: 2209–17.

24 Qadeer MA, Vargo JJ, Khandwala F, Lopez R, Zuccaro G. Propfol versus traditional agents for gastrointenstinal endoscopy: a meta-analysis. *Clin Gastroenterol Hepatol* 2005; 3: 1049–56.
25 Fechner J, Ihmsen H, Schiessel C, Jeleazcov C, Vornov JJ, Schwilden H, Schuttler J. Sedation with GPI 15715, a water soluble prodrug of propofol, using a target-controlled infusion in volunteers. *Anesth Analg* 2005; 100: 701–6.
26 Wilcox CM, Forsmark CE, Cello JP. Utility of droperidol for conscious sedation in gastrointestinal endoscopic procedures. *Gastrointest Endosc* 1989; 36: 112–15.
27 Barthel JS, Marshall JB, King PD, Afridi SA, Gibb LG, Madsen R. The effect of droperidol on objective markers of patient cooperation and vital signs during esophagogastroduodenoscopy: a randomized, double blind, placebo-controlled prospective investigation. *Gastrointest Endosc* 1995; 42: 45–50.
28 Rizzo J, Bernstein D, Gress F. A randomized, double-blind, placebo-controlled trial evaluating the cost effectiveness of droperidol as a sedative for EUS. *Gastrointest Endosc* 1999; 50: 178–82.
29 http://collection.nlc-bnc.ca/100/201/300/cdn_association/cmaj/FDA-Advisory.
30 Yimchareon P, Fogel E, Kovacs R *et al*. Droperidol, when used for sedation during ERCP, may prolong the QT interval. *Gastrointest Endosc* 2006; 63: 979–85.

CHAPTER 4

Endoscopic equipment

GREGORY G. GINSBERG

Synopsis

Gastrointestinal endoscopy applies technology to further the diagnosis and management of disorders of the digestive tract and adjacent structures. This chapter provides a broad overview of the wide variety of endoscopes and accessories now available for diagnostic and therapeutic gastrointestinal endoscopy.

Gastrointestinal endoscopes

Gastrointestinal endoscopes are highly evolved and sophisticated flexible instruments with a broad range of diagnostic and therapeutic applications. Endoscopes incorporate advanced video, computer, material, and engineering technologies [1–4]. The development of modern flexible gastrointestinal endoscopes followed the development of fiber optics and subsequently the charge-coupled device (CCD). Modern endoscopes continue to use fiber optic light guides to transmit light to the endoscope tip. However, fiber-optic image guides have largely been replaced by copper wire that transmits digital information, from a CCD at the endoscope tip to a video processor for display. A variety of endoscope models from several manufacturers are commercially available. Procedure-specific endoscopes are designed to enhance endoscopic diagnosis and therapy.

Endoscope design

Flexible endoscopes are composed of three sections: the control section, the insertion tube, and the connector section (Fig. 4.1). Particular features of any given endoscope are modified to best accomplish the intended use. Endoscopes developed for specific procedures may be used for other applications as clinically indicated (e.g. a thin caliber colonoscope may be used for small bowel enteroscopy) [5]. While there are variations among endoscope manufacturers, there is general uniformity to endoscope design. Endoscope specifications do

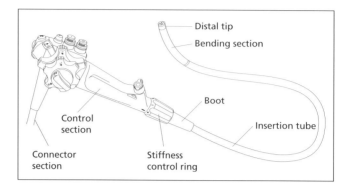

Fig. 4.1 Flexible endoscopes are composed of three sections: the control section, the insertion tube, and the connector section. Particular features of any given endoscope are modified to best accomplish the intended use. The instrument depicted here is a variable stiffness colonoscope, equipped with a stiffness control apparatus.

vary in any given category of endoscope (e.g. colonoscope vs. duodenoscope). Variables include insertion tube length, diameter, and stiffness; instrument channel size and number; and configuration of the distal end of the insertion tube. The control section is modified for specific purposes such as a second instrument channel or an elevator lever control for the duodenoscope. These features affect the endoscope's ergonomics, depth of insertion, and the accessories that can be used adjunctively.

Control section

The control section is held in the operator's left hand (Fig. 4.1). It has two stacked angulation control knobs which direct up/down and left/right deflection of the endoscope tip. These control knobs can be locked in position. Specialty small caliber endoscopes such as the choledochoscope have only one knob, limited to up/down deflection capability. There are air/water and suction valves on the upper front portion of the control section. There are remote switches to modify or capture the video image. The entry port to the instrument channel(s) is (are) located on the lower front portion of the control section. Fiber optic instruments have an eyepiece located at the top of the control section for direct image viewing. Specialty components may include such things as variable stiffness and video magnification controls.

Insertion tube

The insertion tube is attached to the control section, and is the portion of the endoscope that is inserted into the patient (Fig. 4.2). The length, diameter, and degree of stiffness of the insertion tube vary among models. The insertion tube

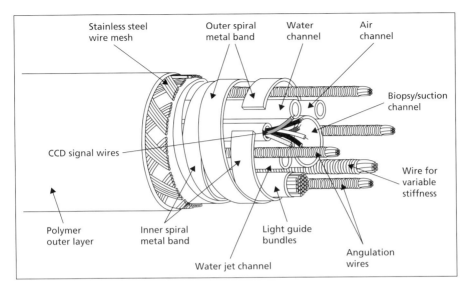

Fig. 4.2 The insertion tube contains one or two instrument channel(s), one or two light guide bundles (incoherent fiber optic), an air channel, a water channel, either an image guide bundle (coherent fiber optic) or a CCD chip with wire connections, and angulation wires. The angulation wires deflect the bending section of the insertion tube. The contents are confined within a mesh tube and covered with an outer polymer layer.

contains one or two instrument channel(s), one or two light guide bundles (incoherent fiber optic), an air channel, a water channel, either an image guide bundle (coherent fiber optic) or a CCD chip with wire connections, and angulation wires. The angulation wires deflect the bending section of the insertion tube. Maximum deflection is 180–230° [6].

The endoscope tip contains (1) an opening(s) to the accessories/suction channel; (2) an air/water nozzle for air insufflation, positioned to wash the lens of debris; (3) light guide illumination system; (4) objective lens system. Instrument models are designed with forward-, side-, or oblique-viewing optics. Insertion tube lengths range from 63 to 2800 cm, with diameters ranging from 2.8 to 13.7 mm. Instrument channel diameters vary from 0.75 to 4.8 mm. Dedicated ERCP and EUS scopes have use-specific modifications at the distal tip.

Connector section

The connector section of the endoscope has a light guide, an air-pipe, and electrical contacts compatible with the processor/light source. This section also has side connectors for a water container, suction, CO_2, insertion tube venting, and an S (safety)-cord connecting mount, which grounds the endoscope, reducing potential for electrical shock hazard to the operator. Some models include a separate lavage port.

Imaging

Endoscopic imaging is achieved through either fiber optic or electronic (video) systems. Fiber optic endoscopes utilize a coherent bundle of glass fibers to transmit an image from the tip of the endoscope to the eyepiece. Some specialty endoscopes are only available in a fiber optic format. A video-adaptor or add-on camera can be used to convert a fiber optic image to video format. Video-endoscopes have a black and white solid state image sensor called a CCD mounted at the tip of endoscope that allows an image to be transmitted via an electronic signal to a video processor for display on one or more video monitors. This signal is converted to a color image by one of two systems.

1   *Color CCD* has a multicolor mosaic filter affixed to the surface of the CCD with illumination by a steady white light.

2   *RGB sequential imaging* has a rotating multicolor wheel filter (red-green-blue) located between the light source and the light guide, yielding a visual strobe effect. The standard magnification is 7× with a 20-inch monitor. Specialty endoscope/processor systems (e.g. Narrow Band Imaging) offer spectral modification and image magnification capabilities (70–150×) [7,8]. Endoscope imaging is detailed in Chapter 5.

Light source/processors

The fiber optic light source is a relatively simple component with or without an air/water pump. High-intensity light bulbs (e.g. halogen) are commonly used as fiber optic light sources. The front panel is equipped with controls and a receptacle for the connector section.

The video-endoscope processor is more complex and expensive than the fiber optic light source as it contains all the circuitry to process the video signal. Some model designs have separate video processors and light source/air–water pump components, while others have combined the components into one chassis. The front panel of a video processor allows for image adjustment, air/water pump control, and a receptacle for the endoscope connector section. A variety of illumination bulb types are used in video processors, including xenon, halogen, and metal halide.

Endoscope equipment compatibility

Fiber optic endoscope equipment from various manufacturers and generations may be compatible and used interchangeably with specially designed adaptors. Compatibility and interchangeability are less feasible with video-endoscopy. The video processor has to be compatible with the endoscope attached to it. For example an RGB sequential endoscope is not compatible with a processor designed for a color chip endoscope. Also, within the same optical family or manufacturer, endoscope generations may or may not be compatible with video processors from newer or older generations. Finally, even when the same color system is used, video-endoscopes are not compatible with video processors from different manufacturers.

Endoscope categories

Esophagogastroduodenoscope (gastroscope)

The esophagogastroduodenoscope or gastroscope is a forward-viewing instrument used primarily for evaluating the esophagus, stomach, and duodenum. Standard feature variables include insertion tube diameter (5.1–12.8 mm), working length (925–1100 mm), and instrument channel size (2.0–6.0 mm) and number (1–2). Specialty features may also include oblique viewing, ultra thin design, and video zoom capability. List prices range from $13 700 to $24 900.

Enteroscope

The enteroscope is similar in design to the gastroscope but is fashioned with a longer insertion tube, allowing for deep intubation of the duodenum and proximal jejunum. Standard feature variables include insertion tube diameter (5.0–11.7 mm), working length (2180–800 mm), and instrument channel size (1.0–3.5 mm). An over-tube may be used to retard gastric looping and enhance insertion depth [5,9]. List prices range from $23 800 to $33 275.

Double balloon enteroscopy (Fijinon Corp, Tokyo) incorporates an iteration of an enteroscope modified with an inflatable/deflatable balloon recessed at its tip used in combination with a flexible overtube similarly balloon-equipped. Under combined endoscopic and fluoroscopic guidance, the double balloon enteroscope and overtube are alternately advanced, fixed in position with their balloons, and undergo a tethered withdrawal. Under ideal circumstances and when advanced via both per-oral and per-rectal routes, the entire small bowel can be accessed for diagnostics and therapeutics [10].

Duodenoscope

The duodenoscope is a side-viewing (90° to the longitudinal access of the insertion tube) instrument designed primarily for ERCP (Fig. 4.3). Duodenoscopes are equipped with an elevator lever that enhances fine movement of devices

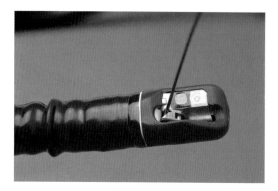

Fig. 4.3 The duodenoscope is a side-viewing (at 90° to the longitudinal access of the insertion tube) instrument designed primarily for ERCP. Duodenoscopes are equipped with an elevator lever that allows deflection of devices passed through the endoscope accessory channel.

passed through the endoscope accessory channel. The elevator lever is positioned at the opening of the accessory channel and is maneuvered by a cable operated from the control section. Standard feature variables include insertion tube length (1030–250 mm), insertion tube diameter (7.4–12.6 mm), and channel size (2.0–4.8 mm). Larger channel instruments allow the passage of larger diameter accessories and even a choledochoscope (see below). List prices range from $19 400 to $30 100.

Choledochoscope

A choledochoscope is a thin caliber endoscope that is passed through the instrument channel of a duodenoscope and inserted intraductally for direct imaging of the biliary and pancreatic ducts (Fig. 4.4). Standard feature variables include insertion tube length (1870–900 mm), insertion tube diameter (2.8–3.4 mm), and instrument channel size (0.75–1.2 mm).

Choledochoscopes are commercially available only in fiber optic format at the time of this writing; however, video choledochoscopes and pancreaticoscopes are under development and have been evaluated as prototypes. List prices range from $18 900 to $22 700. The fragility of these instruments has limited their commercial viability [11]. Spyglass (Boston Scientific Inc., Natick, MA) is a catheter-based image guide that is under development and investigation [12].

Echoendoscopes

The echoendoscope is a hybrid instrument that combines flexible endoscopy with high-resolution ultrasound imaging. Ultrasound imaging elements are affixed to the tip of modified endoscopes to allow close proximity ultrasound imaging of the luminal digestive tract and adjacent organs. Standard feature

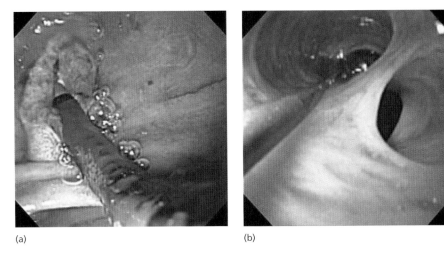

(a)   (b)

Fig. 4.4 A choledochoscope is a thin caliber endoscope that is passed through the instrument channel of a duodenoscope and inserted through the papilla (a), and intraductally for direct imaging of the (b) biliary and pancreatic ducts.

variables include insertion tube length (975–1325 mm), insertion tube diameter (7.9–13.7 mm), instrument channel size (2.2–3.7 mm), and orientation of the optical (forward or oblique) and ultrasound (longitudinal or radial) images. Radial scanning echoendoscopes have a sector scanning ultrasound transducer affixed to the tip of the endoscope providing 270–360° imaging (Fig. 4.5).

Longitudinal imaging is acquired via linear-arrayed piezoelectric ultrasound transducers. The linear array format allows for ultrasound-guided fine-needle biopsy tissue sampling (Fig. 4.6) [13]. List prices range from $33 800 to $71 500. Catheter ultrasound probes, both radial scanning and linear array, are commercially available. These high-frequency devices may be passed through the accessory channel of the endoscope for high-resolution imaging, albeit with limited depth of penetration.

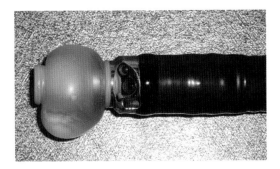

Fig. 4.5 Radial scanning echoendoscopes have a sector scanning ultrasound transducer affixed to the tip of the endoscope providing 270–360° imaging.

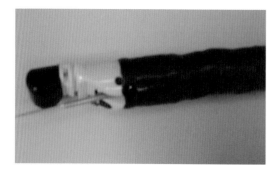

Fig. 4.6 The linear array format allows for longitudinal imaging acquired via linear-arrayed piezoelectric ultrasound transducers and allows for ultrasound-guided fine-needle biopsy tissue sampling.

Colonoscope

The colonoscope is a forward-viewing instrument designed to evaluate the entire colon and the distal terminal ileum. Standard feature variables include insertion tube length (1330–700 mm), insertion tube diameter (11.1–13.7 mm), instrument channel size (2.8–4.2 mm), and number (1–2). List prices range from $11 500 to $25 750. One manufacturer has developed a modification of the standard colonoscope incorporating a control capable of varying the stiffness of the distal portion of the insertion tube [14].

Sigmoidoscope

The sigmoidoscope is a forward-viewing instrument (a shorter version of a colonoscope) used to evaluate the rectum and sigmoid colon. The flexible sigmoidoscope was developed for screening average risk patients for colorectal polyps. Standard feature variables include insertion tube length (630–790 mm), insertion tube diameter (12.2–13.3 mm), and instrument channel size (3.2–4.2 mm). List prices range from $5250 to $15 100. A disposable, sheathed sigmoidoscope is also commercially available [15].

Wireless capsule endoscopy

The wireless endoscopy system has three components: a capsule 'endoscope', an external receiving antenna with attached portable hard drive, and a personal computer workstation for review and interpretation of images [16]. The capsule endoscope is a disposable plastic capsule (Fig. 4.7) which weighs 3.7 g and measures 11 mm in diameter × 26 mm in length. The contents include a metal oxide silicon (CMOS) chip camera, a short focal length lens, four white light-emitting diode (LED) illumination sources, two silver oxide batteries, and a UHF band radio telemetry transmitter.

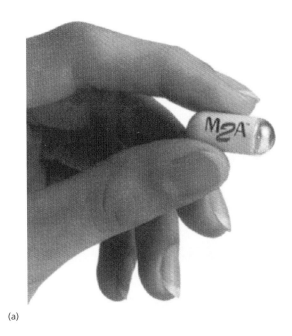

(a)

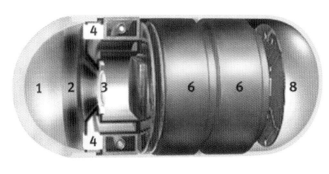

INSIDE THE M2A™ CAPSULE

1. Optical dome
2. Lens holder
3. Lens
4. Illuminating LEDs (Light Emitting Diode)
5. CMOS (Complementary Metal Oxide Semiconductor) imager
6. Battery
7. ASIC (Application Specific Integrated Circuit) transmitter
8. Antenna

(b)

Fig. 4.7 (a) The capsule endoscope is a disposable plastic capsule which weighs 3.7 g and measures 11 mm in diameter × 26 mm in length. (b) The contents include a metal oxide silicon (CMOS) chip camera, a short focal length lens, four white light-emitting diode (LED) illumination sources, two silver oxide batteries, and a UHF band radio telemetry transmitter.

The capsule is activated after removal from a magnetic holder. The wireless capsule endoscope provides image accrual and transmission at a frequency of two frames per second until the battery expires after 7 ($\pm$ 1) h. The capsule is passively propelled through the intestine by peristalsis. The patient wears a shoulder-supported belt pack holding a power supply containing five ('D cell'-sized) nickel-metal 1.2 V batteries, and a small 305 GB hard drive for archiving received images. Data are downloaded from the belt pack recorder to a customized PC work-station. Images are then reviewed at an adjustable rapid scan mode that can display between 1 and 25 frames per second. Interpretation requires 30–120 min. An anticipated software enhancement is intended to provide automated screening for potentially significant findings based on algorithms for image assessment. Wireless capsule systems specifically designed for imaging the esophagus and colon are in development as are real-time image transmission capabilities.

Gastrointestinal endoscopic accessories

Endoscopic accessories are used for tissue sampling, ablation, marking, and resection; object retrieval; image enhancement; injection; hemostasis; enteral access; dilation; and stenting. This section provides an overview of accessory devices used in endoscopy. Specific applications of these accessories are detailed elsewhere.

Tissue sampling

Tissue sampling is used to acquire specimens for histological and cytological inspection. Tissue sampling may be directed or random. The principles of tissue sampling and devices used are fairly uniform throughout the digestive tract. Tissue sampling can be performed with forceps biopsy, brush cytology, fine-needle aspiration, and snare resection. Snare resection will be covered elsewhere, with polypectomy.

Biopsy forceps

Biopsy forceps are used to sample mucosa and mucosal-based lesions. Endoscopic biopsy forceps consist of a flexible, metal-coil outer sheath that houses a steel cable connecting a two-piece plastic handle to opposed metal biopsy cups. Some biopsy forceps sheaths are coated with a synthetic polymer to improve passage through the endoscope accessory channel.

Single-bite cold-biopsy forceps. Single-bite cold-biopsy forceps allow sampling of only a single specimen at a time. *Double-bite* cold-biopsy forceps (most

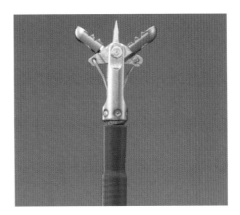

Fig. 4.8 Endoscopic biopsy forceps consist of a flexible, metal-coil outer sheath that houses a steel cable connecting a two-piece plastic handle to opposed metal biopsy cups.

commonly employed) are equipped with a *needle-spike* between the opposing biopsy cups (Fig. 4.8). The needle-spike serves several purposes. First, the spike can be used to impale the tissue of interest, thus stabilizing the forceps cups for selected tissue sampling. Second, needle version forceps obtain deeper biopsies than non-needle versions [17]. Lastly, the spike secures the first specimen on the device while a second specimen is obtained. Without the spike, attempts at multiple tissue sampling with single-bite forceps may result in the loss of specimens and crush artifact.

Biopsy cup jaws. Biopsy cup jaws may be standard oval or elongated, fenestrated or non-fenestrated, and smooth or serrated. Large-capacity cup, or 'jumbo' biopsy forceps obtain a larger volume of tissue than standard capacity forceps, but may require a large channel endoscope for their use. Large-capacity biopsy forceps require a biopsy channel of at least 3.6 mm and yield 2–3× the surface area, but not generally deeper specimens. The use of jumbo biopsy forceps has been advocated by some for surveillance in Barrett's esophagus and for excisional biopsy polypectomy of diminutive colonic polyps [18].

Multi-bite forceps. Multi-bite forceps have been developed that can obtain four or more specimens on a single pass. In a prospective, partially blinded, randomized trial of multi-bite forceps vs. conventional forceps, the multi-bite forceps compared equivalently for diagnostic quality [19]. The multi-bite forceps have the potential to save time when a large number of specimens must be obtained, such as in surveillance of patients with ulcerative colitis.

Other specialty forceps. Other specialty forceps include a variety of innovations for challenging circumstances. 'Swing-jaw' forceps feature a rocking cup assembly action intended to direct the jaws of the forceps toward the tissue of interest.

'Rotatable' forceps are designed to do just that, with variable degrees of control. 'Angled' forceps assume a 90° orientation to the long access of the scope once extended from the accessory channel.

Monopolar hot biopsy forceps. Monopolar hot biopsy forceps were developed for simultaneous tissue biopsy and coagulation. Thermal energy is generated when current, passed through an insulated shaft, is introduced to the tissue at the blunted edges of the forceps jaws [20]. Heat energy is regulated and determined by generator voltage and waveform, current density, and application time [21]. Bipolar hot biopsy forceps have also been developed. Bipolar forceps have insulated biopsy cups except for the cup edges, which are the electrodes [21]. Tissue injury is deeper with monopolar hot biopsy forceps than with bipolar forceps [20].

Hot biopsy became popular for biopsy resection of diminutive colonic polyps. The rationale for coagulative tissue sampling is to destroy neoplastic tissue, thereby preventing residual or recurrent adenoma and the development of carcinoma. However, there is insufficient data to indicate that excisional hot biopsy forceps removal reduces the incidence of colorectal cancer or even complete eradication of all neoplastic tissue [20,22,23]. Furthermore, complications of hot biopsy forceps include hemorrhage, perforation, and postcoagulation (trans-mural burn) syndrome [20]. Based on these observations, routine application of hot biopsy is not recommended.

Reusable vs. disposable biopsy. The relative virtues of reusable vs. disposable biopsy forceps can be debated. Arguments focus on cost, operational performance, and infection control. In two prospective, randomized, pathologist-blinded trials, there were no perceived differences in quality of specimen for histological diagnosis between a variety of commercially available reusable and disposable biopsy forceps [24,25].

Yang *et al.* prospectively measured cost and operational performance of disposable and reusable forceps in 200 biopsy sessions [26]. Reusable costs factored in acquisition and reprocessing. They found that malfunction of reusable forceps increased with number of uses. At up to 15–20 uses, reusable and disposable forceps costs are similar, when the cost of disposable forceps is around $40.00. When reusable forceps can be used more than 20 times, they are less expensive.

However, in their study the performance of reusable forceps deteriorated significantly in this range. Deprez *et al.*, in a much larger study (7740 sessions) using similar design and the lowest available purchase price for disposable forceps at the time ($26.90), reported that total purchase and reprocessing costs for reusable forceps were 25% of those of disposable devices [27]. Further, an average of 315 biopsy sessions were performed with a reusable forceps, extending their mean life to 3 years.

Conversely, in a third study, disposable forceps outperformed their reusable counterparts and offered a cost advantage [28]. These authors also reported a concern over residual proteinacious material observed in reusable forceps, raising an infection control risk. This charge was countered, however, in a study by Kozarek *et al*. who performed an *ex vivo* evaluation of cleaning, and an *in vivo* evaluation of function, performance, and durability of reusable forceps [29]. Their analysis concluded that reusable biopsy forceps are confidently sterilized when accepted cleaning and sterilization protocols are followed. Sterilized reusable biopsy forceps were used a mean 91 times, rendering the potential for significant cost saving, again, depending on acquisition and reprocessing costs. All published cases of transmission of infection associated with reusable biopsy forceps have been attributed to breaches in accepted standards of device reprocessing [30].

The functional performance of reusable biopsy forceps will ultimately deteriorate with increased number of uses. The durability can be extended with care in use and reprocessing. Cost comparisons depend mainly on the cost of disposable devices. Users should also factor in the cost of medical waste disposal and environmental impact associated with disposal of single use devices.

Cytology brushes

A variety of commercially available cytology brushes are used for tissue sampling, especially in the esophagus and pancreatico-biliary ductal systems. Designs include variable brush sizes and stiffness, wire guided and non-wire guided, single and multilumen, and with or without a flexible guide tip. Outer sheaths for brushes used in ERCP are 6–8 Fr [31,32]. A cytology balloon for non-endoscopic esophageal cytological screening and surveillance for infectious and neoplastic diseases has been described [33].

Needle aspiration

Hollow bore needles may be used for aspiration cytological tissue sampling. ERCP aspiration needles consist of a retractable 7.5 mm 22 gauge needle attached to a ball-tipped catheter [34]. The needle is advanced into the target tissue under fluoroscopy and aspiration is applied. Howell *et al*. developed a technique for sampling biliary stricture by endoscopic FNA [35]. Needle aspiration of submucosal lesions under direct endoscopic guidance can be performed; however, this technique and the devices to support it are currently undergoing refinement [36]. EUS-guided fine-needle aspiration is covered in the Endoscopic Ultrasound section.

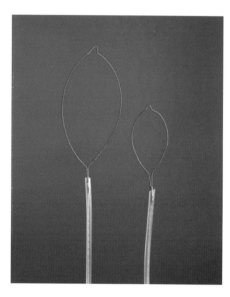

Fig. 4.9 Polypectomy snares are used for resection of sessile and pedunculated epithelial lesions throughout the digestive tract. Polypectomy snares consist of an attached or continuous wire loop housed within a flexible synthetic polymer sheath.

Polypectomy snares

Polypectomy snares are used for resection of sessile and pedunculated epithelial lesions throughout the digestive tract (Fig. 4.9). Snares are used in standard and advanced (often considered under the rubric of endoscopic mucosal resection (EMR)) polypectomy techniques. Polypectomy snares are available in a variety of shapes, sizes, and materials. Specialty snares are designed with special features for specific performance properties.

Snares may be designed and marketed as *disposable* or *reusable*. Reusable snares must be designed so they may be disassembled for cleaning and sterilization and then reassembled, plus have properties that enable them to retain their configuration and performance through multiple use and cleaning cycles. These constraints, plus the availability of cheap materials and production costs, have promoted broad acceptance of disposable snares for endoscopic polypectomy.

Polypectomy snares consist of an attached or continuous wire loop housed within a flexible synthetic polymer *sheath*. This portion of the device is passed through the accessory channel of the endoscope. Sheaths are typically 7.0 Fr in diameter, for a minimal channel size of 2.8 mm, and up to 230 cm or more in length. The wire and sheath are affixed to a moving-parts plastic *handle* at the operator end of the device. The handle controls opening (extension) and closing (retraction) of the wire loop from and within the outer sheath. The snare wire couples to an electrical connector within the handle. The handle has a receptacle for connection to an active cord, thus allowing completion of an electrosurgical circuit.

While bipolar snares have been developed, most snares employ monopolar current. Bipolar snares are designed with each half of the snare loop functioning as an electrode such that current flows across the polyp [37]. In monopolar snares the current flows from the snare to a distant return electrode (grounding pad), generating local thermal energy for cutting and coagulation [21]. There are no comparative trials of bipolar vs. monopolar snares.

Braided stainless steel *wire* is the most commonly used material for polypectomy snares, owing to its strength, conduction properties, and configurational memory. The snare wire typically is 0.30–0.47 mm in diameter. Nitinol wire snares may have superior configurational memory but lack sufficient stiffness, tending to leave them floppier than desired. Monofilament wire snares promote transection over coagulation and are largely limited to use in cold-snare polypectomy of small polyps in patients without coagulation disorders [38].

The standard *shape* of the snare loop is oval or elliptical. Alternative configurations include round, crescent, or hexagonal. A variety of snares are available through device manufacturers and can be viewed in their product catalogues. Selection of snare configuration is based on personal preference. Experienced endoscopists may choose specific snare shapes for removal of individual lesions based on the lesion's location, orientation, size, and configuration. The standard size and shape snare suffices for the vast majority of instances. There are no comparisons of snare shapes to support superiority of one or more snare configurations over others.

While there is some variability among the manufacturers, standard *size* snare loops are typically 2.0–2.5 cm in diameter. Loop lengths vary based on configuration and manufacturer. Mini-snares have loop diameters of 1.0–1.5 cm, and are handy for completion resection of residual adenoma following mucosectomy of a sessile lesion and for resection of diminutive polyps [39]. Jumbo snares have loop dimensions of up to 3×6 cm and are used to transect large pedunculated polyps not accommodated by standard snares.

Other *specialty* snares have been developed to enhance success when circumstances prove challenging to characteristics of ordinary snares. While specialty snares may offer advantages in specific instances, most experienced endoscopists do quite well with standard-loop snares along with the occasional use of mini- and jumbo snares. Nonetheless a familiarity with, and limited stock of, specialty snares may ensure success when faced with the occasional defiant polyp. Duck-bill® and multiangled (Wilson-Cook Medical Inc., Winston-Salem, NC) snares are intended for lesions difficult to access based on their wall location with respect to the tip of the colonoscope. Rotatable snares can be adjusted so that the snare loop opens in an orientation favorable to polyp entrapment.

Needle- or anchor-tipped snares have a short, pointed barb at the tip of the snare. The modified tip is intended to aid in stabilizing the snare for polyp capture. By impaling the barbed tip into the bowel wall just beyond the lesion, the snare tip can be fixed in place while the loop is being flexed to open over and around the polyp.

A variety of snares have been developed and marketed for removal of sessile polyps. These iterations include barbed, spiral, and 'hairy' snares. Each is designed to grip the edges of low profile sessile lesions. There are no studies to indicate superiority of modified over standard snares for resection of sessile colon polyps.

Retrieval devices

An assortment of retrieval devices has been developed for extraction of resected specimens and foreign objects from the luminal digestive tract. These include a variety of graspers, baskets, and nets [40]. Specimen retrieval is critical for histopathological interpretation. The Roth net (US Endoscopy, Mentor, OH) enables the secure retrieval of multiple specimens, thereby reducing the need for repeated withdrawal and reinsertion of the endoscope (Fig. 4.10). The secure handling of the specimen makes this device ideal for retrieval of specimens from the upper digestive tract, wherein unintentional dislodgement in the airway must be avoided.

Many tissue sampling and retrieval devices may be applied to the management of ingested foreign objects. These include: retrieval net, grasping forceps ('Alligator' or 'Rat-tooth'), three-pronged grasper, Dormia basket, polypectomy snare, variceal band-ligation hood, and protector hood [41]. Over-tubes of both standard length that bypass the upper esophageal sphincter and longer 45–60 cm tubes that extend into the stomach should be available. Over-tubes

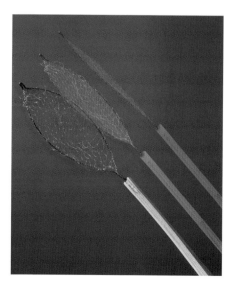

Fig. 4.10 The Roth net (US Endoscopy, Mentor, OH) enables secure retrieval of multiple specimens from the upper and lower digestive tracts.

can protect the esophageal mucosa when retrieving sharp objects, allow multiple passes of the endoscope, and protect the airway during retrieval.

Alternatively, a latex protector hood that can be attached to the end of the endoscope can protect the airway and the mucosa when an object is grasped and pulled tightly against the scope during withdrawal. Knowledge of the type of object and its location prior to endoscopy may permit an *ex vivo* or practice 'dry run', allowing proper equipment selection and improved outcome [42].

Injection devices

Injection devices include injection needles, spray catheters, and ERCP catheters.

Injection needles

Injection needles are devices passed through the accessory channel of the endoscope to enable injection of a solution into tissue. Injection needles are used for injection-assisted polypectomy, hemostasis (variceal, non-variceal, and hemorrhoidal), and tattooing.

Injection needles consist of an outer sheath (plastic, Teflon, or stainless steel coil) and an inner hollow core needle (21–25G) (Fig. 4.11) [43]. The needle tip is typically beveled. Needle tip length should be sufficient to routinely penetrate into the submucosa and not so long as to routinely penetrate through the colon serosa. They are available in colonoscopic lengths and typically have an outside diameter 2.3–2.8 mm. A metal and plastic luer lock handle controls needle extension and retraction to fixed or variable lengths. Some versions allow the needle to be preferentially locked when in the extended position. Most commercially available injection needles are single-use disposable.

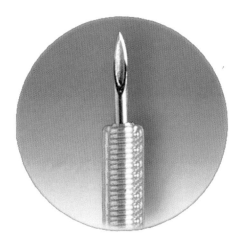

Fig. 4.11 Injection needles consist of an outer sheath (plastic, Teflon, or stainless steel coil) and an inner hollow core needle.

Metal coil-sheathed needles may offer advantages over their plastic-sheathed counterparts in that they are less likely to kink and are more apt to remain fully functional when articulated. This allows use even when there is excessive looping of the colonoscope or when operating with a retroflexed colonoscope position. Metal coil sheaths are also less likely to allow unintended needle puncture through the sheath with the associated risk of scope injury. However, there are no published trials comparing various injection catheters for colonoscopic applications.

An injection needle has also been incorporated into a multipolar electro-cautery device. This device allows combination injection and contact-thermal hemostatic therapy for non-variceal bleeding.

Spray catheters

Spray catheters are used when performing chromoendoscopy. Chromoendoscopy employs a chromic agent to enhance the detection or discrimination of dysplastic epithelia [44]. Chromic agents may be vital stains or contrast agents. Vital stains are selectively taken up by epithelial cell cytoplasm, whereas contrast agents coat the epithelial surface enhancing the contour relief pattern. Contrast agents are commonly employed when performing high-resolution and high-magnification endoscopy [44].

Spray catheters are disposable, flexible, hollow plastic sheaths, with a plastic luer lock handle, and a metal spray nozzle tip (Fig. 4.12). Alternatives to

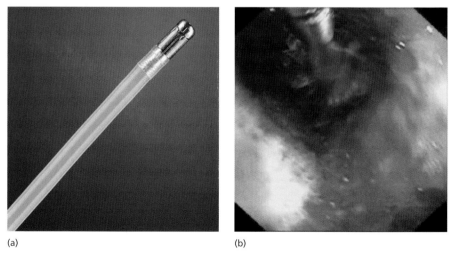

(a)   (b)

Fig. 4.12 (a) Spray catheters are disposable, flexible, hollow plastic sheaths, with a plastic luer lock handle and a metal spray nozzle tip. (b) Vital stains like Lugol's seen here, and contrast agents are applied via spray catheters.

dedicated spray catheters are injection needles, ERCP catheters, and simple injection through the accessory port itself. Spray catheters generally allow the most controlled, precise, and tidy application for chromoendoscopy.

ERCP catheters

A plethora of specially designed catheters are commercially available for cannulation and injection of contrast into the pancreatico-biliary systems. These are single, double, or triple lumen plastic catheters that are passed through the accessory channel of the duodenoscope. In addition to facilitating radiocontrast dye injection, the catheter lumina accept guidewires for access and device exchange. Specialty devices are equipped with adjunctive apparatti to perform specific actions. Sphincterotomes have an electrosurgical wire for transecting the papillary sphincters. Stone retrieval balloon and pneumatic dilating catheters have inflatable balloons specific to their intended purposes.

Hemostatic and ablation devices

Contact and non-contact thermal devices

Thermal devices are used for coagulative hemostasis and ablation. Contact thermal devices include the heater probe and multipolar electrocautery (MPEC) probes [45]. Non-contact thermal devices include laser fibers and argon plasma beam coagulators [45]. Radiofrequency powered contact thermal devices have been developed specifically for mucosal ablation.

Heater probe. The heater probe (Olympus America, Melville, NY) consists of a Teflon-coated hollow aluminum cylinder with an inner-heating coil at the tip of a flexible shaft. A thermocoupling device at the tip of the probe allows maintenance of a predetermined and constant temperature once the pulse has been initiated for a predetermined duration of activation. The mechanism of tissue coagulation is heat transfer. Water for irrigation and cleansing the target tissue passes through a central port. A foot pedal controls coagulation and irrigation. *MPEC* probes deliver thermal energy by completion of an electrical circuit between two or more electrodes on a probe at the tip of a flexible shaft [46]. The electrodes may be arrayed linearly or in a spiral fashion (Fig. 4.13).

The circuit is completed locally and ceases with loss of conductivity as tissue desiccates, limiting maximum temperature (100°C) and depth and breadth of tissue injury. There is a central port for irrigation of water. Foot pedal control is standard. A variety of MPEC probes in colonoscopic lengths are available from

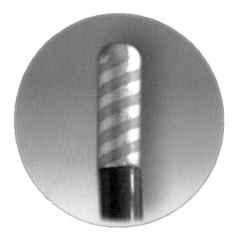

Fig. 4.13 Contact hemostasis probes deliver thermal energy by completion of an electrical circuit between two or more electrodes on a probe at the tip of a flexible shaft. Here the electrodes are arrayed in a spiral fashion.

endoscope device manufacturers with similar specifications but varied characteristics. One device combines an injection needle with the MPEC probe. Both the heater and MPEC probes can be used tangentially and *en face*.

Laser fibers. Laser fibers transmit collimated, highly energized light energy, emitting a focused monochromatic beam [47]. They are flexible glass fibers with coated shafts. The laser light delivered from a focal distance of ~10 mm from the tissue results in coagulation or vaporization. Cylindrical diffuser laser fibers are used in photodynamic therapy (PDT) (Fig. 4.14a).

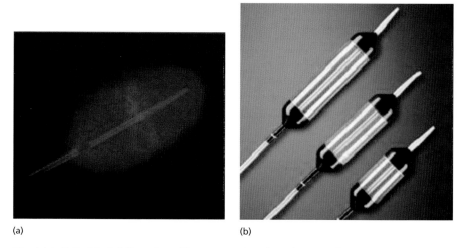

(a)   (b)

Fig. 4.14 Cylindrical diffuser laser fibers are used in photodynamic therapy (PDT).
(a) These flexible glass fibers are modified with a variable length tip that promotes uniform scattering of laser light energy circumferentially along the long axis of the diffuser tip.
(b) A further modification of the cylindrical diffusion catheter used for PDT in the esophagus incorporates an inflatable centering balloon.

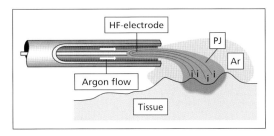

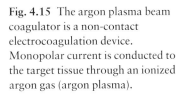

Fig. 4.15 The argon plasma beam coagulator is a non-contact electrocoagulation device. Monopolar current is conducted to the target tissue through an ionized argon gas (argon plasma).

These flexible glass fibers are modified with a variable length tip that promotes uniform scattering of laser light energy circumferentially along the long axis of the diffuser tip. PDT utilizes non-thermal laser energy to interact with a photosensitizing agent present in target tissue. A further modification of the cylindrical diffusion catheter used for PDT in the esophagus incorporates an inflatable centering balloon (Fig. 4.14b).

Argon plasma beam coagulator. The argon plasma beam coagulator is a non-contact electrocoagulation device [48]. Monopolar current is conducted to the target tissue through an ionized argon gas (argon plasma) (Fig. 4.15). As it is monopolar current, a grounding pad is required to complete the circuit. Electrical energy flows through the plasma from the probe tip to the target tissue. Coagulation occurs at the plasma–tissue surface interface. As the target tissue desiccates, the plasma stream shifts to adjacent, non-desiccated tissue. The probes consist of a flexible Teflon tube as a shaft, with a tungsten electrode contained in a ceramic nozzle at its distal tip [49,50].

The operative distance of the probe from the target tissue is 2–8 mm. While mode-specific probes are available, the arch of energized argon plasma to the tissue enables *en face* or tangential coagulation/ablation with the standard probe. An argon plasma beam coagulation unit (ERBE USA, Marietta, GA; ConMed Electrosurgery, Englewood, CO) includes a high-frequency electrosurgical generator, source of argon gas, gas flow meter, flexible delivery catheter, grounding pad, and foot switch to activate both gas and energy.

Contact and non-contact thermal devices are used for hemostasis of bleeding from ulcers, postpolypectomy, angiodysplasia, and diverticulosis. Contact and non-contact thermal devices are also used to ablate residual adenomatous-appearing mucosa at the margins of snare resection of sessile polyps and for ablation of lesions unamenable to endoscopic or surgical resection [51–52]. Non-contact thermal devices have been used to ablate obstructing cancers to achieve recannulation of the lumen, and for hemostasis of inoperable cancers.

Radiofrequency contact thermal ablation. Barrx (BÂRRX Medical, Inc., Sunnyvale, CA) has developed the Halo 360° and 90° systems that are radiofrequency powered contact thermal devices specifically devised for ablation of Barrett's esophageal mucosa. The Halo 360° device consist of a flexible, non-through-the-scope, wire-guided probe equipped with an inflatable balloon covered by a radiofrequency electrode mesh. The balloon is inflated to make uniform contact with the Barrett's involved epithelium. Brief introduction of energy from a radiofrequency generator produces coagulative necrosis [53]. The Halo 90° is a modification for focal endoscopically directed therapy.

Mechanical hemostatic devices

Mechanical hemostatic devices include bands, clips, and detachable loops.

Band ligation. Band ligation devices consist of a transparent, hollow-chamber, friction-fit adapter affixed to the tip of the endoscope, preloaded elastic band(s), and a release mechanism. The target tissue is suctioned into the hollow chamber of the friction-fit adapter (Fig. 4.16). A trigger mechanism deploys an elastic band, ligating the target tissue. Tissue ligation results in hemostasis with subsequent necrosis and sloughing [54,55]. Single and multiple band ligators are available. Variceal band ligation is effective in the control of active hemorrhage in 86–91% of cases [56,57].

Subsequent sessions result in eradication of esophageal varices and decreased rebleeding. Band ligating devices have been used for non-esophageal varices, including gastric, intestinal, and colonic varices, but data are limited. Case reports and small series have described the use of endoscopic band ligation for treatment of bleeding angiectasias, Mallory–Weiss tears, polypectomy sites, Dieulafoy lesions, and duodenal ulcers. Multi-band ligators, all with transparent outer cylinders, carrying 3, 4, 5, 6, or 10 bands, are now available.

There are three commercially available devices on the market: Saeed Multi-Band Ligators (Wilson-Cook Medical, Inc., Winston-Salem, NC), Speedband Multiple Band Ligator (Microvasive, Boston Scientific Corp., Natick, MA), and a new system from Bard (CR Bard, Inc., Billerica, MA). All of these devices have easy to assemble components and vary only slightly in their form and function.

Metallic clip application via flexible endoscopes. Metallic clip application via flexible endoscopes has had considerable appeal for a variety of indications. The most evolved experience has been with the HX series of endoscopic clip fixing devices (Olympus Corp., Tokyo, Japan). This device was first conceived for hemostasis of non-variceal bleeding sources. Other commercially available

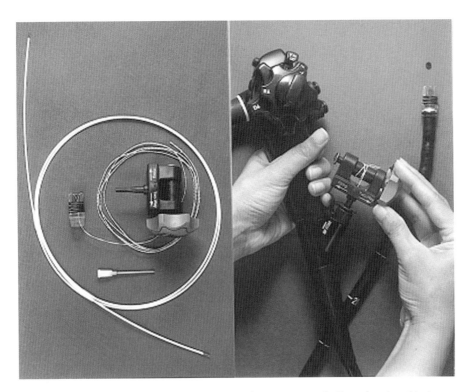

Fig. 4.16 Variceal band ligation devices consist of a transparent, hollow-chamber, friction-fit adapter affixed to the tip of the endoscope, preloaded elastic band(s), and a release mechanism. The target tissue is suctioned into the hollow chamber of the friction-fit adapter. A trigger mechanism deploys an elastic band, ligating the target tissue.

clipping devices are the Triclip (Wilson-Cook Medical, Inc., Winston-Salem, NC) and Resolution Clip (Boston Scientific Inc., Natick, MA).

Endoscopic clip application has been used effectively for hemostasis of immediate and delayed bleeding from polypectomy and hot biopsy forceps sites; diverticular, arteriovenous malformations, and variceal bleeding; and prophylaxis of postpolypectomy bleeding pre- and post snare resection. Such mechanical hemostasis allows localized, directed, and specific therapy, while minimizing tissue injury at the treatment site.

Other applications have included lesion marking (bleeding or tumor site), fixation of endoscopically placed decompression tubes, and primary closure of resection sites and perforations. The clip-fixing device has evolved from its first inception to a relatively easy to use, reliable, and now rotatable delivery device (Fig. 4.17) [58,59].

A single use, preloaded iteration has become available. The clips themselves are configured of a multiangled stainless steel ribbon. Clips are available in a

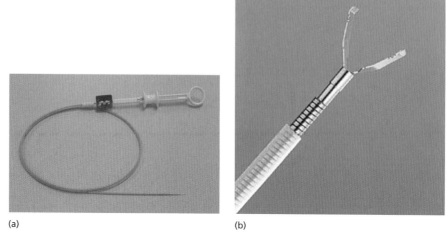

(a)   (b)

Fig. 4.17 (a) The clip-fixing device consists of a control section and an insertion tube. The control section incorporates movable plastic parts that manipulate clip loading and deployment. The insertion tube is made up of a metal coil sheath contained within an outer plastic sheath. A metal cable moves within the coil sheath. (b) The clips themselves are configured of a multi-angled stainless steel ribbon. When fully opened, the predeployment distance between the clip prongs measures 7 mm.

limited variety of lengths and configurations. Clips typically slough off in 3–4 weeks and pass uneventfully in the stool.

In practice, the clip is loaded onto the hooking cable and withdrawn into the outer plastic tube sheath. This procedure is unnecessary when using the preloaded ready-to-use versions. The delivery device insertion tube is then passed through the endoscope working channel. With the target lesion in view, deployment is initiated by exposing the clip from within the tube sheath. Withdrawing the cable within the tube sheath slides the pipe clip up the clip itself, fully opening the clip. With the rotatable version, a rotator-disc located on the control section may be used to turn the clip to the desired orientation. The insertion tube is then advanced so the teeth of the clip engage the target tissue, whereupon further sliding of the pipe clip closes the clip and completes deployment, detaching the clip from the clip connector.

Becoming facile with loading and deployment of endoscopic clips requires practice and regular use. Clips deploy with equal reliability in the *en face*, as well as in retroflexed scope positions. Some models are equipped with the rotating wheel that works surprisingly well. The clip can be rotated to the desired orientation the majority of times. The rotator feature and improved durability are clear advantages over earlier clip designs. An unlimited number of clips can be placed during a single session. Mechanical cleaning followed by gas sterilization can reprocess the reusable-model delivery device.

Endoscopic mucosal clips are highly effective for prophylactic *hemostasis* of polypectomy and mucosectomy sites and for primary or secondary hemostasis of postpolypectomy bleeding [60,61]. Endoscopic hemoclips promote durable hemostasis and do not incur additive tissue injury as is the case with thermal or injection techniques. Among 72 cases of colonoscopic immediate postpolypectomy ($n = 45$), delayed postpolypectomy ($n = 18$), and postbiopsy ($n = 9$) bleeding, effective and durable clip hemostasis was achieved in all but one case [62]. There were no episodes of recurrent bleeding or need for surgery related to bleeding.

Marking with clips. Marking with clips is effective for lesions benefiting from precise localization preoperatively, including tumors and bleeding sites (e.g. diverticulum). Clips can readily be palpated or located with fluoroscopy at the time of surgery. Clips may be used for the *fixation* of colonic decompression tubes to prevent tube migration. Lastly, endoscopic mucosal clips have been used to achieve transient *tissue remodeling* to oppose surrounding tissue at a resection site or luminal defect [63]. The latter application should be limited to use in highly selected instances.

Detachable loops. Detachable loops have been developed for the prevention and management of bleeding from polypectomy sites. Such bleeding is reported to occur in 2% of all polypectomies. Bleeding occurs more frequently with the removal of large polyps with thick stalks and in patients who have underlying coagulopathies or those taking anticoagulation therapy or non-steroidal anti-inflammatory drugs. The detachable loop snare ligature was developed for primary or secondary prophylactic therapy for postpolypectomy bleeding, or as primary or secondary treatment of active or recent postpolypectomy hemorrhage [64–67].

The detachable snare or 'endoloop' (Olympus HX-20Q, Olympus Corp., Tokyo) is composed of an operating apparatus (MH-489) and an attachable loop of nylon thread (MH-477) (Fig. 4.18). The operating apparatus consists of a Teflon sheath 2.5 mm in diameter and 1950 mm in working length, a stainless steel coil sheath 1.9 mm in diameter, a hook wire, and the handle. The nylon loop is non-conductive and consists of a heat-treated circular or elliptically shaped nylon thread and a silicon-rubber stopper that maintains the tightness of the loop.

The optimal application of this device for prevention and management of polypectomy bleeding is yet to be determined. When used for primary prophylaxis, the flexibility of the loop makes it difficult to encircle the large polyps, wherein its use would be most desirable. Entanglement of the subsequent electrocautery snare with the previously placed nylon loop may be a source of frustration. Unintentional transection of the polyp stalk with the detachable loop

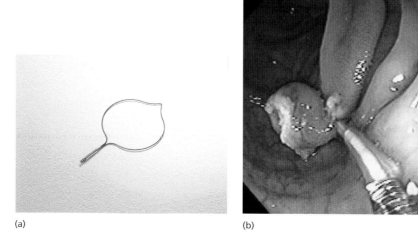

(a)   (b)

Fig. 4.18 (a) The detachable snare or 'endoloop' (Olympus HX-20Q, Olympus Corp., Tokyo). The nylon loop is non-conductive and consists of a heat-treated circular or elliptically shaped nylon thread and a silicon-rubber stopper that maintains the tightness of the loop. (b) Following snare resection of the large pedunculated polyp, a detachable loop was applied to prevent delayed bleeding.

snare, resulting in a frank hemorrhage, is a risk in the hand of an inexperienced assistant. When used as secondary prophylaxis against postpolypectomy bleeding, the loop is placed over the residual pedicle immediately postpolypectomy. This, too, can be challenging in all but the most prominent of residual stalks.

Matsushita *et al.* summarized their experience. They reported primary prophylactic use of a detachable snare for colonoscopic polypectomy of 20 large polyps in 18 patients and secondary prophylactic placement following conventional polypectomy of five polyps in five patients [68]. Four of the 20 polyps were semipedunculated and the loop slipped off after polypectomy in 3 of the 4. Among the 16 pedunculated polyps, bleeding occurred in 4 cases because of transection by the loop of the stalk before polypectomy in one, slipping-off of the loop in one, and insufficient tightening of the loop in two.

Among the five patients in whom the loop placement was attempted following conventional polypectomy, the residual stalk could not be ligated in three of the five lesions because of flattening. These authors concluded that the detachable snare is difficult to apply and subject to operator-dependent error. For the treatment of active bleeding from a polypectomy site again the loop was only effective when there was a sufficient pedicle to allow ensnarement. Iishi *et al.* report a more favorable experience [69].

Primary loop ligation for treatment of postpolypectomy hemorrhage is most apt to occur in the immediate postpolypectomy setting before the stalk has had a chance to flatten. In most instances when postpolypectomy hemorrhage is delayed, there is active hemorrhage or adherent clot obscuring view. Initial attempts at hemostasis with injection of epinephrine or alcohol solution may achieve partial hemostasis and improve visualization. If a sufficient residual stalk is present, loops may well be applied; however, alternatives include additional electrocautery, placement of endoscopic hemostatic clips, or even the placement of a variceal rubber band ligator.

Transparent cap

Plastic transparent caps that affix to and overhang the tip of the endoscope may be used to enhance colonic visualization and to facilitate EMR [70]. These caps are modifications of devices initially used for endoscopic band ligation therapy. The caps consist of a hollow cylinder of fixed or flexible plastic and a snug-fitting adaptor that slides over and is affixed to the tip of the endoscope (Fig. 4.19) [71]. Those devised for cap-assisted EMR may have a built-in rim to house a predeployed, specially designed snare. A commonly used cap size is 16 mm in outer diameter with 2 mm wall thickness, and 15 mm in length. However, they are available in a variety of sizes and configurations, including straight or oblique-angled opening, depending on the intended purpose and endoscope being used (Olympus America Inc., Melville, NY).

For cap-assisted EMR, submucosal injection of saline or other sterile solution is performed to 'lift' the mucosal-based lesion on a submucosal cushion. The scope tip with the attached cap is then placed over the lesion. By applying suction, the cap cylinder becomes a vacuum chamber, drawing the target tissue into a pseudo-polyp within. The predeployed snare is then closed and standard electrocautery excision is performed. This technique has been described for lesions throughout the digestive tract and is safe and effective in experienced hands [72]. Cap-assisted EMR may also be used for completion resection of flat or sessile lesions not amenable to other mucosectomy techniques [73].

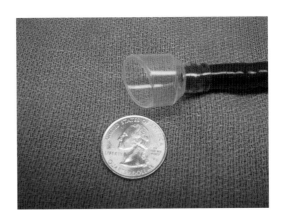

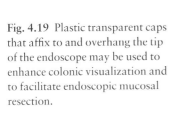

Fig. 4.19 Plastic transparent caps that affix to and overhang the tip of the endoscope may be used to enhance colonic visualization and to facilitate endoscopic mucosal resection.

The transparent cap may also be used to enhance mucosal imaging during colonoscope withdrawal. Using this technique, the semilunar folds can be flattened out for improved inspection. In two series, use of the cap did not interfere with colonoscope insertion or terminal ileal intubation, and enabled identification of small polyps not seen on standard colonoscopy [74,75]. Caps are also used in some applications of magnification endoscopy.

The Duette system (Cook Medical, Winston Sale, NC) is a modification of their multiband variceal ligation device (see above) that permits suction and band ligation of flat mucosa and mucosal-based lesions for snare resection. This enables wide area piecemeal resection.

Dilation devices

Dilatation of strictures is indicated when there is functional impairment or a need to access beyond the stricture for diagnosis or therapy. A variety of devices are available for dilation of digestive tract strictures. Many dilators have indication-specific characteristics; others are relatively generic in design.

Dilation devices can be organized into two categories: fixed-diameter push-type dilators and radial expanding balloon dilators. Fixed-diameter push-type dilators exert axial as well as radial forces as they are advanced through a stenosis [76]. Balloon dilators exert radial forces when expanded within a stenosis.

Dilators can be delivered to strictures in a number of ways based on the dilator design and operator technique, including with or without endoscopic, fluoroscopic, and/or wire guidance. Fixed-diameter and balloon dilator designs include 'through-the-scope' ('TTS') and 'non-TTS' types. The endoscope accessory channel must accommodate TTS dilators. Most push-type dilators are non-TTS devices, except those used for pancreatico-biliary applications.

Guidewires may be used to facilitate delivery of dilating devices to strictures throughout the gastrointestinal tract and can be passed via endoscopy with or without fluoroscopy. Wire-guided TTS dilators are passed over a guidewire and through the endoscope accessory channel. Non-TTS wire-guided dilators are passed over a guidewire following initial endoscopic guidewire placement and subsequent endoscope removal. A variety of specialty wires with flexible coil tips, stiff shafts, and external measurement markers are available.

Push-type fixed-diameter dilators

Push-type fixed-diameter dilators come in a variety of designs, calibers, and lengths. They are sold individually and in sets of varying calibers. Most fixed-diameter dilators are marketed as reprocessable multi-use devices.

Hurst and Maloney dilators. Hurst and Maloney (Medovations, Milwaukee, WI) dilators, also referred to as 'bougies', are fixed-diameter push-type dilators that do not accommodate a guidewire [77–79]. They are internally weighted with mercury or tungsten for gravity assistance when passed with the patient in the upright position. *Hurst* dilators have a blunt rounded tip, while *Maloney* dilators have an elongated tapered tip. Patients may be instructed to use these devices for self-dilation.

Savary-type dilators. Savary-type dilators are flexible taper-tipped polyvinyl chloride cylinders with a central channel for passage over a guidewire. Savary-Gilliard® (Wilson-Cook Medical, Inc, Winston-Salem, NC) dilators have a long tapered tip and a radiopaque marking at the base of the taper designating the point of maximal dilating caliber.

American Dilation System dilators. American Dilation System® (CRBard, Inc, Billerica, MA) dilators have a shorter taper tip and total radiopacity throughout their length.

TTS fixed diameter dilators. TTS fixed diameter dilators are tapered, guidewire-compatible plastic cylinders, developed for ERCP-mediated dilation of pancreatico-biliary strictures. They are passed over a guidewire through the accessory channel of the endoscope. They are equipped with a radiopaque band just proximal to the taper to indicate the point of maximal dilation.

Threaded-tip stent retrievers. Threaded-tip stent retrievers have also been used to dilate very tight pancreatico-biliary and esophageal strictures that otherwise allow only passage of a guidewire [80–82]. The wire-guided screw-tipped device is used to auger through high-grade stenoses. A modified device is now commercially available as a dilator (Wilson-Cook Medical, Inc., Winston-Salem, NC).

Radial expanding balloon dilators

Radial expanding balloon dilators are available in an array of designs, lengths, and calibers for various purposes. Balloon dilators are made of low-compliance, non-latex materials that allow uniform and reproducible expansion to their specified diameter at maximum inflation. One platform of balloon dilator is designed to expand to specific incremental calibers at sequentially higher pressures. Dilating balloons are expanded by pressure injection of liquid (e.g. water, radiopaque contrast), except for those designed for use in achalasia where air is used instead of fluid. The hydraulic pressure of the balloon may be monitored manometrically to gauge radial expansion force. Inflation with full-strength or dilute radiopaque contrast enhances fluoroscopic observation. Most dilating balloons are marketed as single-use items.

TTS dilators. TTS balloon dilators can be used in any accessible region of the gastrointestinal tract including the pancreatico-biliary tree. Non-TTS balloon dilators are wire-guided and primarily intended for use in the esophagus and distal colon.

Achalasia balloon dilators

Achalasia balloon dilators are large diameter (30, 35, and 40 mm), non-TTS, wire-guided radial expansion balloon dilators that are designed for achalasia but have also been used in other disease states [83–85]. A variety of designs used historically have been supplanted by the current non-radiopaque graded-size polyethylene balloons. They are positioned across the esophagogastric junction using fluoroscopic and/or endoscopic guidance. Insufflation with air is monitored manometrically. Some commercially available achalasia dilators are marketed for reuse.

Conclusion

Several manufacturers have developed a variety of endoscope models. Procedure-specific endoscopes are designed to enhance endoscopic diagnosis and therapy. An extensive array of accessory devices have been developed and adopted for diagnostic and therapeutic endoscopy. These innovations and adaptations have enabled the expansion of minimally invasive endoscopic therapies for benign and neoplastic diseases of the digestive tract. Countless lives have been saved, surgical procedures avoided, and societal benefits accrued, as a result of the development and dissemination of endoscope and endoscopic accessories and the techniques they enable. We are indebted to the legions of physician endoscopists and their industry counterparts who contributed to endoscope and device development and evaluation. Continuous creative innovation will see to the further advancement of these tools.

Outstanding issues and future trends

Modern endoscopy has brought forth many advances in direct imaging. The evolution of fiber optic to digital imaging has enabled further image quality enhancement and miniaturization. Efforts are underway to develop *optical biopsy* techniques that would allow accurate and reliable tissue discrimination without the need for tissue sampling. This might better enable identification of dysplastic tissue, otherwise indiscriminate by standard white-light endoscopy. Examples include light immunofluoresence spectroscopy, optical coherence tomography, and narrow-band imaging.

Scope designs are underway that will allow better function of accessories. Examples include attachments to duodenoscopes for fixing guidewires in place and holsters to seat ERCP catheters. Dedicated operating endoscopes will be developed as endoluminal and extraluminal endoscopic therapies emerge. Scope handle ergonomics are apt to evolve to include remote controlled, self-propelling, and power-steered endoscopes. Lastly, miniaturization will permit further reduction in instrument diameters.

Tissue sampling and resection devices continue to evolve and improve. Devices to allow large area *en bloc* mucosal resection are being displayed. Full-thickness resection devices are sure to be developed in our professional life-times. Plicating devices developed for endoluminal antireflux therapies are apt to have broad applications in hemostasis, resection, and bariatric procedures.

We expect to see further application of advanced computing techniques (such as neural networks) incorporated into 'intelligent' endoscopes. Eventually the capsule concept may incorporate automatic therapeutic devices.

Continuing ingenuity and collaboration between physicians and engineers will certainly provide important new tools in the future.

References

1 Sivak MV. Endoscopic technology: is this as good as it gets? 1999; 50: 718–21.
2 Barlow DE. (2000). Flexible endoscopic technology: the video image endoscope. In: *Gastroenterologic endoscopy*, 2nd edn (ed. Sivak MV), pp. 29–49. W.B. Saunders, Philadelphia.
3 Kawahara I, Ichikawa H. (2000). Flexible endoscopic technology: the fiberoptic endoscope. In: *Gastroenterologic Endoscopy*, 2nd edn (ed. Sivak MV), pp. 16–28. W.B. Saunders, Philadelphia.
4 Schuman BM, Kowalski TE. (2002). The history of the endoscope. In: *Gastrointestinal disease: an endoscopic approach*, 2nd edn (ed. Marino AJ, Benjamin SB), pp. 1–13. Slack, Thorofare, NJ.
5 Eisen MD, Dominitz JA, Faigel DO. Enteroscopy. *Gastrointest Endosc* 2001; 53: 871–3.
6 Chen YK, Powis ME. The structure and function of the video image endoscope. In: *Gastrointestinal disease: an endoscopic approach*, 2nd edn (ed. Marino AJ, Benjamin SB), pp. 16–23. Slack, Thorofare, NJ.
7 Nelson DB, Block KP, Bosco JJ. High resolution and high magnification endoscopy. *Gastrointest Endosc* 2000; 52: 864–6.
8 Ginsberg GG. Seeing the light: enhanced endoscopic imaging to glimpse the Holy Grail. *Gastrointest Endosc* 2006; 64: 193–4.
9 Chak A, Koehler MK, Sundaram SN. Diagnostic and therapeutic impact of push enteroscopy: analysis of factors associated with positive findings. *Gastrointest Endosc* 1998; 47 (1): 18–22.
10 Nachbar, MA, Ell C. Double-balloon enteroscopy (push-and-pull enteroscopy) of the small bowel: feasibility and diagnostic and therapeutic yield in patients with suspected small bowel disease. *Gastrointest Endosc* 2005; 62: 62–70.
11 Nelson DB, Bosco JJ, Curtis WD. Technology status evaluation report: duodenoscope-assisted cholangiopancreatography. *Gastrointest Endosc* 1999; 50: 943–5.

12 Chen YK. Results from the first human use clinical series utilizing a new peroral cholangiopancreatoscopy system (Spyglass™ Direct Visualization System). *Gastroinst Endosc* 2006; 63: AB86.

13 Carr-Locke DL, Branch MS, Byrne WJ. Tissue sampling during endosonography. *Gastrointest Endosc* 1998; 47: 576–8.

14 Ginsberg GG. Variable stiffness colonoscope. *Gastrointest Endosc* 2003; 58: 579–84.

15 Nelson DB, Bosco JJ, Curtis WD *et al*. Technology status evaluation: sheathed endoscopes. *Gastrointest Endosc* 1999; 49: 862–4.

16 Ginsberg GG, Barkun AN, Bosco JJ, Isenberg GA, Nguyen CC, Petersen BT *et al*. Wireless capsule endoscopy. *Gastrointest Endosc* 2002; 56: 621–4.

17 Bernstein DE, Barkin JS, Reiner DK, Lubin J, Phillips RS, Grauer L. Standard biopsy forceps versus large-capacity forceps with and without needle. *Gastrointest Endosc* 1995; 41: 573–6.

18 Levine DS. *et al*. Safety of a systematic endoscopic biopsy protocol in patients with Barrett's esophagus. *Am J Gastroenterol* 2000; 95: 1152–7.

19 Fantin AC, Neuweiler J, Binek JS, Suter WR, Meyenberger C. Diagnostic quality of biopsy forceps specimens: comparison between a conventional biopsy forceps and multibite forceps. *Gastrointest Endosc* 2001; 54: 600–4.

20 Gilbert DA, DiMarino AJ, Jensen DM *et al*. Status evaluation: hot biopsy forceps. *Gastrointest Endosc* 1992; 38: 753–6.

21 Carr-Locke DL, Al-Kawas FH, Branch MS *et al*. Technology assessment status evaluation: bipolar and multipolar accessories. *Gastroenterol Nurs* 1998; 21: 187–9.

22 Vanagunas A, Pothen J, Nimcsh V. Adequacy of 'hot biopsy' for the treatment of diminutive polyps: a randomized trial. *Am J Gastroenterol* 1989; 84: 383–5.

23 Peluso F, Golodner F. Follow-up of hot biopsy forceps treatment of diminutive colonic polyps. *Gastrointest Endosc* 1991; 37: 604–6.

24 Yang R, Naritoku W, Laine L. Prospective, randomized comparison of disposable and reusable forceps in gastrointestinal endoscopy. *Gastrointest Endosc* 1994; 40: 671–4.

25 Woods KL, Anand BS, Cole RA *et al*. Influence of endoscopic biopsy forceps characteristics on tissue specimens: results of a prospective randomized study. *Gastrointest Endosc* 1999; 49: 177–83.

26 Yang R, Ng S, Nichol M, Laine L. A cost and performance evaluation of disposable and reusable biopsy forceps in GI endoscopy. *Gastrointest Endosc* 2000; 51: 266–70.

27 Deprez PH, Horsmans Y, Van Hassel M, Hoang P, Piessevaux H, Geubel A. Disposable versus reusable biopsy forceps: a prospective cost evaluation. *Gastrointest Endosc* 2000; 51: 262–5.

28 Rizzo J, Bernstein D, Gress F. A performance, safety and cost comparison of reusable and disposable endoscopic biopsy forceps: a prospective, randomized trial. *Gastrointest Endosc* 2000; 51: 257–61.

29 Kozarek RA, Attia FM, Sumida SE *et al*. Reusable biopsy forceps: a prospective evaluation of cleaning, function, adequacy of tissue specimen, and durability. *Gastrointest Endosc* 2001; 53: 747–50.

30 Bronowicki J-P, Venard V, Botté C, Monhoven N, Gastin I, Choné L *et al*. Patient-to-patient transmission of hepatitis C virus during colonoscopy. *N Engl J Med* 1997; 337: 237–40.

31 De Bellis M. *et al*. Tissue sampling at ERCP in suspected malignant biliary strictures (Part 1). *Gastrointest Endosc* 2002; 56: 552–61.

32 De Bellis M. *et al*. Tissue sampling at ERCP in suspected malignant biliary strictures (Part 2). *Gastrointest Endosc* 2002; 56: 720–30.

33 Casco C. *et al*. A new device for abrasive cytology sampling during upper gastrointestinal endoscopy: experience in infectious and neoplastic diseases. *Endoscopy* 1999; 31: 348–51.

34 Biliary and pancreatic sampling devices during ERCP. *Gastrointest Endosc* 1996; 43: 775–8.

35 Howell DA. *et al*. Endoscopic needle aspiration biopsy at ERCP in the diagnosis of biliary strictures. *Gastrointest Endosc* 1992; 38: 531–5.

36 Hwang JH, Kimmey MB. The incidental upper gastrointestinal subepithelial mass. *Gastroenterology* 2004: 126: 301–7.

37 Forde KA, Treat MR, Tsai JL. Initial clinical experience with a bipolar snare for colon polypectomy. *Surg Endosc* 1993; 7: 427–8.

38 Tappero G, Gaia E, De Giuli P *et al*. Cold snare excision off small colorectal polyps. *Gastrointest Endosc* 1992; 38: 310–13.

39 McAfee JH, Katon RM. Tiny snares prove safe and effective for removal of diminutive polyps. *Gastrointest Endosc* 1994; 40: 301–13.

40 Nelson DB, Bosco JJ, Curtis WD *et al*. ASGE technology status evaluation report: endoscopic retrieval devices. *Gastrointest Endosc* 1999; 50: 932–4.

41 Ginsberg GG. Management of ingested foreign bodies and food bolus impactions. *Gastrointest Endosc* 1995; 41: 33–8.

42 Faigel DO, Stotland BR, Kochman ML, Hoops T, Judge T, Kroser J *et al*. Device choice and experience level in endoscopic foreign object retrieval: an in vivo study. *Gastrointest Endosc* 1997; 45: 490–2.

43 Nelson DB, Bosco JJ, Curtis WD *et al*. Injection needles. *Gastrointest Endosc* 1999; 50: 928–31.

44 Brooker JC, Saunders BP, Shah SG, Thapar CJ, Thomas HJ, Atkin WS *et al*. Total colonic dye-spray increases the detection of diminutive adenomas during routine colonoscopy: a randomized controlled trial. *Gastrointest Endosc* 2002; 56: 333–8.

45 Nelson DB, Barkun AN, Block KP *et al*. Endoscopic hemostatic devices. *Gastrointest Endosc* 2001; 54: 833–40.

46 Laine L. Bipolar/multipolar electrocoagulation. *Gastrointest Endosc* 1990; 36 (Suppl.): S38–S41.

47 Carr-Locke DL, Conn MI, Faigel DO, Laing K, Leung JW, Mills MR *et al*. Developments in laser technology. *Gastrointest Endosc* 1998; 48: 711–16.

48 Ginsberg GG, Barkun AN, Bosco JJ *et al*. The argon plasma coagulator. *Gastrointest Endosc* 2002; 55: 807–10.

49 Cipolletta L, Bianco MA, Rotondano G, Piscopo R, Prisco A, Garofano ML. Prospective comparison of argon plasma coagulator and heater probe in the endoscopic treatment of major peptic ulcer bleeding. *Gastrointest Endosc* 1998; 48: 191–5.

50 Zlatanic J, Waye JD, Kim PS, Baiocco PJ, Gleim GW. Large sessile colonic adenomas: use of argon plasma coagulator to supplement piecemeal snare polypectomy. *Gastrointest Endosc* 1999; 49: 731–5.

51 Brooker JC, Saunders BP, Shah SG, Thapar CJ, Suzuki N, Williams CB. Treatment with argon plasma coagulation reduces recurrence after piecemeal resection of large sessile colonic polyps: a randomized trial and recommendations. *Gastrointest Endosc* 2002; 55: 371–5.

52 Low DE, Kozarek RA. Snare debridement prior to Nd:YAG photoablation improves treatment efficiency of broad-based adenomas of the colorectum. *Gastrointest Endosc* 1989; 35: 288–91.

53 Fleischer *et al*. Circumferential RF ablation for non-dysplastic Barrett's esophagus (NDBE) using the HALO360 Ablation System (AIM) Trial: one-year follow-up of 100 patients. *Gastrointest Endosc* 2006; 63: AB127.

54 El-Newihi HM, Achord JL. Emerging role of endoscopic variceal band ligation in the treatment of esophageal varices. *Dig Dis* 1996; 14: 201–8.

55 Slosberg EA, Keeffe EB. Sclerotherapy versus banding in the treatment of variceal bleeding. *Clin Liver Dis* 1997; 1: 77–84.

56 Laine L, Cook D. Endoscopic ligation compared with sclerotherapy for treatment of esophageal variceal bleeding: a meta-analysis. *Ann Intern Med* 1995; 123: 280–7.

57 Stiegmann GV, Goff JS, Sun JH, Hruza D, Reveille RM. Endoscopic ligation of esophageal varices. *Am J Surg* 1990; 159: 21–5.

58 Hachisu T. Evaluation of endoscopic hemostasis using an improved clipping apparatus. *Surg Endosc* 1988; 2: 13–17.

59 Hachisu T, Yamada H, Satoh S, Kouzu T. Endoscopic clipping with a new rotatable clip-device and a long clip. *Digestive Endoscopy* 1996; 8: 127–33.

60 Cipolletta L, Bianco MA, Rotonano Gcatalano M, Prisco A, De Simone T. Endoclip-assisted resection of large pedunculated colon polyps. *Gastrointest Endosc* 1999; 50: 405–6.

61 Uno Y, Satoh K, Tuji K *et al*. Endoscopic ligation by means of clip and detachable snare for management of colonic postpolypectomy hemorrhage. *Gastrointest Endosc* 1999; 49: 113–15.

62 Parra-Blanco A, Kaminaga N, Kojima T *et al.* Hemoclipping for postpolypectomy and post-biopsy bleeding. *Gastrointest Endosc* 2000; 51: 37–41.

63 Yoshikane H, Hidano H, Sakakibara A *et al.* Endoscopic repair by clipping of iatrogenic colonic perforation. *Gastrointest Endosc* 1997; 46: 464–6.

64 Pontecorvo C, Pesce G. The 'safety snare': a ligature placing snare to prevent hemorrhage after transection of large pedunculated polyps. *Endoscopy* 1986; 18: 55–6.

65 Hachisu T. A new detachable snare for hemostasis in the removal of large polyps or other elevated lesions. *Surg Endosc* 1991; 5: 70–4.

66 Uno Y, Satoh K, Tuji K, Wada T, Fukuda S, Saito H, Munakata A. Endoscopic ligation by means of clip and detachable snare for management of colonic post polypectomy hemorrhage. *Gastrointest Endosc* 1999; 41: 113–15.

67 Rey JF, Marek DA, Cotton P. Endoloop in the prevention of post polypectomy bleeding: preliminary results. *Gastrointest Endosc* 1997; 46: 387–9.

68 Matsushita M, Hajiro K, Takakuwa H *et al.* Ineffective use of detachable snare for colono-scopic polypectomy of large polyps. *Gastrointest Endosc* 1998; 47: 496–9.

69 Iishi H, Tatsuta M, Narahara H, Iseki K, Sakai N. Endoscopic resection of large pedunculated colorectal polyps using detachable snare. *Gastrointest Endosc* 1996; 44: 594–7.

70 Tada M, Inoue H, Yabata E, Okabe S, Endo M. Feasibility of the transparent cap-fitted colono-scope for screening and mucosal resection. *Dis Colon Rectum* 1997; 40: 618–21.

71 Nelson DB, Block KP, Bosco JJ *et al.* Technology status report evaluation: endoscopic mucosal resection. *Gastrointest Endosc* 2000; 52: 860–3.

72 Tada M, Inoue H, Yabata E, Okabe S, Endo M. Colonic mucosal resection using a transparent cap-fitted endoscope. *Gastrointest Endosc* 1996; 44: 63–5.

73 Oshitani N, Hamasaki N, Sawa Y, Hara J, Nakamura S, Matsumoto T *et al.* Endoscopic resec-tion of small rectal carcinoid tumors using an aspiration method with a transparent overcap. *J Int Med Res* 2000; 28: 241–6.

74 Matsushita M, Hajiro K, Okazaki K, Takakuwa H, Tominaga M. Efficacy of total colonoscopy with a transparent cap in comparison with colonoscopy without the cap. *Endoscopy* 1998; 30: 444–7.

75 Dafnis GM. Technical considerations and patient comfort in total colonoscopy with and with-out a transparent cap: initial experiences from a pilot study. *Endoscopy* 2000; 32: 381–4.

76 Abele JE. The physics of esophageal dilatation. *Hepatogastroenterology* 1992; 39: 486–9.

77 Patterson DJ, Graham DY, Smith JL, Schwartz JT, Lanza FL, Cain GD. Natural history of benign esophageal stricture treated by dilatation. *Gastroenterology* 1983; 85: 346–50.

78 Cox JG, Winter RK, Maslin SC, Dakkak M, Jones R, Buckton GK *et al.* Balloon or bougie for dilatation of benign esophageal stricture? *Dig Dis Sci* 1994; 39: 776–81.

79 Wesdorf IC, Bartelsman JF, den Hartog Jager FC, Huibregtse K, Tytgat GN. Results of con-servative treatment of benign esophageal strictures: a follow-up study in 100 patients. *Gastroenterology* 1982; 82: 487–93.

80 Faigel DO, Ginsberg GG, Kochman ML. Innovative use of the Soehendra stent retriever for biliary stricture recanalization [Letter]. *Gastrointest Endosc* 1996; 44: 635.

81 Ziebert JJ, Disario JA. Dilation of refractory pancreatic duct strictures: the turn of the screw. *Gastrointest Endosc* 1999; 49: 632–5.

82 Parasher VK. A novel approach to facilitate dilation of complex non-traversable esophageal strictures by efficient wire exchange using a stent pusher. *Gastrointest Endosc* 2000; 51: 730–1.

83 Vaezi MF, Richter JE. Current therapies for achalasia: comparison and efficacy. *J Clin Gastroenterol* 1998; 27: 21–35.

84 Vaezi MF, Richter JE. Practice guidelines: diagnosis and management of achalasia. *Am J Gastroenterol* 1999; 12: 3406–12.

85 Virgilio C, Cosentino S, Favara C, Russo V, Russo A. Endoscopic treatment of postoperative colonic strictures using an achalasia dilator: short-term and long-term results. *Endoscopy* 1995; 27: 219–22.

CHAPTER 5

Digital documentation in endoscopy

LARS AABAKKEN

Synopsis

Gastrointestinal endoscopy is a visual clinical discipline. All examinations, findings, descriptions, and recommendations are based on the images that are created during the endoscopy. In interventional work, the images are our sole guiding material for correct procedures. Images are becoming an integral part of our documentation, and hence the selection and quality of those images are of paramount importance.

Fiberoptic imaging

Fiberoptic imaging was introduced into endoscopes in the 1960s. The mere view into the intestine was a revolution. However, the revolution was a very private one, conveyed through the eyepiece of the endoscope, without dissemination, sharing, or storing options. Endoscopic teaching and clinical practice was somewhat anecdotal and inconsistent, simply because the endoscopists had little or no means of communicating what they saw, apart from the written endoscopy report—already an *interpretation* of the images. Furthermore, no standards were set even for that written document.

Teaching attachments and photography

Twin eyepieces and mountable cameras (still and video) were steps in the right direction, allowing exchange and discussion of image information, but these were cumbersome gadgets with limited dissemination, and archiving solutions were mostly non-existent.

Videoscopes

The introduction of video-based imaging systems created a host of new opportunities. The eyepiece was replaced with the greatly enhanced viewing experience of a large monitor screen. The endoscopic examination became a shared experience with colleagues and assistants, and, in some cases, even with the patients themselves. Important findings could be recorded in print form, and the facility for image and video recordings was greatly enhanced.

Image capture

The video signals that are received and processed in the endoscopy rack can be utilized further: they can be stored *electronically*—as captured electronic images, or as digital video. In combination with other existing technologies, this enables access and utilization of our endoscopic images far beyond what was previously feasible (Fig. 5.1).

The increasing availability of electronic image-capturing systems opens up new ways for documenting our procedures. Where we were previously confined to the endoscopist's concept of a 'large ulcer', 'profuse bleeding', or 'moderate inflammation' in a text report, the addition of images allows the reader of the endoscopy report to get a better understanding of what is actually being described, sometimes even take part in the interpretation. Radiologists have long since supported their diagnostic considerations directly by demonstrations of their image material. There is no compelling reason why the endoscopist should not now be doing the same thing.

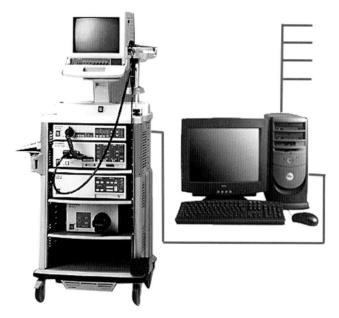

Fig. 5.1 The marriage between video endoscopy racks and PCs paves the way for the new world of digital image documentation.

Standardized image terminology

This enhanced information *flux* has a very interesting side-effect: we are beginning to understand what our colleagues are talking about. The exposure of how we label our findings with medical terms has brought to attention the need for language standardization; the same words should have the same meaning. The content of a written report will be of value only if the 'image-to-word' coding algorithm is the same. The task of establishing a common language for gastrointestinal endoscopy has been taken on by the OMED, and later by the European and US Endoscopy Societies.

Structured reporting

Once the lexicon is agreed upon, the collected information needs also to be structured. The endoscopy report should be composed in a standardized way, similar to what we have come to expect for other encounters, e.g. the medical history and physical findings of a patient on admission. The introduction of computerized reporting systems for endoscopy likewise calls for this type of structuring. The use of these systems for cumulative reporting and statistics requires rigorous coding. Even more standardization is required if our endoscopy reports and images are to be implemented in a complete electronic medical record.

The opportunities and challenges of the digital revolution

The digital revolution in endoscopy has the potential to change the way we work and communicate, offering great improvement in the service we can give our patients and referring doctors. However, this pay-off requires a significant investment of money, time, and thought on the part of the endoscopist. This chapter deals with some of these issues.

Digital imaging

Imaging the gastrointestinal tract using a videoendoscope requires several steps

- Illumination by fiberoptic light transmission
- Surface reflectance
- Magnification
- CCD conversion of the reflected light to an electrical signal
- Reconstruction of the signals to an image
- Display on a monitor.

PCs with image capture cards and network capabilities permit these images to be captured, stored, printed, and transmitted.

Color models

The physical quantities of the colors that represent an image are defined chromatically by wavelength, and the *luminance* is defined by the amount of light. The colors detected by a videoendoscope are continuous values. In the digital domain, color must be converted from this continuous or analog value to a discrete digital value.

The representation of color can be based on one of three color models:

RGB

Most of the visible color spectrum can be represented by mixing the three primary colors, Red, Green and Blue, known as the RGB color model. This model is the one used by most computer monitors, TV screens, graphics cards, and lighting effects. Color mixing is analogous to illumination of an area with red, green, and blue bulbs of different intensity. Mixing different amounts of the red, green, or blue creates different colors, and each can be measured on a scale ranging from 0 to 255. If red, green, and blue are all set to 0, the color is black; if all are set to 255, the color is white (Fig. 5.2).

CMYK

The CMYK color model is based on printing ink being absorbed into paper. It gives the greatest number of printable colors from the fewest number of inks. By using varying amounts of cyan, magenta, yellow, and black, a great number of

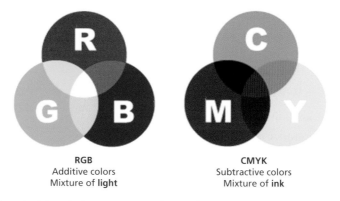

RGB
Additive colors
Mixture of **light**

CMYK
Subtractive colors
Mixture of **ink**

Fig. 5.2 The principles of mixing primary colors in the two main color models.

colors can be printed. Most full-color printed materials, including magazines, posters, and packaging, are printed using just the four CMYK inks. Here the level of ink is measured from 0% to 100%. As an example, orange would be represented by 0% cyan, 50% magenta, 100% yellow, and 0% black.

HSB

With the HSB model all colors are described in terms of three fundamental characteristics, hue, saturation, and brightness. This is a useful model for image processing, because calculations need be applied only to one HSB axis as opposed to three RGB axes. Therefore, it is often used in imaging software in computers.

Hue is the wavelength of light reflected or transmitted from an object, although more commonly, hue is known as the actual color, such as red, yellow, or blue. Hue is measured as a position on the standard color wheel, and is described as an angle in degrees, between 0 and 360.

Saturation is the amount or strength of the color (or hue). It is measured as a percentage. At 0% the color would contain no hue, and would be gray; at 100%, the color is fully saturated.

Brightness is the lightness or darkness of the color, again measured as a percentage. If any hue has a brightness of 0%, it becomes black; with 100% it becomes fully light (Fig. 5.3).

Each of these three models has advantages and shortcomings, but there is good reason to know they exist, in particular to understand the pitfalls in

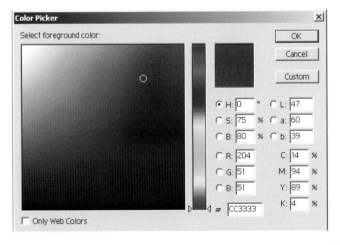

Fig. 5.3 A typical color panel of computer software, which allows adjustment of the various parameters of either color model.

converting computer screen images to printed images. To accurately match a color print with what you see on screen, special expertise from a print-shop is usually recommended. Practical experience and trial-and-error exercises make a good alternative approach.

Digitization of color

The number of unique colors that can be represented by the coordinate system depends on the length of each axis. Because the digital world is binary, the number of possible values is represented by an exponential exponent of 2 or 2^x. If a color is represented in RGB space by 8 unique binary digits (bits), then there are only $2^8 = 256$ colors to choose from. Increasing the number of digits representing a color increases the color range, i.e. 16 or 24 bits define $2^{16} = 65\ 536$ and $2^{24} = 16\ 777\ 216$ colors, respectively. Computer screens are typically able to display 2^{24} colors ('millions of colors'), but the color range still has an impact on file size.

An image is presented as a continuous signal, which is converted or transduced by an analog-to-digital device. To create a digital image, a specific device in the computer called a frame grabber or capture board converts the video signal into a digital form. The resulting digital values are mapped to specific locations and stored as a two-dimensional array of numbers.

The frame grabber performs two functions: sampling and quantification.
- *Sampling* captures evenly spaced data points that represent the image.
- *Quantification* assigns each data point a binary value. The evenly spaced data points for an image represents specific two-dimensional locations called picture elements or pixels. The pixel is the basic unit of a digital image and each pixel stores the value produced by the quantification described above.

Color depth

The number of discrete colors available to present an image is the *color depth* or *color resolution*. A grayscale image digitized by an 8-bit image capture card is represented by assigning values to each pixel making black = 0 and white = 256, because $2^8 = 256$. Color is more complex. The range of colors depends on the number of bits that can be stored at the pixel location. Thus, an 8-bit frame grabber can capture 8 bits/pixel or 256 colors/pixel. Most frame grabbers today capture 24 bits per pixel (i.e. 8 bits for each of the three colors red, green, and blue). This allows a total of 2^{24} combinations, 'millions of colors'. It is important to recognize that the actual color range (number of discrete colors) of an endoscopic image is small. This is the reason why the appreciable difference between 16 and 24 bits/pixel images is minimal. The limited range of

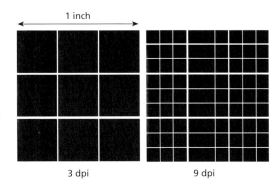

Fig. 5.4 The illustration shows how an image area is divided into equally sized pixels. The smaller the pixels, the more you can fit per area unit (e.g. inch), and the higher the resolution.

colors present in an endoscopic image also affects how such an image can be compressed.

Pixel density

Pixel density (sampling density) is the number of pixels into which an image is divided by the frame grabber. The greater the number of pixels/unit area the higher the resolution of the image (Fig. 5.4). For an image of a given size, sampling density can be defined by the dimension of the image in pixels. For example, 640×480 represents an image that is 640 pixels wide and 480 pixels high (VGA resolution). If this same image is sampled at 1024×768 (XGA resolution) then the number of pixels/unit area is higher and the resolution is greater (Fig. 5.5). Sampling becomes important when images are enlarged because there is a discrete separation between adjacent points in the image. Thus, zooming an image which has been sampled at a low density quickly reveals the individual pixels, a phenomenon called pixelation. On the other hand, pixel resolution beyond that of your viewing mechanism (e.g. an 800×600 computer screen (SVGA)) requires extra storage space without any utility.

File size

The final size of an uncompressed image is calculated simply by the formula width (in pixels) by height by color depth. A VGA resolution 24-bit image (typical for an endoscopic image) would be $640 \times 480 \times 8 \times 3 = 7\ 372\ 800$ bits, approximately 900 kilobyte (1 byte = 8 bits).

File size affects storage requirements, display delays, and transfer times, and so becomes important in the everyday use of the images. Transferring a 900 kbyte image with a 28.8 kbyte modem requires 4.3 min, and a 1 gigabyte disk drive would be filled with 1100 such images [2].

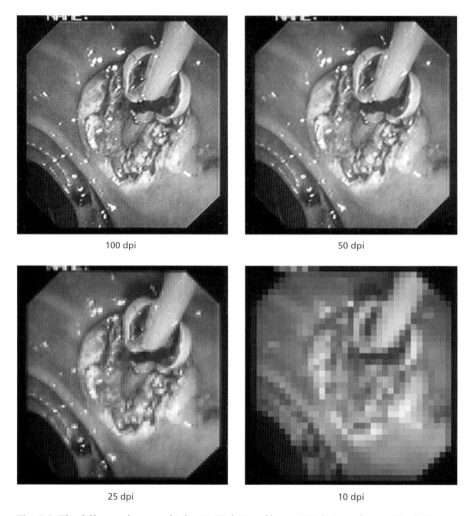

100 dpi

50 dpi

25 dpi

10 dpi

Fig. 5.5 The difference between higher (100 dpi) and lower (10 dpi) resolution. Pixelation is clearly seen at lower resolutions. The same phenomenon is seen if a picture is zoomed beyond its generic resolution.

Thus, all the factors determining the file size should be considered to optimize the composition of endoscopic images.

What detail is needed?

In some clinical situations resolution is not important, e.g. a large mass or a pedunculated polyp may be easily identified as such even at low resolution. On the other hand, subtle findings such as mucosal erythema, the granularity or disruption of the vascular pattern may require a higher pixel ratio. It is also of interest how the image will be utilized. To show the image on a computer screen, the resolution of the screen determines the optimal resolution (e.g. SVGA), but for printing with a high-quality printer (e.g. glossy prints for a journal manuscript), a higher resolution is needed, typically 2–3 times the screen requirements for optimal printing quality.

At the present time, there is definitely an upper limit to the resolution that is feasible for endoscopic images. The CCD chip in the tip of the endoscope has a pixel resolution in the SVGA range. Thus, even with higher resolution capture cards, the image quality would be but marginally better. However, high-resolution endoscopes will change this situation.

File compression

For practical purposes, uncompressed images are almost theoretical relics of the past. With the increasing utility of network-based and internet-based computer applications, the need for smaller files is indisputable.

File compression is a computational processing technique that effectively reduces the size of a file by removing redundancies in large binary data sets. Full motion video requires a display rate of 30 frames/s. If each frame is 0.5 megabytes then one second of digital video contains 15 megabytes of data. Disk storage would be rapidly exceeded and image transmission even on high-speed networks would be slow. Compression is measured as a ratio of the size of the original data divided by the compressed data.

Compression techniques

There are two general categories of compression techniques: lossless and lossy.

Lossless compression

Lossless compression techniques preserve all the information in the compression/decompression process. This may be vital for compressing documents or computer program files, but these techniques can only achieve moderate compression ratios, which may not be sufficient for medical images, especially for radiological grayscale images. However, when images are used as a means of primary diagnosis, they require lossless compression, storage, and transmission. Most PACS systems utilize lossless compression, but require high-end hardware and dedicated high-speed networks.

Lossy compression

For the purpose of practical archival storage and transmission of medical images, compression ratios of 20 : 1 or higher are required. In order to achieve this amount of file size reduction, lossy compression techniques need to be employed. Lossy compression implies that some information is lost in the compression/decompression process, but algorithms can be designed to minimize the effect of data loss on the diagnostic features of the images.

Image file formats

JPEG (Joint Photographic Experts Group) compression is one of the three file formats used for graphical images on the World Wide Web (the others being GIF (Graphical Interchange Format) and PNG (Portable Network Graphics)). JPEG files have the advantage of retaining 24-bit true color files during compression, while GIF files are limited to 8-bit color (256 colors). The PNG file format shows promise as a lossless compression method for the Web, but has not yet gained acceptance. The issue of standard Web formats is an important one, because an increasing number of relevant software solutions rely on browser technology for screen display (Figs 5.6 & 5.7).

Color and black and white compression

While color images using JPEG can typically achieve 10 : 1 to 20 : 1 compression ratios without visible loss and can compress to 30 : 1 to 50 : 1 with small to moderate defects, black and white (grayscale) images do not compress so well by such large factors. Because the human eye is much more sensitive to brightness variations than to hue variations, JPEG can compress hue (color)

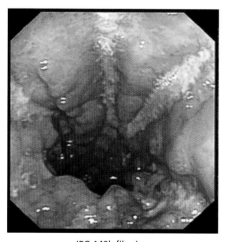 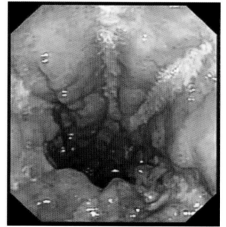

JPG 140k file size   JPG 12k file size

Fig. 5.6 Compressing a typical endoscopic image from 140 kbyte (already compressed from around 800 kbyte) to 12 kbyte is hardly noticeable.

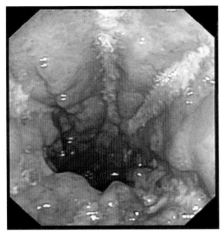 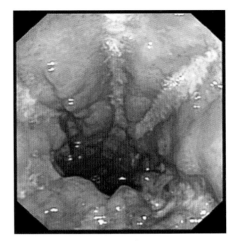

JPG millions colors   GIF 256 colors

Fig. 5.7 Intelligent reduction of the number of colors in an endoscopic image does not ruin the image, because the color range is limited to the gray–yellow–red hues.

data more heavily than brightness (grayscale) data. A grayscale JPEG file is generally only about 10–25% smaller than a full-color JPEG file of similar visual quality. But the uncompressed grayscale data is only 8 bits/pixel, or 1/3 the size of the color data, so the calculated compression ratio is much lower. The threshold of visible loss is often around 5 : 1 compression for grayscale images, substantially different from color images [1].

JPEG 2000 and beyond

The importance of image handling and compression for Internet applications creates a huge momentum for development. The JPEG working group has developed a new standard which is only just becoming available (accepted as an ISO standard December 2000). This standard is called JPEG 2000, with the file extension jp2. This standard offers a host of advantages over the existing JPEG standard, the most significant being lack of pixelation at high compression rates, and significantly more effective compression (Fig. 5.8).

Although the file sizes of individual endoscopic images are not a major issue at this point, we should keep in mind that when the display and transfer of large numbers of images and videos becomes a significant part of our daily workflow, even minute delays for every picture will have an impact. Further developments for more efficient file compression will be of major significance for medical imaging. PACS development currently suffers from the heavy cost of high-end workstations and networks to handle huge image data sets.

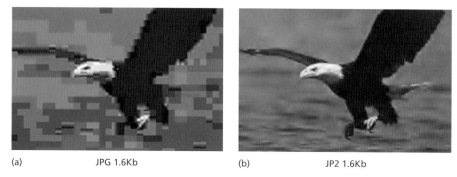

(a)   JPG 1.6Kb   (b)   JP2 1.6Kb

Fig. 5.8 Comparison between maximum compression with regular JPG (a) and with the JPEG 2000 standard (b). The file size is the same: minute.

DICOM standard

DICOM (Digital Imaging and Communications in Medicine) is a standard for imaging that contains very specific information about the images, as well as the images themselves. DICOM relies on explicit and detailed models of how the features (patients, images, reports, etc.) of an imaging operation are described, how they are related, and what should be done with them. This model is used to create Information Object Definitions (IODs) for all of the imaging modalities covered by DICOM.

Information Objects

An Information Object is a combination of Information Entities and each Entity consists of specific modules. A Service Class defines the service that can take place on an Information Object, e.g. print, store, retrieve. In DICOM a Service is combined with an Information Object to form a Service/Object Pair, or SOP. For example, storing a CT scan or printing an ultrasound is an SOP. A device that conforms to the DICOM standard can perform this function. Thus, in a DICOM-conforming network the devices must be capable of executing one or more of the operations the SOP definition prescribes. Each imaging modality has an IOD. The result is that different imaging modalities such as CT, MRI, digital angiography, ultrasound, endoscopy, pathology; imaging workstations; picture archiving systems; and printing devices can be networked and execute a high level of cooperation. In addition, these imaging networks can be connected to other networks found in a hospital or facility.

The modules that comprise an Information Entity (IE) are precisely defined and may be common to multiple entities. The Patient Entity is common to all IODs. However, the Image Entity must be capable of supporting different imaging modalities. An IOD that supports endoscopy will of necessity include modules

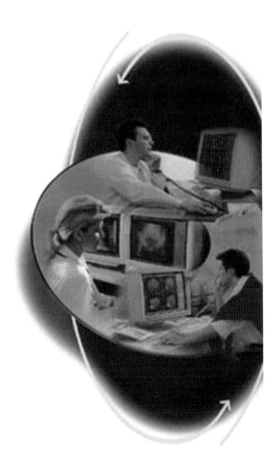

Fig. 5.9 Commercial PACS products rely heavily on the DICOM standard for image handling.

unique to endoscopy and be distinct from a CT IOD. The Patient IE defines the characteristics of a Patient who is the imaging subject of one or more procedures that produce images. The Patient IE is modality independent, i.e. it is common to all imaging modalities. The Patient IE consists of only one module, which is illustrated in Fig. 5.9. Each module is a table consisting of four attribute elements:

- Name
- Tag
- Type
- Description.

The *attribute name* and *description* define the attribute precisely.

The *attribute tag* uniquely identifies that attribute among all of the many other attributes present. The tag (0010,0010) always identifies the fact that this is the patient name. The *attribute type* specifies whether this attribute is mandatory or optional. For example, it is not necessary for an image to be transmitted with the patient's name. In fact, DICOM requires only a few mandatory attributes that give the study a unique identifier, define the modality, e.g. CT, MRI, ultrasound, and provide information about the image, e.g. pixel data, number of rows and columns. DICOM also provides a dictionary that specifies the form in which the value of each attribute must be presented.

Patient name attributes

The patient name attribute (0010,0010) uses Person Name (PN) as its value representation. PN contains five components in the following order: family name, given name, middle name, name prefix, and name suffix. Thus, any system that complies with DICOM knows that (0010,0010) is a person name and that the format of the information transmitted is defined by the DICOM standard.

DICOM conformance

It is not sufficient simply to define a standard. It is also necessary to develop a mechanism to enable vendors and purchasers to understand whether a particular system conforms to the standard. DICOM defines a conformance statement that must be associated with a specific implementation of the DICOM standard. It specifies the Service Classes, Information Objects, Communication Protocols, and Media Storage supported by the implementation.

DICOM in endoscopy

The American Society for Gastroentestinal Endoscopy (ASGE), in collaboration with other medical and surgical societies such as the European Society for Gastrointestinal Endoscopy (ESGE), American College of Radiology, the College of American Pathologists, the American Academy of Ophthalmology, and the American Dental Association, has defined a new Supplement to the DICOM standard [2]. This specifies a DICOM Image Information Object Definition (IOD) for Visible Light (VL) images. This standard enables specialists to exchange color images between different imaging systems using direct network connections, telecommunications, and portable media such as CD-ROM and magneto-optical disk.

The DICOM standard for endoscopy is part of a larger standard for color images in medicine which has been provisionally approved by the DICOM Committee. The current version will go through a process of public comment and testing. This period ensures that any interested party may review the document and suggest changes to a committee that is responsible for creating the final version. This process is time-consuming but it ensures that the standard is comprehensive and meets the needs of a broad group of users.

Expanding the scope of DICOM

The endoscopy community, through the ASGE and ESGE, has also suggested that the DICOM standard be expanded to incorporate other information associated with the imaging study. These expanded standards would include image labels and overlays, sound, and waveform. The goal of a true multimedia report will be achieved only when these standards have been thoroughly tested and implemented as part of the daily clinical activities of endoscopists throughout the world. The cooperation of endoscopists, professional societies, and industry is absolutely necessary for improved endoscopic information systems and will result in improved patient care.

How much compression is clinically acceptable?

Because of the specific nature of endoscopic images, the amount of compression that can be employed without compromising important information must be determined by the endoscopist. The acceptable compression rate when we are looking at a polyp would likely differ substantially from that for a case of mild gastritis. These issues have major impact on the utility of digital images. We have to be involved in deciding what imaging is required to be useful for clinical purposes.

Studies of compression acceptability

The topic was excellently reviewed by Kim [1], but very few relevant studies have been published.

Vakil and Bourgeois

Vakil and Bourgeois [3] conducted a trial to determine the amount of color information required for a diagnosis from an endoscopy image. The least amount of color information in an endoscopic image that carries sufficient diagnostic information was unknown. Ten lesions of upper gastrointestinal lesions were presented in an 8-bit format, 16-bit format, and a 24-bit format blindly side-by-side on a Macintosh II system with a 19 inch monitor that could display 24-bit color. Eleven observers (6 nurses and 5 endoscopists) were asked to rank each format for each lesion (i.e. which of the two was the higher quality one). There were a total of 330 observations, and for each format and total the results were similar: the observers could not tell a difference on 41% of the images; identified the best image correctly in 22%; and identified incorrectly in 37% of the images. All the lesions were correctly diagnosed from both images. From

Table 5.1 Clinical acceptability of compressed GI images

Lesion	Original file size (kbyte)	Mean compressed file size (kbyte)
AVM	903.3	14.1
Barrett's	903.6	10.6
Chromoscopy polyp	904.7	18.4
Arterial bleed	182.2	2.4
Pseudomembranous	185.7	6.6
Duodenal ulcers	183.6	5.6

Adapted from Kim [1].

this study for endoscopic images, the color resolution does not appear to affect an endoscopist's ability to make a diagnosis.

Kim

Kim presented a set of six images to 10 expert gastroenterologists using software that allowed them to determine their personal cut-off level of acceptable compression for each of the images. Different types of lesions were studied. The acceptable compression ratio varied markedly, as expected, but in general, a compression ratio of between 1:40 and 1:80 was deemed acceptable (Table 5.1).

This type of study gives us important information concerning the order of magnitude of acceptable compression. However, the clinical context is of interest as well—the arterial bleed in the above study was probably identified easily as such at a high rate of compression, but a therapeutic endoscopist would likely need additional details as to the exact location, structures next to the vessel, etc. (Kim, personal communication).

Developments in compression

Compression schemes are evolving quickly and, at the same time, the requirements for minute files are becoming less crucial. Storage space is rapidly becoming cheaper, and networks faster. The 28.8 kbyte modem is no longer a reasonable yardstick for download time. The virtue of compressing our images remains, but there is no reason to compromise the quality of our images to achieve the tiny file sizes that yesterday's technology urged us to aim at. The endoscope manufacturers have been struggling hard to offer us high-resolution endoscopes, structure enhancement, and magnification, and it would be counterproductive to take that advantage away for a few kilobytes of file size reduction.

As for clinical utility, we will need to establish a general standard for compression and formats that will work across diagnoses. This will have to aim at a quality sufficient for our most difficult diagnoses, e.g. subtle, diffuse lesions like mild gastritis or tiny erosions, or delineation of the vascular pattern in colitis.

Still pictures or live video?

Digital *video* is increasingly becoming an option for endoscopic documentation. Many capture cards have the capability of storing video as well as still images, and in certain situations, video may definitely offer an advantage. This is particularly true for teaching purposes, but even clinical documentation can be enhanced by live footage in certain situations. Obvious examples are documentation of distensibility or propagating waves of the stomach, spasticity of the colon, or imaging in difficult areas (the cardia).

However, video clips come at a cost in terms of processing, storing, and even presentation. While still images can be vividly reproduced in our printed endoscopy report together with our recommendations, a video clip is forever tied to the computer or network. Down the road—when electronic medical records become mainstream and wide area networks (WANs) a tool for medical purposes—these concerns may vanish, but for now a paper-based report is a prerequisite in most endoscopy labs.

Then there is the issue of storage and transfer. Studio quality video shows at 25 or 30 frames per second (fps). Although we can get reasonable quality video at 10–15 fps, this still produces enormous files quickly, and we need to determine if and when the value of digital video justifies the cost.

For the time being, images will be preferable in most clinical contexts. It has been shown that for example, documentation of ulcerative colitis, images convey information very similar to high quality video clips, allowing correct grading of the lesions [4].

Video storage developments

Again, fortunately, things are moving rapidly in the right direction. Compression algorithms allow significant compression of digital video file size with acceptable results. Best known to date are probably the Quick Time and MPEG-1 formats, but this is a field of continuous development, MPEG-4 being one of the most promising options at the moment.

Most of the compression algorithms utilize similar techniques to those discussed above for still images. For example: if a segment of the movie image is unchanged for a period of time (the sky, or the black portion to the left of the endoscopic picture), all the information that needs to be stored is the boundaries of the area, the color value, and the start and stop timecodes.

With this type of compression, a video, for example, of a news reader can be reduced to a still picture with a small moving segment representing the mouth. This technique, in addition to a multitude of others, allows for increasing compression of video clips, offering efficient storage, as well as network-based distribution, with no or minimal depreciation of the diagnostic value.

What images should be recorded in practice?

In parallel to the technological developments in digital imaging and video, there are important decisions that need to be made by the endoscopic community. A crucial one is: What pictures are needed?

Lesion documentation

If we want to report a polyp in the sigmoid colon, a single picture might be sufficient if it is a good one—showing the size and shape, stalk, amount of luminal obstruction, surface texture, etc. But what about a distal rectal lesion? Maybe an extra picture of the relation to the anal verge would be important, not least if a surgeon is to remove it. A retroflexed view, as well as a standard forward-viewing depiction, would be reasonable for that. For diffuse pathology, typically more than one image might be preferable, and maybe high resolution becomes an issue for minimal changes.

Recording negative examinations

More complex still are the issues raised by 'negative' examinations. Which images are needed to *rule out* a lesion, e.g. to document a normal colonoscopy? We obviously cannot picture every single fold, let alone behind them, but there may still be reasons to document normality, e.g. to show what kind of view, cleansing, and distension was available to the endoscopist and to confirm that the examination was complete (e.g. by digital images of the ileocecal value).

The virtue of this becomes even more obvious in the context of referrals and second-opinion cases. When we are asked to evaluate a patient who has had a procedure at another hospital, too often we distrust the results because the images that we receive are inadequate for independent assessment, or even lacking. Standardization of documentation will reduce the need to repeat many procedures. In addition, the availability of relevant images from a prior examination will make follow-up studies much more meaningful (e.g. in the assessment of the activity of colitis or esophagitis).

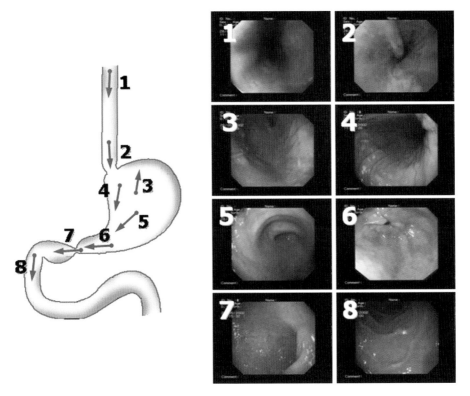

Fig. 5.10 Initial suggestion for standard imaging of upper endoscopy. Will this be part of our future endoscopy report?

Structured image documentation

The ESGE has made an attempt to establish guidelines for image recording, proposing fixed sets of images for various procedures [5]. Figure 5.10 illustrates the standard set of images for upper endoscopy, and a similar set has been prepared for colonoscopy. The requirements are similar for ERCP and EUS, but may be slightly more complex to describe. This is obviously a process that will continue, but the importance of initiating this work in parallel with the implementation of digital documentation systems in the endoscopy lab cannot be over-emphasized.

Costs of image documentation

Previously, the cost of color reproduction of a large number of pictures for every procedure was a concern. However, with electronic storage and display, this concern is diminishing, and picture documentation should be the rule now rather than the exception. Having these images in a readily searchable management system is essential.

Image enhancement

The impact of video endoscopes has been substantial, but the images produced are still just natural light images showing the gastrointestinal mucosa in a life-like manner. Novel technologies are now emerging, offering modification of the original images that may increase the diagnostic output of the endoscopic procedure. These technologies do not relate to the digital imaging as such, but they all rely on such imaging as the core technology for endoscopy.

Color manipulation

Color manipulation methods deal primarily with the color characteristics of the pixels representing the image. This is a simple way of enhancing the contrast features of the image, but sometimes at the cost of resolution. These methods are so far available only for manipulation of still images, and a live version of the technology would be needed to make this applicable clinically (Fig. 5.11).

Narrow band imaging and spectroscopy

Narrow band imaging and spectroscopy are just two examples of a host of other technologies that will enhance our diagnostic yield. In these technologies, parallel 'imaging' is utilized to extract information about the imaged tissue, and the regular digital images are used primarily to guide the process of advanced tissue characterization.

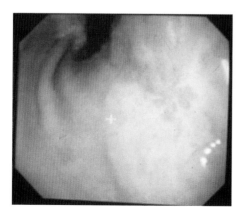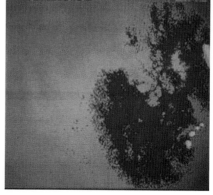

Fig. 5.11 Pure color manipulation can be used to amplify the subtle differences in mucosal color in the original picture (*left*), revealing an early gastric cancer.

Terminology standardization

Endoscopic findings are conveyed with words, although the findings themselves are images. Thus, the coupling between what we see and how it is described becomes crucial, and standardization of our endoscopic *language* is an integral part of this concept.

Endoscopic teaching includes descriptions of what is found, but the definitions of terms used have been weak or non-existent. If the conclusion of the endoscopy report is the only item of value then the specifics of the findings are of less importance. However, if the findings themselves are important, then the descriptive language becomes interesting too. For research purposes, in particular collaborative research, the utility of this is obvious, but even for general clinical purposes the objective description of lesions may be of interest, e.g. in the situation of a second-opinion referral of a case where the referral center needs to decide whether a repeat endoscopy is needed. Likewise, follow-up endoscopy in a patient with a known lesion will profit from an unequivocal initial description of what was seen, at least when no image documentation is available.

OMED standardized terminology

The world organization of digestive endoscopy (OMED) initiated the efforts to standardize our language based on the pioneer work of Professor Zdenek Maratka who developed the first 'Terminology, definitions and diagnostic criteria in digestive endoscopy.' This terminology is a codified list of terms with explicit definitions that allow endoscopic findings to be fitted into a hierarchical nomenclature and assigned a code, thus enabling international collaboration. This terminology has since been supplemented with images to exemplify the various terms. Despite deficiencies, this remains the *de facto* standard for describing the various findings of digestive endoscopy.

Minimal standard terminology—MST

The OMED terminology, while defining the framework for the terminology efforts within digestive endoscopy, proved too complex for practical utilization in everyday endoscopy. A simplification was needed, and the European Society for Digestive Endoscopy (ESGE) teamed up with its US counterpart (ASGE) to develop *minimal standard terminology* (MST) for endoscopy [6]. This terminology is completely based on the OMED terminology, but the term lists are limited, aimed at covering 95% of the terms needed for typical endoscopic practice, and omitting the definitions, which are available when needed in the OMED terminology book. The MST is meant to be a standardizing prerequisite

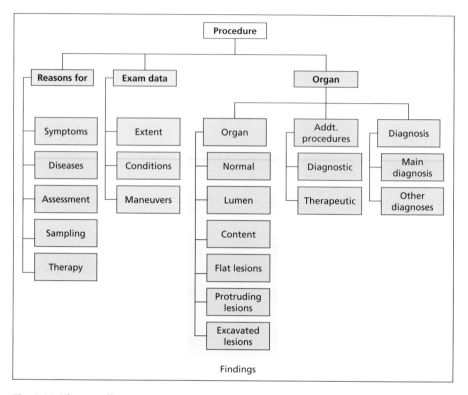

Fig. 5.12 The overall MST structure covering all core aspects of the endoscopy report.

for software companies developing reporting software for digestive endoscopy, ensuring that a joint language is used in the various available software solutions. The MST work has been endorsed and supported by all the major vendors of such systems (Figs 5.12 & 5.13).

The initial version of the MST was thoroughly tested within the GASTER project [7] and this experience led to a number of adjustments as to the selection and definition of terms. The present version of the MST is coined 2.0, but further revision work is already underway.

In addition, term definitions are now being included, and an image library is being developed through a joint European effort, to help illustrate the various terms of the MST by high-quality sample pictures.

Problems with MST

The principles of the MST work have been endorsed almost universally, and the utility of a joint standardized language of endoscopy is readily acknowledged. Still, the knowledge, dissemination, and implementation of the MST is at the present time insufficient, even disappointing. Why is this?

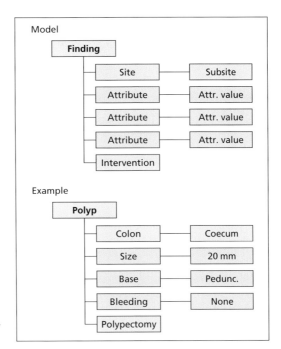

Fig. 5.13 The MST model for describing findings, assigning attribute values to predefined lesion-specific attributes.

One issue is that the MST term lists are still not perfect. They are designed to be 'minimal lists', and this means you may not find the precise term that you need. This is partly a software issue, because the lists were never meant to be all-inclusive, and individual additions will be needed in most centers. Still, incomplete choice lists are difficult to accept.

More fundamental, though, is the whole concept of structuring the language of the endoscopist. We are used to formulating our findings and recommendations in natural language, and any superimposed structure may take extra time, be considered cumbersome and limiting, and even as something that yields less informative reports.

The solution to this has not yet been found, and the MST is at present primarily an excellent initiative. The utility of standardized terms is indisputable, but the challenge is to embed them in software that allows their use to be sufficiently transparent. Also, it is probably unnecessary that the endoscopy report be produced exclusively by 'point-and-click'. Certain segments should probably remain free text blocks with natural language.

Outstanding issues and future trends

Endoscopic recording has come a long way since Rudolph Schindler employed an artist to paint watercolor pictures of the images he saw with his semiflexible gastroscope. We are now on the threshold of easy and comprehensive digital (still and video) documentation of all of our procedures. This should provide enormous enhancement of the clinical value of our examinations, and of our ability to both teach and communicate with colleagues. Tele-endoscopy (distance diagnosis) has been tested, and could have substantial clinical and educational benefits.

Image manipulation and automated analysis eventually will add another dimension to our practice. Image data, when collected, stored, annotated, and validated, will provide a memory bank far greater than the human brain can handle, or perhaps even contemplate. Our endoscopes will soon start to recognize pathology ('optical biopsy'), and will provide instant differential diagnoses, along with access to examples of similar conditions (and a comprehensive knowledge base about them). Integrated image atlases may even be able to help suggest possible differential diagnoses for us.

It will be some time before the brain of the endoscopic processor replaces the brain of the endoscopist, but the potential for development is enormous. Neural networks and artificial intelligence will facilitate and optimize our effectiveness. Initially these developments will have greatest impact in diagnostic endoscopy. Already the video capsule maximizes the digital information whilst minimizing endoscopic expertise. Eventually these concepts will be applied to therapeutic procedures; endoscopes may recognize lesions (and even their depth), and apply therapy automatically. The future is as exciting as it is unpredictable.

Acknowledgments

I would like to thank Doctors Louis Korman and Chris Kim for valuable input to specific segments of this manuscript, and for their efforts in the field in general.

References

1 Kim CY. Compression of color medical images in gastrointestinal endoscopy: a review. *Medinfo* 1998; 9 Part 2: 1046–50.
2 Korman LY, Bidgood WD Jr. Representation of the Gastrointestinal Endoscopy Minimal Standard Terminology in the SNOMED DICOM microglossary. *Proceedings of the AMIA Annu Fall Symp*, 1997: 434–8.
3 Vakil N, Bourgeois K. A prospective, controlled trial of eight-bit, 16-bit, and 24-bit digital color images in electronic endoscopy. *Endoscopy* 1995; 27 (8): 589–92.
4 de Lange T, Larsen S, Aabakken L. Image documentation of endoscopic findings in ulcerative colitis: photographs or video clips? *Gastrointest Endosc* 2005; 61 (6): 715–20.
5 Rey JF, Lambert R. ESGE recommendations for quality control in gastrointestinal endoscopy: guidelines for image documentation in upper and lower GI endoscopy. *Endoscopy* 2001; 33 (10): 901–3.
6 Delvaux M, Korman LY. The minimal standard terminology for digestive endoscopy: introduction to structured reporting. *Int J Med Inf* 1998; 48 (1–3): 217–25.
7 Delvaux M, Crespi M, Armengol-Miro JR, Hagenmuller F, Teuffel W, Spencer KB *et al.* Minimal standard terminology for digestive endoscopy: results of prospective testing and validation in the GASTER project. *Endoscopy* 2000; 32 (4): 345–55.

CHAPTER 6

Principles of electrosurgery, laser, and argon plasma coagulation with particular regard to endoscopy

GUENTER FARIN AND KARL E. GRUND

Editor's note

This contribution is an updated and expanded version of the chapter by the same authors, from the textbook *Colonoscopy: Principles and Practice*, by Waye JD, Rex DK, and Williams CB, Blackwell Publishing, 2003, and is reproduced by kind permission of the authors and editors.

Introduction

Hemostasis and the ablation of pathologic tissues are the most important indications for thermal techniques in flexible endoscopy. However, because the wall of gastrointestinal organs is thin (especially the colon), it is very important to know the different thermal effects in biologic tissue, and also how to apply electric or electromagnetic energy to cause therapeutic thermal effects in the target tissue, whilst avoiding unintended effects in lateral tissue. The colon especially is not an ideal organ for the application of thermal techniques. The three layers (mucosa, submucosa, and muscularis propria) are only 1.5 to 3 mm thick (Fig. 6.1), and can be even thinner following insufflation. Since damage to the muscularis propria of the colon should be avoided during endoscopic interventions, thermal injury must not extend beyond the submucosa in order to avoid complications. As a consequence, only about half of the 1.5–3.0 mm constituting the thin wall of the colon is accessible to the endoscopist for thermal interventions. The necessity that endoscopically applied thermal techniques do not damage the muscularis propria of the colon makes their application within the colon difficult, especially when the lesion to be treated is large.

Safe and effective application of thermal techniques in the gastrointestinal tract requires knowledge of thermal effects in biologic tissues. In addition, the endoscopist must have sufficient training and master the available endoscopes, instruments, and peripheral equipment. This article deals with the theoretical principles concerning the application of thermal techniques.

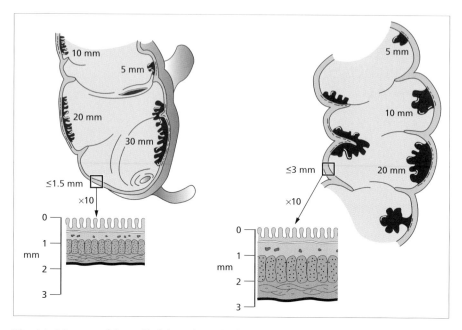

Fig. 6.1 Diagram of the wall of the right and left colon with scale representation of thickness as well as small, medium, and large adenomas.

Relevant thermal effects in biological tissues

All thermal effects in and on biological tissues—whether intentional or unintentional—depend on the level and duration of temperature in the tissue (Fig. 6.2) almost regardless of the way in which this temperature is reached.

Thermal treatment is among the oldest of therapeutic techniques. Although high-frequency (HF) surgery was introduced about 100 years ago, and laser surgery about 30 years ago, the terminology is centuries old. Some words do not adequately describe the various thermal effects nor their intended purpose. As an example, coagulation is the only term used currently to describe thermal hemostasis, even though several different thermal effects and techniques can be used for this purpose. The term actually encompasses many different tissue effects, such as devitalization, coagulation and desiccation. We should define and use relevant terms more precisely and consistently.

Thermal devitalization

Thermal devitalization is defined as irreversible death of biologic tissue, which occurs if its temperature reaches 41.5°C. The higher the temperature, the faster devitalization occurs. Unfortunately, devitalization is not a visible phenomenon and hence difficult to control. Even if it is not employed intentionally, some degree

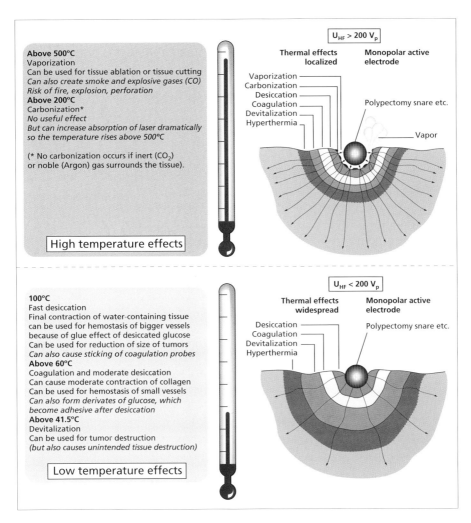

Fig. 6.2 Thermal effects in biological tissue resulting from application of high or low (peak) voltage high-frequency current.

of thermal devitalization occurs outside the border of the coagulation zone. The depth of the invisible thermal devitalization zone depends on many different parameters. For the sake of safety, it should be assumed that it occurs in direct proportion to the visible coagulation effect, as described in more detail below.

Thermal coagulation

Thermal coagulation is defined as conversion of colloidal systems from solid state to a gel, which occurs at approximately 60°C. When this temperature is exceeded, the structure of the cell changes causing the following effects:

- change of the color of the tissue;
- formation of derivatives of collagen, e.g. glucose;
- contraction of collagen.

The change in color of the tissue can be used to visually control intended as well as unintended coagulation. Unfortunately, color changes can only be seen on the surface, but not within the tissue.

Because thermal devitalization can not be controlled visually, the change of tissue color caused by the coagulation effect can be used as indicator of devitalization. It should be noted that an invisible thermal devitalization zone of variable depth is unavoidable outside the border of the coagulation zone.

The formation of derivatives of collagen, e.g. glucose, can become adherent after desiccation.

The contraction of collagen can cause some narrowing of the lumen of blood vessels and hence cause hemostasis. Even though the term 'coagulation' is used as a synonym for thermal hemostasis, thermal coagulation alone is only efficient for hemostasis of very small vessels (< about 0.5 mm diameter). Larger vessels can become closed thermally by desiccation of the vessel and/or adjacent tissue, as described in more detail below. Big vessels must be compressed mechanically during thermal coagulation or desiccation to achieve hemostasis.

Thermal desiccation

Thermal desiccation is defined as heat-induced dehydration of tissue, which occurs at the boiling temperature of intra or extracellular water. (c. 100°C). Thermal desiccation can cause:

- shrinkage of tissue, by dehydration;
- an adhesive effect of glucose;
- a dry layer that acts to insulate tissue electrically.

Thermal desiccation causes significant shrinkage by drying and shrinkage of vessels and/or adjacent tissue, resulting in hemostasis of *small* vessels. Larger vessels (> about 1 mm) must be mechanically compressed during thermal coagulation or desiccation to achieve hemostasis.

Desiccation of glucose as a derivative of collagen results in a glue effect, which in turn causes sticking of desiccated tissue to the tip of electrodes, heater probes, laser fibers, polypectomy snares and sphincterotomes.

Desiccated tissue has a relatively high specific electric resistance. A layer of desiccated tissue functions like an electric isolating layer. This can cause a problem during polypectomy and sphinterotomy if the tissue adjacent to the snare becomes desiccated. When this occurs, there is no cutting effect and the electrode can get stuck within the desiccated tissue and cannot be moved forward or backward. During use of the argon plasma coagulator (APC) the desiccated and hence electrically isolating layer automatically limits the (maximum) penetration depth of the thermal effects, described in more detail below.

Thermal carbonization

Thermal carbonization is defined as partial oxidation of tissue hydrocarbon compounds if the temperature exceeds 200°C and the tissue is within an atmosphere containing oxygen. Because tissue which contains water does not exceed approx. 100°C, only desiccated (and relatively dry) tissue can become heated to higher temperatures and become carbonized. Dry tissue will achieve temperatures above 100°C only via an electric arc or laser.

If the temperature of desiccated tissue increases above 200°C in the presence of oxygen, it becomes carbonized after desiccation. However, if the target tissue is bathed by a noble gas such as argon, the tissue does not become carbonized.

Even though carbonization of tissue is not a goal in therapeutic endoscopy, it is relevant during tissue vaporization by laser, because the absorption of light increases when the tissue becomes blackened.

Carbonization of tissue can cause smoke, which can interfere with endoscopic vision. Smoke may contain gases like CO, which can cause fire when mixed with oxygen, and ignited by electric sparks or laser.

Thermal vaporization

Thermal vaporization is defined as combustion of desiccated and/or carbonized tissue, when the temperature increases to approximately 500°C in the presence of oxygen-containing gas, e.g. air. If the target tissue is within an inert gas (e.g. CO_2) or noble gas (e.g. argon), the tissue does not become vaporized (see argon plasma coagulation).

Thermal vaporization can be used directly for the ablation of pathologic tissues as well as indirectly for tissue cutting. In flexible endoscopy only laser energy, especially the Nd:YAG laser, is used for tissue ablation by vaporization, and only high-frequency surgery is used for thermal cutting of tissue.

Possibilities for increasing the temperature of target tissue in the GI tract

Various energy forms, and their respective sources, applicators and application techniques are available for thermal intervention in the gastrointestinal tract (GI tract) (Fig. 6.3). A description of these possibilities and their relevance for endoscopic applications in the GI tract follow.

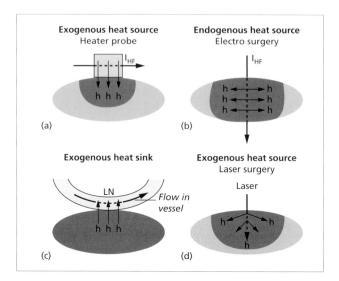

Fig. 6.3 Modalities of heat surgery. (a) Heat (h) from a heat source flows into tissue. (b) Heat (h) from the tissue flows into a heat sink such as a blood vessel. (c) Electric current I_{HF} becomes converted to heat (h) within the tissue. (d) Laser becomes converted to heat (h) within the tissue.

The temperature of tissue can be increased either exogenously, e.g. by means of a heater probe, or endogenously, e.g. by means of electric current or laser; it can also be increased by a combination of both, as in high-frequency surgical cutting, where endogenous heat is caused by electric current and exogenous heat is caused by electric arcs between the active electrode and tissue. A combination of exogenous and endogenous heat also increases the temperature when using argon plasma coagulation (APC). For thermal interventions in the GI tract, it is important that the temperature required for an intended thermal effect is delivered only into the target tissue.

Unintentional thermal damage to adjacent lateral tissues must be avoided. This stipulation is difficult to achieve since it is not possible to heat part of a tissue to a desired temperature without at the same time heating adjacent tissue. Although it is not possible to avoid heat transfer, it may be possible to keep thermal damage of adjacent tissues to a minimum. Where possible, the distance between the target tissue and deeper surrounding tissue can be increased for the purpose of limiting thermal damage by submucosal injection with physiological saline or other solution (Fig. 6.4).

Some coagulation and/or desiccation effect to adjacent (deeper or surrounding) tissue may be desired in some cases, especially during cutting of vascularized biologic tissue, such as during polypectomy, mucosectomy or sphincterotomy. During cutting, the tissue becomes vaporized in front of a cutting electrode and

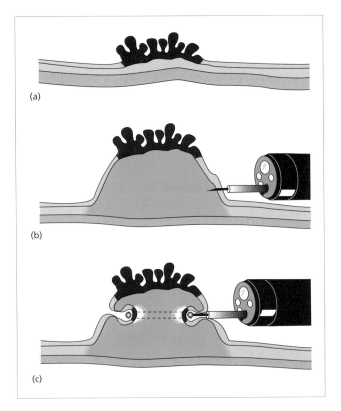

Fig. 6.4 Injection of fluid into the submucosa will increase the distance between a target tissue which is to be heated and adjacent tissue which should not be heated.

heat spreads to the adjacent tissue (the cut edges), which can be intended (to promote hemostasis) but also unintended, with damage to adjacent tissues. In order to avoid unintentional damage to tissues adjacent to the target, it is necessary to know the maximum depth of the tissue injury and how to control the effect produced by the various thermal techniques. All of these aspects should be taken into account when choosing the primary energy form, its source, applicators, and application techniques for thermal intervention in the GI tract.

Heater probe

Heater probes belong to the family of cautery instruments, which have a very long history. Cautery instruments consist of a handle with a distal tip, which can be heated to a temperature appropriate to cause a specific thermal effect. The heater probe consists of a catheter with a special heat-generating device built into the tip, which converts electric energy to heat energy [1,2]. The heat generated outside the tissue (exogenously) can be applied to a target tissue by touching it with the hot tip.

The temperature of heater probes for flexible endoscopy is adjustable and automatically controlled. Modern probes are provided with irrigation from a nozzle on the tip, which can be used to clear blood from the site to facilitate a clear view and for accurate positioning. A special coating on the tip prevents it from sticking to desiccated tissue.

Because heater probes can be pressed against the target tissue during heat application, even bleeding from medium size vessels can be treated by simultaneously compressing and coagulating the vessel (Fig. 6.5a). However, this should be done very carefully to avoid thermal damage to the muscularis propria (Fig. 6.5b).

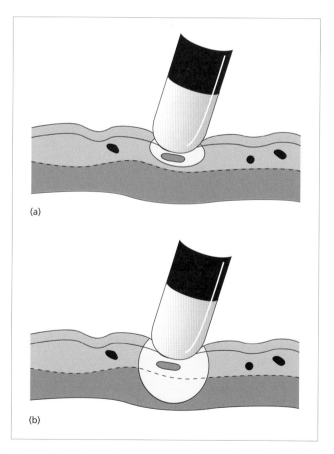

(a)

(b)

Fig. 6.5 (a) Heater probe can be used to compress and coagulate medium-sized vessels. (b) Thermal damage to the muscularis propria may result from several factors such as temperature, pressure, and duration.

High-frequency surgery

General principles of high-frequency electric devices

High-frequency surgery is a thermal technique where the required temperature in the target tissue is reached by conversion of electric energy into heat energy (endogenously) and/or exogenously by electric arcs between an active electrode and the target.

High-frequency alternating current with frequencies greater than 300 kHz (ICE 6001-2-2) is well suited for the heating of vital biologic tissues because it does not stimulate nerves or muscles. The electric energy (E) in tissue caused by the HF current becomes converted endogenously into heat energy (Q). The amount of heat energy (Q) measured in watt-seconds (Ws) produced in the tissue is a function (f) of the electric resistance (R) and the square of the averaged value (Iav^2) and the effective duration (Δt) of the HF current (Iav).

$$E \rightarrow Q = f(R, Iav^2, \Delta t) \text{ (Ws)}$$

If electric sparks exist between the active electrode and target tissue, which is the case during cutting (actually a prerequisite for the cutting effect), the electric energy becomes converted into thermal energy partially within the electric arcs and partially within the target. The temperature of a biologic material rises proportionally to the amount of heat and inversely proportionally to the specific heat capacity of the tissue in question.

As mentioned above, a requisite for the application of thermal techniques in the gastro intestinal tract, especially in the colon, is that the temperature required for an intentioned purpose is reached and becomes effective only at the target tissue, and unintentional thermal damage to adjacent or lateral tissues must be avoided. In HF surgery, this objective is achieved via the current density (j) and the current flow duration (Δt) in the target tissue. The current density (j) is a function (f) of the amount of current (i) measured in amperes (Amp) which flows through a defined area (A) measured in square centimeters (cm^2) at a certain point in time (t) or averaged over a defined time interval (Δt).

$$j = f(i/A) \text{ (A/cm}^2)$$

The partial amount of heat (q) generated endogenously through electric current at an arbitrary point within the tissue is proportional to the specific electric resistance (ρ), the square of the current density (j^2), and the effective current flow duration (Δt) at that point.

$$q = f(\rho, j^2, \Delta t) \text{ (Ws)}$$

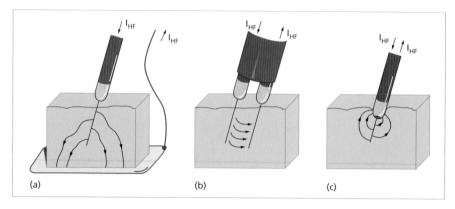

Fig. 6.6 Application techniques of electrosurgery: (a) monopolar; (b) bipolar; (c) quasi-bipolar.

Conduction of an electric current through a target tissue requires that both poles of the electric source be connected to the target tissue in an electrically conductive manner. The electrodes at the target tissue are called active electrodes. The electrodes through which the electric current is conducted away from the tissue (the patient), back to the energy source, without any thermal damage of the tissue at this electrode, are called neutral electrodes. Applications which use an active and a neutral electrode are called monopolar applications, and the instruments used for these applications are called monopolar instruments (Fig. 6.6a). Applications which use both electrodes simultaneously as active electrodes are called bipolar applications, and the instruments used for these applications are called bipolar instruments. As a rule, both active electrodes of bipolar instruments are located close by on the same instrument (Fig. 6.6b).

The density of current within the target tissue can be varied in proportion to the size and shape of the contact surfaces of the active electrodes of HF instruments. Most active electrodes used in flexible endoscopy are in the shape of a needle, loop, or ball (Fig. 6.6c).

Apart from the shape, the size of the contact surface plays an important role as regards the current density and its distribution both in the target tissue and in adjacent tissue. A smaller contact surface results in a steep reduction in the current density and in the temperature profiles in the tissue independent of the distance from the contact surface (Fig. 6.7).

HF current can flow through biological tissue only when the tissue contains water and electrolytes. As a consequence, the temperature of tissue containing water cannot rise above the boiling point of water (approx. 100°C). Tissues that contain less water and/or electrolytes have a lower electric conductivity and less HF current can flow through this tissue if the voltage does not increase

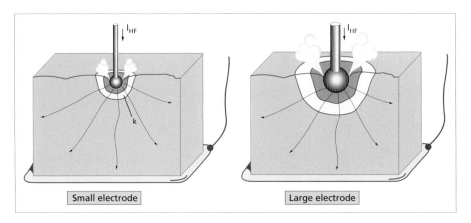

Fig. 6.7 Current density and the resulting penetration depth of thermal effect in the tissue is dependent on the size of the contact surface.

simultanously. Completely dry biologic tissue is an electric insulator, hence no electric current can flow through it, and the temperature cannot rise (Fig. 6.2). This fact is of importance during use of argon plasma coagulation.

Electric arcs

Electric arcs are ignited between an active electrode and tissues when the peak value of the HF voltage is equal to or greater than 200 V, which is typical if the active electrode consists of metal and the tissue contains water (Fig. 6.2). Since these electric arcs reach temperatures far above 300°C, they generate exogenous heat, which raises the temperature of desiccated and hence dry tissue above 100°C, thus causing carbonization and vaporization.

In flexible endoscopy, carbonization (and vaporization) of tissue caused by electric arcs is not only unnecessary, but also annoying, since it generates smoke which impedes visibility. Because the depth of heat penetration cannot be controlled during electric arcing, it is not used as a therapeutic tool in endoscopy.

Even if the vaporization effect caused by electric arcs is not directly used in endoscopy, it is useful indirectly for cutting tissue (see below: Principle of HF-surgical cutting).

Principles of high-frequency surgical coagulation

In flexible endoscopy, HF surgical coagulation can be used for thermal devitalization of pathologic tissue and for hemostasis. Thermal devitalization is performed by argon plasma coagulation (APC) or laser and is described in more detail below. Thermal hemostasis can be used to stop spontaneous bleeding as well as to prevent iatrogenic bleeding, for example during resection of pathologic mucosa, such as polyps.

There is a wide variety of techniques and instruments available for thermal hemostasis, some of which have been developed or designed especially for application in flexible endoscopy. Because the wall of the GI-tract, especially the colon, is relatively thin, thermal hemostasis is a compromise between efficiency and potential damage.

The best method and instrument for thermal hemostasis is dependent on the size of the vessels causing bleeding. In small vessels, hemostasis can be achieved by thermal coagulation or desiccation alone. Control of bleeding from larger vessels requires mechanical compression during heat application. This principle is also applicable for hemostasis during polypectomy.

Monopolar coagulation instruments

In their most simple form, monopolar coagulation instruments for flexible endoscopy consist of a catheter at the distal end of which is an electrode, often ball-shaped. Because this electrode can be pushed against the target tissue, this instrument is useful for hemostasis not only of small but also of larger vessels. In the colon the risk of deep thermal wall damage has to be taken into consideration. During hemostasis, coagulated or desiccated tissue can stick to the electrode, so bleeding can be restarted when the electrode is pulled off the site. This problem was addressed by the development of the electro-hydro-thermo probe and by addition of a coating to reduce sticking.

Electro-hydro-thermo probes

Electro-hydro-thermo (EHT) probes for flexible endoscopy (Fig. 6.8) consist of a catheter with an electrode at the distal end (usually ball-shaped). On this electrode is a hole through which water or saline solution can be instilled between the electrode and target tissue. When the electric current is applied the contact surface between electrode and tissue does not become dry and the electrode does not stick [3,4]. The instillation of fluid can also be applied for the irrigation of bleeding sources. When applying EHT, the depth of the thermal effect cannot be well controlled. This problem has been addressed with the development of bipolar coagulation probes for flexible endoscopy.

Bipolar coagulation instruments

In their most simple form bipolar coagulation instruments for flexible endoscopy consist of a catheter, at the distal end of which are at least two closely placed

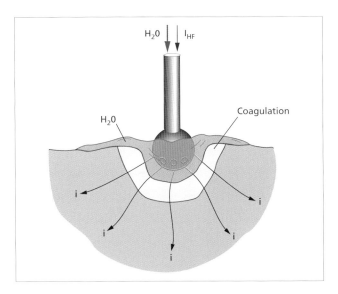

Fig. 6.8 Schematic of electro-hydro-thermo (EHT) probes.

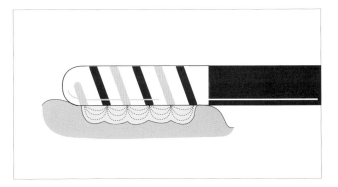

Fig. 6.9 Schematic depiction of current flow of bipolar coagulation probes.

electrodes (Fig. 6.9). The HF current flows through the tissue only between these two electrodes. They can be applied either axially or laterally. The depth of the thermal effects which can be reached is relatively small, decreasing the risk of penetration; however, the efficacy is also limited, i.e. the instruments are useful only for small lesions. Bipolar instruments often have irrigation capacity and some have integrated injection needles [5,6].

Principles of high-frequency surgical cutting

Biologic tissue can be incised electrosurgically when the HF voltage between an electrode and tissue is sufficiently high to produce electric arcs between the

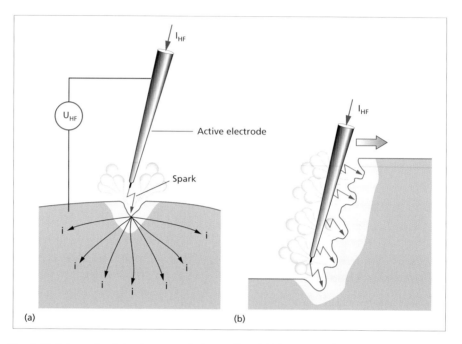

Fig. 6.10 Schematic of the electrosurgical cut effect. (a) Electric sparks ignite between an electrode and tissue if the HF voltage U_{HF} is sufficiently high. (b) The high temperature of the electric sparks evaporates the tissue adjacent to the electrode which will cause a cut if moved through tissue.

electrode and the tissue; this concentrates the HF current at specific points of the tissue (Fig. 6.10a). The temperature produced at the interface where the electric arcs contact the tissue (like microscopic flashes of lightning) is so high that the tissue is immediately evaporated or burned away. As the active cutting electrode passes through the tissue, electric arcs are produced wherever the distance between the cutting electrode and the tissue is sufficiently small, producing electric arcs and hence the cut (an incision) (Fig. 6.10b). As mentioned previously, a minimum peak voltage (Up) of 200 Vp is required in order to produce electric arcs between a metal electrode and biological tissue containing water. The intensity of the electric arcs increase in proportion to the peak voltage. Experience has shown that the depth of thermal coagulation along the cut edges increases with increasing peak voltage (Fig. 6.11).

In the system of HF surgical cutting, the electric power (P) increases by the square of the voltage $(P = f(U^2))$, so it is necessary to modulate the amplitude of the voltage.

The higher the peak voltage (Up) and the degree of amplitude modulation, the deeper the thermal coagulation of the cut edges. If the voltage is not modulated

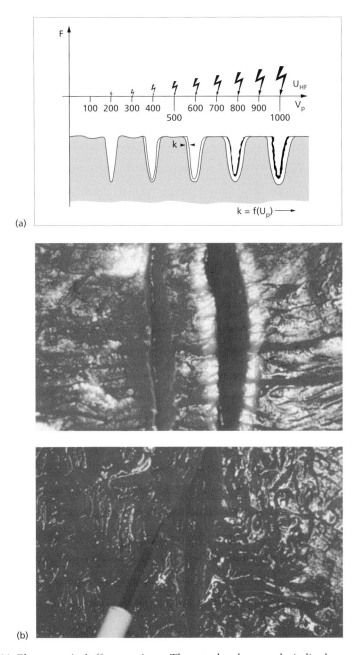

(a)

(b)

Fig. 6.11 Electrosurgical effects on tissue. The cut edges become devitalized, coagulated (k) and carbonized in proportion to the peak voltage (U_{HF}) and the intensity of the electric sparks (F). (a) Graphic depiction. (b) Photograph of effect on tissue with low and high voltage.

and its peak value is low, the coagulation depth at the cut edges is minor or nil, it is called 'cut mode', and the HF current caused by this voltage is called 'cutting current.' If the voltage is strongly modulated and its peak value is high, resulting in deep coagulation of the cut edges, it is called 'coagulation mode', and the HF current caused by this voltage is called 'coagulation current.' One reason for this confusing terminology is the fact that conventional HF surgical generators do not have the capacity for setting the output voltage, only the output power. Setting of the output power of HF generators is not the best option for polypectomy, mucosectomy or sphincterotomy, but it is the standard at the present time.

Especially in colonoscopy the depth of thermal coagulation and also the possibility of thermal devitalization outside the coagulation zone must be considered. If deep thermal damage occurs, tissue histology may be interfered with. A useful aspect is that coagulation of the cut edge of the colon wall can cause hemostasis, which can be used advantageously. Hence, coagulation of the cut edges always is a compromise between these three aspects in colonoscopy.

Another problem with regard to the adjustability, reproducibility and constancy of the depth of coagulation common to all conventional HF surgical generators is the greater or lesser generator impedance Ri, making the HF output voltage Ua dependent on the HF output current Ia. The greater the generator impedance Ri, the more the HF output voltage Ua depends on the HF output current Ia. Conventional HF surgical generators have a generator impedance of between 200 and 1000 ohms.

$$Ua = U0 - Ri \times Ia$$

The output voltage Ua, and hence also the intensity of the electric arcs and ultimately the depth of coagulation, vary considerably, since the load resistance Ra and current Ia vary from one cut to the next and also during each cutting process. During polypectomy for example the load resistance Ra, which is the electric resistance between a polypectomy snare and a polyp, depends among other things on the size of the polyp and increases during closing the snare because the contact between the snare and tissue becomes smaller and smaller.

Another special problem of HF surgical resection of polyps is that HF surgical cutting can be done with minor mechanical force, as long as the HF voltage between the polypectomy snare and the tissue to be cut is above 200 Vp. Because the speed of the snare while cutting through the polyp has a major influence on the degree of hemostasis of the cut edges, the speed should be appropriate to the size of the polyp's attachment. Control of closure speed can be very difficult if there is mechanical friction in the device (Fig. 6.12). Poor control can cause uncontrolled or insufficient hemostasis, especially if the snare zips through the polyp.

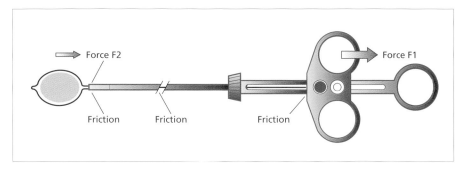

Fig. 6.12 Depiction of mechanical friction at different parts of the polypectomy snare.

Technical aspects of polypectomy

Polypectomy is one of the most important applications of HF surgery in the GI tract, and especially in the colon [7–11] and hemostasis is one of the main problems. If the problem of post-resection bleeding did not exist, it would be possible to resect polyps in a purely mechanical fashion with a thin wire snare in the absence of heat. This would have the advantage that neither the resected specimen (with regard to the histology) nor the wall of the colon (with regard to the risk of perforation) would be thermally damaged. This is possible for tiny polyps, but the endoscopist must tread the path between application of sufficient heat for hemostasis and yet to avoid deep thermal damage. For safe polypectomy, the endoscopy team should be familiar with the equipment available for polypectomy [12–14].

Polypectomy snares

The ideal polypectomy snare should cut cleanly, and not too deeply, and should not coagulate the cut edge of the polyp, to permit adequate histologic examination. For a perfect cut and minor thermal coagulation of the cut edge on the polyp margin the snare wire should be as thin as possible, but, for effective coagulation of the cut edge the snare wire should be as thick as possible. For easy and safe application on all different polyps the snare should be both flexible as well as stiff and should assume the optimal size for small as well as big polyps. In reality, available polypectomy snares offer only a compromise of all these features.

A special problem can be caused by the nose at the distal end of polypectomy snares. If this nose is too long, because it is out of endoscopic view, it can touch the mucosa behind the polyp without the operator's knowledge and cause inadvertent damage when electrically activated.

Polypectomy snare handles should be designed ergonomically for both male and female hands, and should have minor friction between the slider bar and the slider. This is important to provide even loop closure allowing a consistent cut quality and even coagulation.

Polypectomy snare catheters should be flexible enough to pass through the working channels of twisted and looped endoscopes, but have sufficient stiffness to prevent shortening when removing large polyps.

Safety aspects of high-frequency surgery

Monopolar HF surgery can cause unintended thermal effects outside the target tissue [15]. This can happen in tissue directly adjacent to the target tissue or remote from it, when the HF current density is higher outside the target tissue.

To prevent thermal damage to the patient's skin, the neutral electrode must be firmly in contact with the skin as recommended in the instruction manual of the specific HF surgery generator.

HF surgery can cause interference with other electronic devices, such as a pacemaker where it can cause reversion of synchronous to asynchronous pacing or possibly pacemaker inhibition.

During polypectomy, the head of a big or stalked polyp must not touch the colon wall because HF current can flow through this contact resulting in uncontrolled thermal effects (Fig. 6.13a).

If an endoloop is used to prevent bleeding and is placed on the stalk of a polyp between the colon wall and where the polypectomy snare is placed, the HF current density in the smaller diameter compressed by the endoloop can be much higher compared with the HF current density at the polypectomy snare; this will cause the narrowest part to become heated (within the endoloop) instead of the tissue within the polypectomy snare (Figs 6.13b,c).

If metallic hemoclips are used for hemostasis, the snare must not touch the clips as HF current will be conducted through it.

CAUTION: HF surgery must not be used within the colon before potentially explosive gas is eliminated.

Argon plasma coagulation

The principle of argon plasma coagulation

The principle of argon plasma coagulation (APC) is relatively simple [16]. When an electrode (E) is placed at a distance (d) from the surface of a tissue (G) and a HF voltage (U_{HF}) is applied between the electrode and the tissue, the gas between the electrode and the tissue becomes ionized and hence electrically

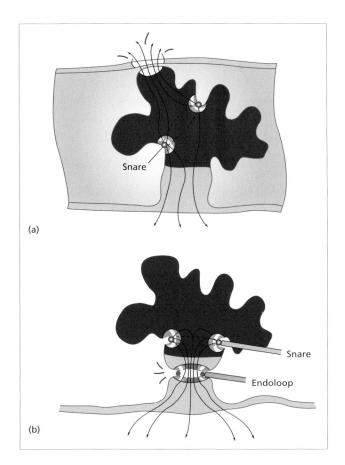

(a)

(b)

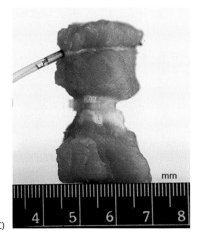

(C)

Fig. 6.13 Unintended thermal effects. (a) If part of a polyp touches the colon wall during polypectomy HF current can flow through this contact point into the colon wall. The closer the snare to this point, the higher the flow of HF current through it. (b) If an endoloop is placed around the polyp the HF current must flow through the strangulated part of the polyp and heat will increase at the point of constriction because of the higher current density. (c) Photographic demonstration of (b) with increased heat damage at point of narrowing.

conductive when the electric field strength (U_{HF}/d) exceeds a critical level. If the gas between the electrode and the tissue is a noble gas (argon, helium, etc.), an electric field strength of about 500 V/mm is needed for ionization. Argon is preferred because of its relatively low cost. The ionized argon forms argon plasma beams between the electrode and the tissue, which can be visualized as small sparks that conduct the HF current to the tissue. An important advantage of argon in comparison to air is its inert character, which neither carbonizes nor vaporizes biologic tissue so that the thermal effects of APC are limited to the devitalization (zone 1), coagulation (zone 2), desiccation (zone 3), and shrinking of tissue (zone 4) as a result of coagulation and desiccation (Fig. 6.14).

A special aspect of APC is that the direction of the argon plasma beams follows the direction of the electric field between the electrode and the tissue. The electrically active beams are directed from the electrode to electrically conductive tissue closest to the electrode, regardless of whether the tissue is in front of or lateral to the electrode. As soon as the target tissue becomes desiccated and hence loses its electric conductivity, the beams automatically move from desiccated to non-desiccated tissue until a large area of the target tissue is desiccated. As a result of the loss of electric conductivity at a treated site, the depth of desiccation, coagulation, and devitalization is limited.

Equipment for argon plasma coagulation

The argon source is an argon cylinder with a pressure-reducing valve (Fig. 6.15). For safety reasons, the argon source must have automatically controlled flow rates and limitation of the pressure. The HF current source must provide both sufficiently high HF voltage for the ionization of argon as well as sufficiently high HF current to generate adequate heat within the target tissue.

APC probes for flexible endoscopy basically consist of a non-conductive flexible tube (Fig. 6.16) through which argon flows. An electrode within the distal end is connected to the HF generator by a wire through the lumen of this tube. For safety reasons, the electrode is recessed from the distal end of the tube so that it cannot come into contact with tissue.

As shown in Fig. 6.17, the depth of coagulation depends on power setting and on application time. In addition, the application technique has a significant influence on the depth. Movement of the activated probe tip will result in a shallower depth of thermal effect than is produced by directing the tip at one point.

When the probe is held at one site for between about 3 and 10 s, the depth of thermal coagulation is up to about 2 mm. Above 10 s the depth increases slowly to its maximum of about 3–4 mm.

Touching the foot pedal activates the flow of argon gas and simultaneously starts the flow of electric current. The time that the foot pedal is depressed

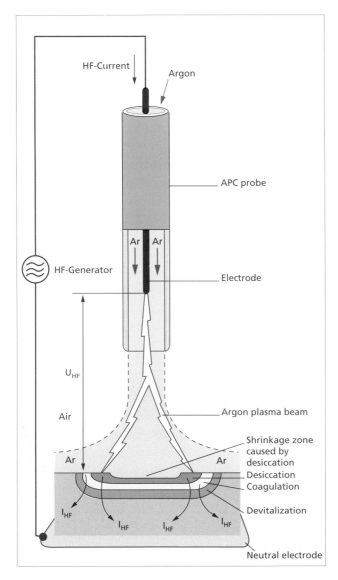

Fig. 6.14 The principle of argon plasma coagulation (APC).

may not be the same as the activation time, which refers to the interval when the argon plasma sparks actually touch the target tissue. There may be no or intermittent sparks if the distance between the probe and the tissue is too great.

Figure 6.18 shows that the shape of an argon gas beam consists of a zone of laminar argon flow, a zone of divergent argon flow and a zone where the flow becomes turbulent. Argon plasma beams can only reach the target tissue when

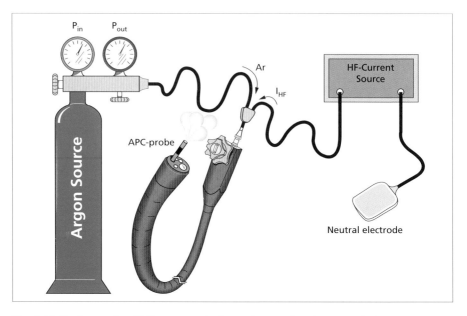

Fig. 6.15 Equipment for APC: argon tank, flow valves, probe, electrosurgical generator.

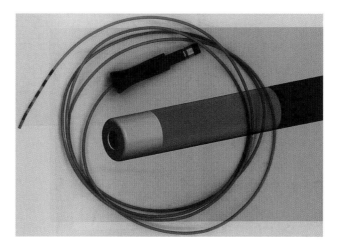

Fig. 6.16 An APC probe and its distal end.

there is argon gas between the distal end of the APC probe and the target tissue. This is the case when the argon gas beam is directed to the target tissue as shown in Fig. 6.19a (axial APC probe) and Fig. 6.19b (lateral APC probe). APC probes can be used laterally as well, but the lumen must be filled with argon. The ignited spark will direct itself to the nearest grounded tissue (Fig. 6.19c). If the target tissue is not within the argon gas beam or within an argon-filled

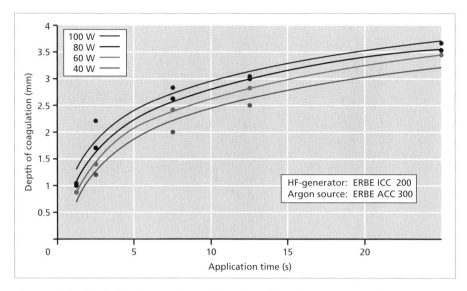

Fig. 6.17 The depth of APC coagulation depends on the application time and power setting.

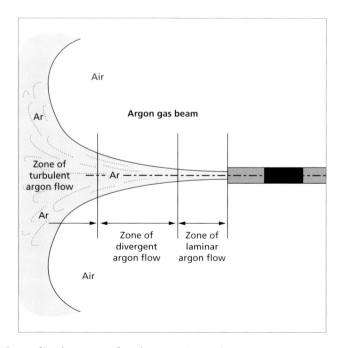

Fig. 6.18 The profile of argon gas flow from an APC probe.

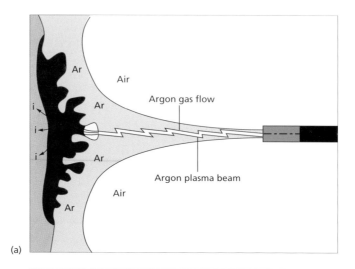

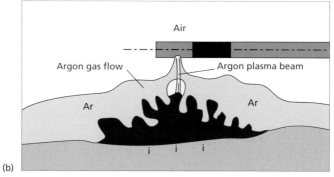

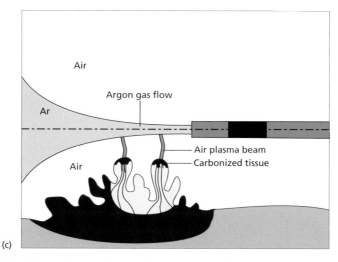

Fig. 6.19 The effects of forward- and side-firing APC probe application.

lumen the argon plasma beams will not ignite, or plasma beams of air will ignite instead. Air plasma beams do not look very different from argon plasma beams; however, air plasma beams can cause carbonization as well as vaporization of tissue and hence can cause deep damage and perforation of organs. Endoscopists typically use air plasma beams when using the tip of the snare wire to 'spark' a polypectomy site to stop bleeding or destroy residual polyp fragments. Air plasma beams, consisting of ionized air, only travel over extremely short distances, and are uncontrollable.

Safety aspects of argon plasma coagulation

As in any monopolar electrosurgical procedure, the neutral electrode must be applied to the skin surface.

Because argon gas is insufflated into the colon during APC, extensive distension of the colon can occur. The distal end of the APC probe must never be pressed against the mucosa or perforation can occur. If the superficial mucosal layer is destroyed by the probe pressure against the colon wall, the flow of argon gas will create instantaneous submucosal emphysema.

CAUTION: APC must not be used within the colon before potentially explosive gas is eliminated.

Laser

Principle of Nd:YAG laser

'Light Amplification by Stimulated Emission of Radiation (LASER)', first described theoretically by Albert Einstein in 1917, and put into practice by T.H. Maiman 5 years after Einstein's death, made possible the generation of electromagnetic radiation in the range of optical wavelengths (light) with an extremely high power density. For about 50 years, the high energy of the laser has been used in medicine. The endoscopic application of laser began in 1975 [17], and following the successful development of a flexible light conductor. Of all the different laser sources, only the argon laser ($a = 488/515$ nm, $P_{max} = 20$ W), and the Nd:YAG laser ($a = 1064$ nm, $P_{max} = 100$ W) can be used endoscopically because their wavelengths can be conducted through thin flexible light guides without significant loss of energy.

Specific characteristics of Nd:YAG lasers in flexible endoscopy

With an adjustable power of up to approx. 100 W, Nd:YAG laser sources are able to generate light with a wavelength of 1064 nm, which is located in the

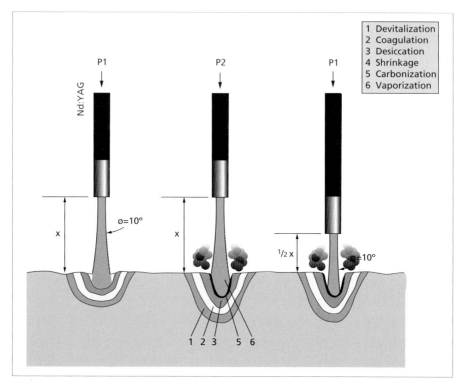

Fig. 6.20 The influence of power as well as the distance between the distal end of the laser fiber and tissue, where P2 > P1 and X1 > X2.

infrared range and is thus invisible to the human eye. With a light guide of 0.6 mm, this light can be guided through an instrumentation channel of a flexible endoscope. The laser light emanates from the light guide in an axial direction with a divergence of about 10°. The invisible Nd:YAG laser is combined with a 'pilot light' in the visible range to see where the beam is directed.

The thermal effects within the radiated tissue are primarily dependent on the density of absorption (W/mm^2) in the tissue and the duration of effect (Δt). The density of absorption refers to the power of light (W) which is absorbed by the tissue per mm^3. The density of absorption is dependent on several variables: the distance (x) of the distal end of the light guide from tissue (Fig. 6.20), the angle with which the light radiates onto the surface, and the absorption and reflection characteristics of the tissue. The parameters may change rapidly due to coagulation, desiccation, or even carbonization. The latter can cause a dramatic increase in absorption or a decrease in reflection, leading to intentional or unintentional vaporization of tissue or even a perforation of the colon.

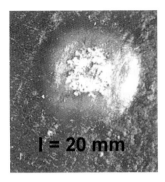 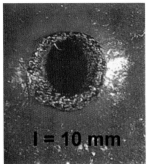 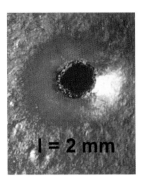

Fig. 6.21 Tissue effect is related to the distance between the distal end of the laser fiber and the tissue.

For intentional vaporization of larger tumor masses, the distal end of the light guide has to be placed close to the target tissue and the power of the laser has to be set sufficiently high.

When using lasers for thermal hemostasis, the experience of the operator is most important; if the light guide is too far away the density of power could be too low for hemostasis, and if too close, the source of bleeding could be started by vaporization rather than stopped by coagulation (Fig. 6.21).

The introduction of APC into flexible endoscopy has reduced the need for lasers in endoscopy [18,19].

Safety aspects of Nd:YAG laser in flexible endoscopy

Lasers can cause unintended thermal effects outside the target tissue during applications. During Nd:YAG laser applications all persons, including the patient, must protect their eyes, even when the distal end of the laser fiber is within the colon, because the light guide can break outside the endoscope. Since Nd:YAG laser is invisible, a break of the laser fiber can damage the retina of unprotected eyes.

Summary

All the different thermal modalities described in this chapter have their special advantages and disadvantages. None of the methods or equipment can yet be regarded as ideal for all cases. A modern endoscopy facility should have adequate equipment to provide optimum treatment for each case as listed in Table 6.1. Endoscopists should also be familiar with the physical background as well as with the advantages and disadvantages of all modalities. This, combined

Table 6.1 Optimum treatment required by case

Treatment required	Thermal method
Thermal ablation of pathologic tissue	
By resection	HF
By devitalization	APC
By vaporization (only in the rectum, not in the colon)	Laser
Thermal haemostasis	
By coagulation (desiccation) (applicable for small vessels only)	HF, APC, HP, laser
By coagulation and mechanical compression (applicable for bleeding of larger vessels)	HF, HP, BICAP
Polypectomy	HF

with practical skill and experience, and competent assistants, is the prerequisite for obtaining optimal results.

References

1 Protell RL, Rubin CE, Auth DC *et al.* The heater probe: a new endoscopic method for stopping massive gastrointestinal bleeding. *Gastroenterology*, 1978; 74: 257–62.
2 Jensen DM, Machicado GA. Principles, technical guidelines, and results of arterial hemostasis with coagulation probes. In: Classen, M, Tytgat, GNJ, Lightdale, CJ, eds. *Gastroenterological Endoscopy*. Stuttgart: Thieme Verlag; 2002: 274–83.
3 Matek W, Frühmorgen P. Electrocoagulation—animal experiments. *Endoscopy* 1986; 18 (Suppl. 2): 58–60.
4 Frühmorgen P, Matek W. Electro-hydro-thermo and bipolar probes. *Endoscopy* 1986; 18 (Suppl. 2): 62–4.
5 Auth DC, Gilbert DA, Opie EA, Silvfristin FE. The multipolar probe—a new endoscopic technique to control gastrointestinal bleeding. *Gastrointest Endosc* 1980; 26: 63.
6 Jensen DM, Machicado GA, Cheng S *et al.* A randomized prospective study of endoscopic bipolar electrocoagulation and heater probe treatment of chronic rectal bleeding from radiation telangiectasia. *Gastrointest Endosc* 1997; 45: 20–5.
7 Deyhle P, Seubert K, Jenny S, Demling L. Endoscopic polypectomy in the proximal colon. *Endoscopy* 1971; 2: 103.
8 Shinya H, Wolff W. Therapeutic application of colonofiberscope polypectomy via the colonoscope. *Gastroenterology*, 1971; 60: 830.
9 Wolff WI, Shinya H. Colonofiberoscopy: diagnostic modality and therapeutic application. *Bull Soc Int Chir* 1971; 5: 525–9.
10 Wolff WI, Shinya H. Colonoscopic management of colonic polyps. *Dis Col Rectum* 1973; 16: 87.
11 Wolff WI, Shinya H. Polypectomy via the fiberoptic colonoscope. *New Engl J Med* 1973; 288: 329–32.
12 Waye JD. New methods of polypectomy. *Gastrointest Endosc Clin N Am*, 1997; 7: 413–22.
13 Waye JD. Colonoscopic polypectomy. In: Classen, M, Tytgat, GNJ, Lightdale, CJ, eds. *Gastroenterological Endoscopy*. Stuttgart: Thieme Verlag, 2002: 302–21.
14 Inoue H, Kudo S. Endoscopic mucosal resection for gastrointestinal mucosal cancer. In: Classen, M, Tytgat, GNJ, Lightdale, CJ, eds. *Gastroenterological Endoscopy*. Stuttgart: Thieme Verlag; 2002: 232–3.

15 Farin G. Möglichkeiten und Probleme der Standardisierung der Hochfrequenzleistung (possibilities and problems of standardizing electrosurgery). In: Lux, G, Semm, K, eds. *Hochfrequen-
zdiathermie in der Endoskopie*. Berlin: Springer-Verlag; 1987: 33–57.

16 Farin G, Grund KE. Technology of argon plasma coagulation with particular regard to endoscopic applications. *Endosc Surg Allied Technol* 1994; 2: 71–7.

17 Barr H. Laser application. In: Classen, M, Tytgat, GNJ, Lightdale, CJ, eds. *Gastroenterological
Endoscopy*. Stuttgart: Thieme Verlag; 2002: 284–9.

18 Mathus-Vliegen EMH, Tytgat GNJ. Analysis of failures and complications of neodymium:
YAG laser photocoagulation in gastrointestinal tract tumors. *Endoscopy* 1990; 22: 17–23.

19 Canard JM, Védrenne B. Clinical application of argon plasma coagulation in gastrointestinal
endoscopy: has the time come to replace the laser? *Endoscopy* 2001; 33: 353–7.

CHAPTER 7

Infection control in endoscopy

ALISTAIR COWEN AND DIANNE JONES

Synopsis

The prevention of infections associated with endoscopy is complex and requires meticulous attention to detail. Practical limitations of applying recognized sterilizing and high-level disinfection processes to endoscopes must be understood, as must the mechanisms of infection and the organisms which provide the greatest clinical risks. Antibiotic prophylaxis will depend not only on the particular endoscopic procedure undertaken but also on a variety of host factors. Detailed endoscope reprocessing protocols are discussed with particular emphasis on the problems of biofilms and the difficulties of providing rinse water of adequate quality. Automatic flexible endoscope reprocessors are widely used but the numerous problems associated with these machines are often inadequately addressed. Part of any quality control program must be adequate microbiological surveillance of endoscopes.

Sterilization and disinfection

Sterilization

Sterilization is defined as the complete elimination or destruction of all forms of microbial life [1]. Sterility is a state more easily conceived of than demonstrated in a practical way. How can the sterility of a batch of medical devices be proven? Microbiological examination of a few items of a batch does not exclude a 1/100 000 or a 1/1 000 000 possibility that the batch contains an article which is unsterile. In practice safety assurance levels (SAL) are used [2]. This technique studies a selected microorganism (usually a resistant bacterial spore) under fixed conditions in a sterilizing process and extrapolates the chance of remaining organisms from the inactivation curve. The usual convention is for a medical device labeled as 'sterile' to have an SAL of 10^{-6}, i.e. there is one in one million chance or less that the item is unsterile. This is an arbitrary definition which has no intrinsic scientific merit. For example, there is no evidence that items with an SAL of 10^{-3} have more adverse patient outcomes than items with an SAL of 10^{-6}.

High-level disinfection

High-level disinfection is defined as the elimination or destruction of all forms of microbial life except high concentrations of some spores [3].

What level of disinfection is required?

Earle H. Spalding devised a practical approach to patient safety and medical device usage.

Critical items

Critical items are those which enter sterile tissues, including body cavities and vascular spaces, and should be sterile.

Semi-critical items

'Semi-critical items' are those which come into contact with mucous membranes or 'skin that is not intact', and should undergo at least high-level disinfection.

This has proved to be a workable, practical, and largely safe classification. In clinical practice the boundaries are not so clearly defined. Where does 'non-intact skin' end and 'sterile tissue' begin? Who can know with certainty that an endoscope will 'come into contact' with intestinal mucosa but not breach it?

It is generally accepted that endoscopes should undergo high-level disinfection and that accessories which breach mucosa, or may breach mucosa, should be sterile [4]. These will include biopsy forceps, snares, injecting needles, dilators, ERCP equipment, and implantable devices such as stents.

The practical problem

There is a curious belief that if endoscopes are subjected to a 'sterilizing process' then many of the problems of endoscopy associated infections will disappear. Unfortunately, this attitude reveals a basic ignorance of the fundamental problem faced in endoscope reprocessing. Endoscopes cannot be subjected to reliable, easily validated, high temperature disinfecting or sterilizing systems because of the heat sensitive nature of the materials from which they are constructed. In addition the complexity of long, fine, interconnecting channels which are difficult to clean, impossible to inspect, and which cannot be adequately assessed for channel surface irregularities and damage, make endoscope reprocessing a special challenge for any system of sterilization or disinfection [4].

These physical characteristics of endoscopes have dictated that time consuming manual cleaning by well trained staff is necessary. It has been demonstrated on numerous occasions that any attempt to achieve high-level disinfection or sterilization by any of the currently available techniques, including ethylene oxide exposure and all chemical sterilants, will be ineffective if appropriate meticulous manual cleaning has not been completed [5,6].

Biocides

Chemical biocides which are used for endoscope reprocessing throughout the world include glutaraldehyde, peracetic acid, chlorine dioxide, hydrogen peroxide, ortho-phthalaldehyde and electrolytic water. None of these chemicals or processes can be considered ideal.

In most developed countries biocides used for high-level disinfection of endoscopes must receive appropriate government approval after submission of extensive validation data. It must be recognized that the effect of biocides on microorganisms is a complex process where variation in temperature, concentration, and remaining organic material on devices, markedly alter efficacy and it is therefore critical that the agent be used strictly as directed by the manufacturer.

The organisms

The level of intrinsic microbial resistance to chemical sterilants varies widely [4]. Spore forming organisms are relatively resistant. Fortunately the common microorganisms of greatest concern to endoscopy, particularly HBV and HIV, are among the most sensitive of all microbiological agents to some chemical sterilants. HCV, being a lipid containing virus, is predicted to have a similar sensitivity to HBV. Intermediate levels of resistance are shown by common vegetative bacteria. Some increased resistance is present with mycobacteria and non-lipid containing viruses, e.g. polio virus, hepatitis A virus. These levels of resistance are far less than for bacterial spores.

The critical points in reprocessing

The critical points of any endoscope reprocessing system:
- Adequate cleaning is by far the most important part of any endoscope reprocessing system.
- Numerous studies show that no disinfecting or 'sterilizing' process capable of use with current flexible endoscopes will achieve even high-level

disinfection, let alone sterilization, if adequate cleaning has not been undertaken.
• Currently there are no studies in peer reviewed journals that consistently show that totally automated machine cleaning of endoscopes can achieve satisfactory removal of biological material.

Risks of infections associated with endoscopic procedures

Mechanisms of infection

• An infectious disease may be transmitted from a patient to subsequent patients because infected biological material is not totally removed from the endoscope or accessories during reprocessing.
• Endemic health care facility pathogens, including those present in the water supply, may contaminate and colonize endoscopes, automatic flexible endoscope reprocessors (AFERs), storage areas, or water feed systems.
• Endoscopic manipulation may result in bacteremia from the patient's endogenous gut flora.

Clinical infections

The American Society for Gastrointestinal Endoscopy has estimated that the overall risk of patient to patient transmission of a serious infection at endoscopy is 1 in 1.8 million examinations. Since this estimate is based on retrospective rather than prospective studies, it is almost certainly a significant underestimation, but it does indicate the rarity of patient to patient transmission of serious infectious diseases. The risk of endoscopy associated infections due to the contamination of instrument or accessory items by health care facility environmental pathogens, or infection with the patient's own flora, is very significantly higher.

Whether or not a clinical infection occurs as a result of an endoscopic procedure will depend upon:
• infecting organisms
• the endoscopic procedures
• host factors.

Infecting organisms

A vast array of microorganisms could be associated with endoscopy transmitted infections. In practice a relatively limited number of infective agents have been transmitted by endoscopy. The more important agents together with those that are of major theoretical concern are considered here.

Bacteria

Vegetative bacteria. Numerous reports in the older literature of transmission of salmonella and related species were associated with cleaning and disinfection protocols which would be totally inadequate today [7]. Transmission of such infections indicates serious deficiencies in cleaning and disinfection which would be cause for major concern and investigation.

Clostridium difficile. Clostridium difficile is a spore forming organism and therefore might be expected to be highly resistant to chemical disinfectants. There is clear evidence of person to person transmission by environmental contamination at hospital ward level. Fortunately, *Clostridium difficile* spores are much less resistant to chemical disinfectants than most other spore forming organisms. To date there is no definite evidence of endoscopic transmission of *Clostridium difficile*. The rapid rise of serious clinical pseudomembranous colitis in hospital inpatient populations is a cause for serious concern. Many strains of *c. difficile* are now resistant to vancomyin.

Mycobacterium tuberculosis. There is no proven case of transmission of *Mycobacterium tuberculosis* by gastrointestinal endoscopy. Numerous infections have been transmitted as a result of bronchoscopy [8,9]. Contaminated suction valves, damaged biopsy channels, contaminated topical anesthetic sprays, and colonized AFERs have all been implicated.

Hanson *et al.* [10] have shown that proper cleaning of bronchoscopes deliberately contaminated with *Mycobacterium tuberculosis* reduced the bacterial bioburden by at least 3.5 $\log_{10}$ and subsequent immersion in 2% glutaraldehyde for 10 min rendered the instrument free of infective material. Nicholson *et al.* [6] dramatically illustrated the critical role of cleaning by showing that a deliberately contaminated flexible bronchoscope which was cleaned inadequately still had remaining viable *Mycobacterium tuberculosis* after *10 sequential full disinfection cycles.*

An additional hazard is the development of multidrug resistant tuberculosis (MDRTB). Infection transmission has largely been by aerosol. An outbreak with deaths in the southern United States was convincingly traced to inadequate reprocessing of flexible bronchoscopes.

The Center for Disease Control and Prevention recommends bronchoscopy should not be performed on patients with active TB unless absolutely necessary. Bronchoscopy should not be regarded as the first line investigation in the diagnosis of TB. Patient to patient and patient to staff transmission of mycobacterium tuberculosis by aerosols associated with coughing during and after bronchoscopy is a significant hazard.

Scrupulous, mechanical cleaning by properly trained and certified endoscope reprocessors remains the best defense against the transmission of mycobacterial disease by flexible bronchoscopy. (See also section on pseudomonas).

Atypical mycobacteria. A variety of atypical mycobacteria may be present in the hospital water supply. These organisms frequently colonize AFERs and are prone to develop serious chemical resistance. Some strains of atypical mycobacteria (particularly *Mycobacterium chelonei*) have developed almost total resistance to glutaraldehyde. Atypical mycobacteria contaminating flexible bronchoscopes have caused pseudo-epidemics. Positive specimen cultures taken at bronchoscopy have been wrongly assumed to be patient infections, leading to potentially seriously toxic and prolonged drug therapy [11].

Serratia marcescens. There are several reports of *Serratia marcescens* being transmitted by flexible bronchoscopy. In an outbreak involving three fatalities the instrument had been inadequately cleaned but then subjected to a full ethylene oxide sterilizing cycle [5].

Helicobacter pylori. *Helicobacter pylori* has been transmitted by endoscopy biopsy forceps which were inadequately cleaned [12]. Given the high background prevalence of *Helicobacter pylori* infection it is likely that disease transmission by endoscopy has been significantly under reported. There is conflicting evidence about whether endoscopists and endoscopy nurses have an increased risk of helicobacter infection.

Pseudomonas. *Pseudomonas aeruginosa* and related species are common environmental contaminants which may be present in tap water. Clinical endoscopy associated infections due to *Pseudomonas* spp. have largely been confined to ERCP and related procedures [13,14]. There are several reports of transmission by ordinary endoscopy in severely immunocompromised patients. *Pseudomonas* spp. frequently colonize AFERs and may be difficult to eradicate. Kovacs *et al.* [15] have reported a strain of *Pseudomonas aeruginosa* which appeared to have developed chemical resistance. The organism was responsible for several ERCP-related chemical infections. A disturbing feature of ERCP-associated pseudomonas infections has been the frequent failure by endoscopy units to recognize the problem. Pseudomonas transmission during bronchoscopy has become a major problem with outbreaks reported from the United States and France [16–20].

Serious clinical infections and even fatalities have been linked to the contaminated bronchoscopes. The mechanisms of contamination include a poorly designed port valve and defective or wrong connectors between bronchoscopes and AFERs during reprocessing [16,18,21]. The valve port in question was designed as a non-removable part of the bronchoscope (this in itself would seem to be a seriously flawed concept). Microbiological cultures of the bronchoscope channels taken using samples collected by perfusion of the channels from the control head to the distal tip were negative but samples collected with reverse flushing grew pseudomonas. The episodes associated with AFER connectors yet again emphasize the risk of AFERs which do not have flow alarms on individual channels and do not test rinse water quality.

Viruses

Human immunodeficiency virus (HIV). The transmission of HIV to a number of patients undergoing minor surgical procedures has created major public concern that medical procedures including endoscopy may be a serious source of disease transmission. Inflammatory articles in popular magazines in the USA, e.g. 'Do scopes spread sickness?' 'Medicine's dirty little secret', and 'Blood money' have all resulted in increasing public scepticism concerning the self-regulation of the medical profession. There is increasing demand for greater official regulation and accountability. Despite these concerns there is no proven case of transmission of HIV by endoscopy. However, the extremely long latent period before the development of clinical AIDS increases the difficulty of detecting transmission. High concentrations of viral particles may be present in the blood during most stages of HIV infection. Fortunately the virus is very sensitive to most chemical disinfectants including glutar-aldehyde [22].

Elegant 'in use' studies by Hanson *et al.* [23,24] have demonstrated that endoscopes used in patients with HIV infection have had all infectious material removed by standard cleaning and disinfection protocols. There have been some reports suggesting that artificially contaminated endoscopes had remaining viral material after standard reprocessing. However, in all of these reports detection has used PCR techniques which do not distinguish between live infective viral particles and non-infective degraded viral material. Deva *et al.* [25] have shown in the duck hepatitis model that PCR positive material remaining after reprocessing is not infective.

Hepatitis B. Despite the highly infectious nature of this virus there is only a single proven case of hepatitis B transmission by endoscopy [26]. The reprocessing protocol used on this instrument was clearly inadequate. A number of studies have followed patients undergoing endoscopic procedures with instruments and accessories used on known hepatitis B positive patients and none have found evidence of disease transmission [27].

Hepatitis C (HCV). Hepatitis C has been transmitted to a patient undergoing ERCP and endoscopic sphincterotomy [28]. HCV transmission occurred during colonoscopy from a known infective patient to the two subsequent patients [29]. A French National blood transfusion study suggested that endoscopy was a significant risk factor for HCV acquisition. Another French study, however, could find no evidence of increased prevalence of hepatitis C amongst patients undergoing endoscopy. Transmission of Hepatitis C during simple endoscopy has been proven by detailed viral analysis [30]. In this case it was claimed that the reprocessing protocol was adequate. In this report it remains unclear whether disease transmission was associated with the endoscopic procedure or anaesthetic administration. Seven cases of hepatitis C transmitted at a Brooklyn endoscopy clinic were unrelated to the endoscopy procedure [31]. The infections were due to reuse of syringes or needles used for the administration of sedation during the procedures. A large number of hepatitis C infections appear to have been transmitted in an American day surgery center by the same mechanism [32].

Prions

Prion diseases include Creutzfeldt–Jakob disease (CJD), new variant CJD (vCJD), and kuru in human beings. Animal diseases include bovine spongiform encephalopathy (BSE) and scrapie. Prions are unique amongst infectious agents because nucleic acid (DNA or RNA) has not been detected. The disease is characterized by an abnormal isoform of a cellular protein called prion protein (PrP^c). Mutations in the PrP^c gene on chromosome 20 may result in transformation into the pathological isoform (PrP^{sc}).

CJD. CJD occurs in sporadic, familial, iatrogenic, and occupational forms. Less than 200 cases worldwide of iatrogenic or occupational acquired CJD have been reported [33]. The majority of these relate to dura mater transplants or the use of human cadaveric growth hormone. Rarer sources include contaminated neurosurgical instruments, cadaveric pituitary gonadotrophin, brain electrodes, and corneal transplants.

The risk of infection transmission depends on the concentration of abnormal prion in the tissue examined. High concentrations exist in the brain (including the dura mater), spinal cord, and eye. Low levels are present in liver, lymphoid tissue, kidneys, lungs, and spleen. Prions are undetectable in intestine, bone marrow, whole blood, white cells, serum, nasal mucus, saliva, sputum, urine, feces, and vaginal secretions. Attempts to transmit CJD by blood and blood products from humans to primates have consistently failed [34].

Prions unfortunately display a markedly increased resistance to conventional methods of sterilization. Commonly used disinfectants including glutaraldehyde are ineffective. Steam sterilization (standard gravity displacement at 120°C) is only partly effective even after exposure times as long as 2 h.

What to do in practice about CJD? The dilemma faced by endoscopists is whether extraordinary precautions in reprocessing endoscopes need to be taken because of the risk of CJD. The approach described by Rutala and Webber [35] is recommended—that endoscopes which are exposed to essentially 'no risk tissues' will not be exposed to detectable levels of prion and therefore should be reprocessed by conventional disinfection protocols. Clearly this does not apply to any endoscopic device used in neurosurgery. This appears to be sound scientific advice. However, given the widespread emotional and press reactions to this devastating disease, few will be able to resist taking additional precautions. Many will believe that patients with known Creutzfeldt–Jakob disease, Gerstmann–Straussler–Scheinker syndrome, and fatal familial insomnia, and patients with undiagnosed rapidly progressive dementia should not undergo endoscopic examination unless there is no acceptable diagnostic or therapeutic alternative. If endoscopy is necessary in proven cases then examination should be undertaken with an endoscope reserved for this purpose. For those with a high suspicion of disease many would prefer to use endoscopes which have reached the point of retirement from clinical service and not to reuse the scope. This may be an argument for retaining some older endoscopes, at least in large facilities.

New variant CJD (vCJD). Variant CJD in humans appears to be due to the transmission of the identical prion strain causing bovine spongiform encephalopathy in cattle [36]. The disease has a different clinical course with a much earlier age of onset, presentation with psychiatric symptoms, and a rapid downhill progression. In complete contra-distinction to other forms of CJD large quantities of the abnormal prion (PrP^{sc}) are found in lymphoid tissue [37]. In fact vCJD can reliably be diagnosed by tonsil biopsy. This obviously raises concerns that endoscopes exposed to lymphoid tissue in the alimentary tract may become contaminated with tissue in which significant concentrations of abnormal prions exist. Currently quantification of risk transmission is hampered by a lack of knowledge about relative prion titres in alimentary lymphoid tissues. Recent development of a highly sensitive immunoblotting assay for vCJD may allow a clearer understanding of transmission risks associated with endoscopy [38]. The UK is the only country with a large number of vCJD affected patients—150 deaths to 1st July 2005 [39]. The Health Department guidelines have been updated in March 2007 [40]. Countries not currently affected by vCJD will choose not to introduce a number of their recommendations.

Other infections

A wide variety of other bacteria, viruses, fungi, protozoa, and helminths could potentially be transmitted by endoscopy. Candida infections in immunocompromised patients have been related to endoscopy. Pseudo-infection with *Rhodotorula rubra* was associated with bronchoscopy. Strongyloides infection of the esophagus and cryptosporidial infection have been linked to upper endoscopy. Claims that tropheryma whipplei (Whipple's Disease) is resistant to glutaraldehyde and could be transmitted by endoscopy [41] has not been confirmed and appears unlikely. Many of these infectious agents are likely to represent a greater hazard to immunocompromised patients.

The endoscopic procedures

Bacteremia may be associated with simple everyday events such as teeth cleaning. The significance of the bacteremia will depend on the particular types of organisms present, the numbers of organisms, whether the tissues are inflamed, and the degree of mucosal trauma.

Upper gastrointestinal endoscopy

Simple diagnostic endoscopy and biopsy are associated with low levels of bacteremia, usually with non-virulent organisms. Clinically significant bacteremia may, however, occur in patients with compromised immune status and severe mucositis (e.g. bone marrow transplantation, leukemia).

Disruption of the esophageal mucosa almost invariably occurs during esophageal dilatation. This procedure is associated with high levels of bacteremia [42] and a number of serious clinical infections have been reported.

Endoscopic sclerotherapy, particularly where there is a significant submucosal injection, is associated with high levels of bacteremia. In addition these patients are often severely immunocompromised [43].

Endoscopic banding is associated with significantly lower rates of bacteremia [44].

Lower gastrointestinal endoscopy

Somewhat surprisingly, only low levels of bacteremia have been reported in association with diagnostic colonoscopy. However, manipulation of the sigmoid colon in patients with acute peridiverticular inflammation or abscess formation undergoing colonoscopy may result in gross bacteremia.

Endoscopic retrograde cholangiopancreatography

ERCP is the one endoscopic procedure which has consistently been associated with significant clinical infection rates. Clinical infections may be due to the patient's endogenous flora, particularly if duct obstruction is not totally relieved at the time of the procedure. However, the vast majority of clinical infections have been with *Pseudomonas aeruginosa* or closely related species and have been due to contamination of the endoscope or accessory equipment [13,14,45,46]. AFERs, contaminated water feed systems, inadequate cleaning and disinfection of the forceps elevating channel, and failure to alcohol rinse and air dry *ALL* duodenoscope channels have been the most common underlying causes.

Percutaneous endoscopic gastrostomy

Bacteremia during the procedure and wound infection have led to significant procedure related complications [47].

Endoscopic ultrasound

There have been conflicting reports on the degree of bacteremia occurring during endoscopic ultrasound.

Mucosectomy

Significant rates of bacteremia have been reported following endoscopic mucosectomy particularly where large quantities of tissue are removed.

Host factors

Immune competence

Patients with compromised immune status are significantly more susceptible to endoscopy associated infections. A wide variety of disorders can affect immune competence. These will include infections (e.g. HIV), neoplastic disorders (particularly hematological malignancies), chemotherapy, radiotherapy, bone marrow transplantation, advanced diseases of the liver and kidney, and specific disorders of immune response. These patients are not only more susceptible to infections with conventional organisms but may also be susceptible to a variety of other organisms not usually associated with human disease (e.g. atypical mycobacteria infection). In addition they may harbour unusual organisms. In most cases these organisms will not pose a clinical threat to other patients with normal immune status but may be a hazard to those with compromised immune systems. It is important to remember that hospital water contamination with atypical mycobacteria, pseudomonas, or even cryptosporidia may pose a particular hazard to the immunocompromised.

The degree of tissue damage

The greater the procedural damage caused during an endoscopic procedure, the greater the risk of subsequent infection. Significant tissue disruption can occur during esophageal dilatation. Chemical and ischemic damage to tissues occurs with injection sclerotherapy. Endoscopic sphincterotomy and stone extraction, removal of foreign bodies, endoscopic placement of stents, mucosectomy, and removal of large sessile polyps are all associated with significant tissue damage.

Intrinsic sources of infection

Intrinsic sources of infection within the patient may contribute to clinical infection. Poor oral hygiene with severe bacterial gingivitis will ensure greater contamination of instruments and accessories in the upper GI tract. Peri-diverticular abscess, infected pseudocysts, and intra-abdominal collections may be traumatized during endoscopic procedures.

Damaged valves and implants

There is a significant risk that bacteria present during periods of bacteremia will lodge on damaged or foreign tissues. The most important factor here is endovascular integrity. Colonization can occur with indwelling vascular devices, vascular grafts, and coronary artery stents before complete re-epithelialization. Mechanical heart valves, valve abnormalities which create turbulent flow, and other irregular endovascular surfaces are prone to bacterial lodgement. Artificial joints and other indwelling foreign devices may be slightly more prone to infection following endoscopic procedures but the risk is very small and mainly within the first few months following insertion.

Antibiotic prophylaxis for endoscopic procedures

There are three situations where antibiotic prophylaxis may be considered for endoscopic procedures:
* Patients at increased risk of bacterial endocarditis.
* Patients at increased risk of general infections following particular procedures.
* ERCP.

Principles of prevention of bacterial endocarditis

The American Heart Association stresses that 'there are currently no randomised and carefully controlled human trials in patients with underlying structural heart disease to definitively establish that antibiotic prophylaxis provides protection against development of endocarditis during bacteremia inducing procedures. Further, most cases of endocarditis are not attributable to an invasive procedure' [48]. There is no definite consensus on which patients should receive antibiotic prophylaxis for which endoscopic procedures and indeed there is no real consensus on the preferred antibiotic regimen [49]. Nonetheless, some general guidelines may be offered. There is a consensus that some comorbid cardiovascular conditions pose a greater risk than others.

High risk cardiovascular conditions [48]

- Prosthetic heart valves.
- Previous history of endocarditis.
- Complex cyanotic congenital heart disease.
- Surgically constructed systemic pulmonary shunts or conduits.

Moderate risk cardiovascular conditions [48]

- Uncorrected shunt defects.
- Bicuspid aortic valves.
- Coarctation of the aorta.
- Acquired valvular dysfunction.
- Hypertrophic cardiomyopathy.
- Mitral valve prolapse without regurgitation is considered a low risk condition but a moderate risk where regurgitation exists.

Recommendations for antibiotic prophylaxis

Who should receive antibiotics?

The perceived need for antibiotic prophylaxis varies also by the type of endoscopic procedure. General recommendations are given in Table 7.1.

Clinical problems where opinions diverge. Indwelling vascular devices. Antibiotic prophylaxis may be of value for patients undergoing endoscopic procedures with a high rate of bacteremia, particularly if they have a compromised immune system.

Table 7.1 Recommendations for antibiotic prophylaxis in endoscopy

Endoscopic procedure	Cardiac conditions		Other situations requiring special consideration
	High risk	Moderate risk	
Diagnostic endoscopy	No	No	Yes Chemotherapy/bone marrow transplant
Oesophageal dilatation	Yes	Yes	Yes Severely immunocompromised
Injection sclerotherapy	Yes	Yes	Yes Severely immunocompromised
Oesophageal banding	Yes	±	± Severely immunocompromised
Mucosectomy	Yes	Yes	Yes Severely immunocompromised
Endoscopic ultrasound	Yes	±	± Severely immunocompromised
PEG	Yes	Yes	Yes All patients
Routine colonoscopy	Yes	Yes	Yes Ascites/severely immunocompromised
Colonoscopy with peridiverticulitis	Yes	Yes	All patients
Traumatic procedures, e.g. foreign body removal, difficult stent placement	Yes	Yes	Yes Immunocompromised

- Recent coronary artery stenting. Antibiotic prophylaxis has been recommended by some authorities in the first 3–4 months following stenting until epithelialization has occurred.
- Orthopedic prostheses. There are isolated case reports of orthopedic prosthetic infection associated with endoscopic procedures. However, the risk is extremely low.

The risk is presumably higher immediately after joint replacement and many would recommend antibiotic prophylaxis for the first few months after joint replacement, particularly if the patient has any impairment of immune competence.

New recommendations from the American Heart Association (ASA). The ASA has recently stated that routine GI endoscopy procedures do not justify endocarditis prophylaxis [50]. No doubt the Gastroenterology Societies will take this into account when they update their recommendations.

What antibiotic regimen? While there is little agreement on details of prophylactic regimens, the general principles are accepted. It is important to ensure

Table 7.2 Commonly used prophylactic antibiotic regimens

Standard regimen—not allergic to penicillin	
Adults	Amoxycillin 1–2 g IM/IV *and*
	Gentamicin 80–120 mg IV
	Before commencement of procedure
Children	Amoxycillin 50 mg/kg IM/IV *and*
	Gentamicin 2 mg/kg IV
	Before commencement of procedure
Allergic to penicillin/On long-term penicillin/Recent penicillin	
Adults	Vancomycin 1 g over 90 min *and*
	Gentamicin 80–120 mg
	IV 1 h before procedure
Children	Vancomycin 20 mg/kg *and*
	Gentamicin 2 mg/kg
	IV 1 h before procedure
	or
	Replace Vancomycin with Teicoplanin 6 mg/kg up to
	a maximum dose of 400 mg

adequate antibiotic concentrations in the serum during and after the procedure. To reduce the likelihood of microbiological resistance it is important that prophylactic antibiotics are given only during the operative period. Commonly used antibiotic regimens are detailed in Table 7.2.

Antibiotic prophylaxis for ERCP

The value of antibiotic prophylaxis for ERCP is also controversial [51]. Some of this confusion has arisen because of the inappropriate use of the term 'prophylactic'. There can be little argument that patients with clinical cholangitis or other evidence of biliary or pancreatic sepsis should be on appropriate antibiotics. There is also general consensus that patients who have undergone traumatic procedures with major tissue manipulation, incomplete drainage of obstruction, or widely dilated duct systems should continue to receive appropriate antibiotics.

The area of controversy is whether patients with minimal or no bile duct dilatation undergoing simple procedures such as endoscopic sphincterotomy and stone removal require antibiotics commencing before the procedure. A meta-analysis of studies examining antibiotic prophylaxis prior to ERCP concluded that while it may reduce the instance of bacteremia, it did not substantially reduce the incidence of clinical sepsis/cholangitis. One of the difficulties in deciding for or against antibiotic prophylaxis commencing before the procedure is that the complexity and outcome of the procedure cannot always be accurately predicted.

Optimum benefit of antibiotics will only be obtained if therapeutic levels are present in the bile and tissues at the time of examination. Patients should commence antibiotic prophylaxis at least 1–2 h before the procedure. The common pathogenic organisms encountered in the biliary tree are *Pseudomonas aeruginosa*, *Klebsiella* spp., *E. coli*, *Bacteroides* spp., and *Enterococci*.

Prophylactic antibiotic regimens for ERCP

Ciprofloxin oral 750 mg—2 h before procedure
IV 200 mg—2 h before procedure
Piperacillin—before procedure

OR

Piperacillin + tazobactam

The reason for giving antibiotics needs to be clearly borne in mind. Is the risk simply of cholangitis or is there also a significant risk of endocarditis because of valvular damage or other abnormalities? Cephalosporins and ureidopenicillins (e.g. piperacillin) have very poor activity against enterococci and are generally considered inappropriate for endocarditis prophylaxis.

Principles of effective decontamination protocols

Cleaning is essential

The most important step in the process of endoscope decontamination is scrupulous manual cleaning prior to disinfection.

Manual cleaning refers to the physical task of removing secretions and contaminants from the endoscope with appropriate brushes, cloths, detergents, and water. This is a two-stage process, beginning immediately upon removal of the endoscope from the patient in the procedure room, and continuing once the instrument has been taken to the specific reprocessing area. This area should be separate to the procedure room.

Automated industrial processes used for cleaning have yet to be shown to be effective in endoscope reprocessing. All instruments currently need to be manually processed prior to chemical disinfection. It is desirable that in future automated systems be developed which physically lift the soils present and then remove them by fluid flow [52–54].

In order for manual cleaning to be effective it must:
- Be performed by a person conversant with the structure of the particular endoscope and trained and certified in cleaning techniques.
- Be undertaken immediately after the endoscope is used so that secretions do not dry and harden.
- Follow a protocol which, using appropriate detergents and cleaning equipment, allows all surfaces of the endoscope, internal and external, to be cleaned. Recommended protocols produced by respected authors are detailed in references [55–61].
- Be followed by thorough rinsing to ensure that all debris and detergents are removed prior to disinfection.

Effectiveness of recommended protocols

A standard for testing of cleaning efficacy in endoscope reprocessing procedures has not yet been developed. Several studies have examined methods such as ATP bioluminescence in an endeavor to provide an accurate marker of cleanliness [62].

Recommended reprocessing protocols remove microbiological contamination. However, even minor deviations from cleaning protocols have resulted in persistent microbiological contamination after disinfection. This emphasizes that present reprocessing techniques are less than ideal and have a lower margin of safety than is desirable. It reinforces the need for all steps in reprocessing protocols to be carried out meticulously.

Endoscope structure

There are at least 50 different models of flexible endoscopes available, with each manufacturer constantly expanding their range. The manufacturer supplies an instruction book with each endoscope.

It is essential that every person responsible for endoscope decontamination reads these instruction books and is familiar with the particular characteristics of each model of endoscope required to be cleaned. This is particularly important where staff are reprocessing loan instruments which may differ in the configuration of the internal channels to the instruments with which they are familiar.

Common features

- *External features.* All flexible endoscopes have a light guide plug, an umbilical cable (cord), a control head, and an insertion tube.

- *The light guide plug.* The light guide plug fits into the light source. The air/water and suction channels have ports in the light guide plug. The light guide plug of a video endoscope is heavier than that of a fiberoptic endoscope and needs to be handled with care. Most light guide plugs have electrical connections that need to be sealed by a protective cap prior to immersion in liquid.
- *The umbilical cable/universal cord.* The umbilical cable connects the light guide plug to the endoscope's control head. The external surface may be contaminated by splashes or hand contact during endoscopic procedures.
- *The control head.* The control head contains the control handles, which allow the operator to flex the distal portion of the instrument and valves to access the suction and air/water functions. Fiberoptic endoscopes have an eyepiece on the control head. Video endoscopes are similar in construction to fiberoptic endoscopes, except that they do not have an eyepiece—the image is seen on a video screen. The control head is contaminated during endoscopic procedures by the operator's hands. The control handles have grooved surfaces, which must be carefully brushed during cleaning. The hollow structure of some control handles should be noted and care taken to ensure that the under-surface is thoroughly rinsed and emptied of fluids. The seats which house the suction and air/water valves (buttons) must be thoroughly cleaned. The biopsy channel port is located at the base of the control handle near its junction with the insertion tube. This port must be brushed carefully during the cleaning process.
- *The insertion tube.* The insertion tube enters the patient's body and is grossly contaminated during the procedure. The distal tip of the insertion tube houses the microchip (in video endoscopes), the openings for the suction and air/water channels, and the lens covering the flexible fiberoptic light guides. The section of the insertion tube adjacent to the distal tip is known as the bending section. Its covering is made from soft flexible material and is particularly vulnerable to damage and material deterioration.

Common internal features. The suction and air/water channels and the fiberoptic light guide extend from the light guide plug to the distal tip. In non-video models an additional fiberoptic bundle, the image guide, extends from the control head to the distal tip. Wire cables, which allow the tip to be flexed, run through the insertion tube. Any damage to either the umbilical cable or the insertion tube can potentially damage any of the internal structures. Care must be taken during cleaning procedures to ensure that the umbilical cable and insertion tube do not become kinked or acutely bent. Kinks in biopsy channels trap debris and lead to failure of the cleaning process. Suspected damage should be referred to the supplier for assessment and repair. A negative leakage test does *NOT* preclude damage to internal endoscope structures.

Special internal features. Most duodenoscopes have an additional channel—the forceps elevator (raiser) which is extremely fine (capacity 1–2 ml) and requires scrupulous attention during the cleaning process. Cleaning adaptors for this channel are provided with each duodenoscope.

Therapeutic endoscopes often have a second biopsy/suction channel which is usually different in diameter to the other suction channel. There may be a connection between the two channels at the access point for accessory items. Each channel and any connecting section needs to be specifically and independently brushed and flushed during cleaning, irrespective of its use during the procedure.

Some colonoscopes have a carbon dioxide (CO_2) channel that may be connected to the air channel. Cleaning protocols must include flushing of this channel.

Jet (washing) channels are found in many endoscopes. These are contaminated during procedures and must be independently flushed during cleaning, whether or not they have been used.

Cleaning equipment

All endoscopes are supplied with appropriate cleaning adaptors. It is vital that persons cleaning endoscopes are conversant with these adaptors and use them correctly. Serious clinical infections and epidemics of pseudoinfection have been associated with incorrect adaptors and worn adaptors. Rubber 'O' rings on the adaptors must be inspected regularly for defects or looseness and should be replaced as required.

Cleaning brushes for both channels and valve ports are also supplied. These have a limited life. They should be inspected regularly and replaced when worn or kinked. Metal wear from abrasion by cleaning brushes and other endoscope accessories may occur on the edge of the biopsy valve port or the suction button port. Alternative items for removal of material from the channels have recently been developed. These include flexible bladed cleaning devices which are designed to be used by a single passage pull through the lumen. An enzyme impregnated sponge affixed to a plastic stem has also been developed.

Soft toothbrushes are useful to clean grooved control handles and to brush the distal tip and biopsy ports. Cotton buds may be used to clean biopsy valve caps but should not be used in the air/water port as threads can become caught and cause blocked channels.

Adequate supplies of disposable cloths or swabs should be available.

Cleaning fluids

The desirable properties of detergents include loosening of particulate and other soil and microorganisms so that they are removed by the flushing process. Enzyme products promote protein lysis and enhance the efficacy of brushing and flushing and are the preferred detergent [63]. Where an enzyme product is not immediately available, a neutral instrument detergent can be used. Household detergent is NOT suitable. Cleaning products specifically for removing biofilms from instruments have also been developed [64].

Manufacturers of enzymatic solutions report optimum efficacy when used in warm water. However, enzymes will continue to be active in water that has cooled to room temperature (20°C). The use of hot water (>60°C) denatures proteins, inactivating the enzyme, and may fix both the enzyme from the detergent and any protein soil onto the instrument. *Heavy contamination may exceed the enzyme capacity.* Enzymatic detergents must be diluted and used exactly according to manufacturers instructions [65].

Rinsing

Rinsing should take place under running water so that all traces of detergent and disinfectant are flushed away. Failure to adequately rinse glutaraldehyde from endoscopes has been reported to cause severe post colonoscopy colitis and may be responsible for some cases of post ERCP pancreatitis. Ortho-phthaldehyde [OPA] can cause marked skin staining in both patients and staff if not thoroughly rinsed off equipment. In more severe cases blistering and skin necroses have occured. Static rinsing, i.e. rinsing in bowls of water, is not recommended.

The amount of water required to thoroughly rinse an endoscope after disinfection will vary according to the design and length of the instrument and the chemical used for disinfection. Manufacturers' instructions for volume of rinse water should be followed. See also 'Problem areas—rinsing water', p. 156.

Disinfectants

Disinfectants for endoscope reprocessing need to have wide bacteriocidal properties, together with the ability to kill relevant viruses including HIV, HBV, and HCV. Testing should have been conducted under clinical operating conditions as well as under laboratory conditions. Many disinfectants have either a restricted spectrum of activity or have not been adequately tested.

Worldwide, glutaraldehyde is the most frequently used chemical disinfectant for use in unsealed systems. The most common formulation used is 2% activated alkaline glutaraldehyde. Other products used include mildly acidic glutaraldehyde, peracetic acid, hydrogen peroxide, chlorine dioxide, and ortho-phthalaldehyde (OPA). A safety alert has been distributed advising against use of OPA for cystoscopes used on patients with bladder cancer as anaphylaxis as occurred with repeated exposure.

Soaking time. Effective manual cleaning of the item to be soaked is critical in determining the effectiveness of chemical disinfection.

Endoscopes which are not adequately cleaned will not be adequately disinfected even with prolonged soaking times.

Chemical manufacturers are legally required to indicate disinfectant contact times on the product label. Some professional organizations have published guidelines which recommend a shorter soaking time. Those recommendations are based on evidence that significantly less time is needed if the instrument has first been manually cleaned. Soaking times of 10–45 min for 2% alkaline glutaraldehyde are common.

Other issues which effect soaking time include temperature and concentration of the disinfectant for example, high level disinfection using acidic glutaraldehyde is achieved with a contact time of 10 minutes when used at 35 degrees Celsius. Automatic flexible endoscope reprocessors also use elevated temperatures.

Staff required to chemically disinfect endoscopes must be provided with education in the safe use of hazardous chemicals, and with personal protective clothing which includes impervious gowns (or gowns and plastic aprons), gloves which have been approved for use with the specific chemical, and face shields.

General maintenance

Leak testing of endoscopes should be performed after use as per manufacturers' instructions. Failure to detect a leak prior to thorough cleaning and disinfection may result in major damage to the instrument or transmission of infection [9].

Examination of the instrument lens and outer sheath should be performed following each session to detect any signs of cracking or damage. The function of angulation cables should be checked.

Inspection of 'O' rings on valves for signs of wear should be performed at the end of each session. 'O' rings should be changed when signs of wear are detected. Biopsy caps should be checked for signs of wear and replaced as required.

Lubrication

Lubrication is used to ensure optimal functioning of both endoscopes and accessories. The 'O' rings on suction and air/water control buttons require lubrication to prevent the buttons sticking in the depressed position. Traditionally silicone oil supplied with the endoscope has been used. Silicone oils can be either petroleum based or in a water soluble base. There is evidence that both preparations may impair reprocessing. Biological fluid can be entrapped within oil globules and protected from disinfectant action. The choice is therefore to either take particular pains to ensure complete removal of silicone based lubricants or to use surgical instrument lubricant.

Recommendations

• Accessory items processed in ultrasonic cleaners should be lubricated with an instrument lubricant following completion of the ultrasonic cleaning. They should then be wiped with a clean, lint-free cloth and allowed to air dry prior to packaging for steam sterilization.
• Where silicone oil lubricants are used for suction and air/water control buttons, they should be applied immediately before use (*after* chemical disinfection). It is essential to remove lubricant residue to allow germicide contact. Ultrasonic cleaning will remove any small amounts of lubricant that remain following manual cleaning.

Work areas

Endoscopy should not be performed in centers where adequate facilities for cleaning and disinfection are not available. Instrument reprocessing should be performed in an area separate to the procedure room. Work flow should be from dirty to clean and endoscopes prepared ready for use should be stored separately to those awaiting processing. Recently designed large units have incorporated a total separation of dirty and clean sections within the reprocessing area, with pass through facilities reinforcing the one-way flow.

Chemical disinfection must take place in an area with adequate physical controls such as forced air extraction. Soaking bowls must have close fitting occlusive lids. Forced air extraction should extend to the rinsing sink.

Work areas should be planned carefully. The areas should be well ventilated and the reprocessing area should include the following:
• At least one sink designated for the cleaning of instruments, referred to as the 'dirty' sink. This should be made of materials which are impervious to chemicals. Suitable materials include stainless steel, porcelain, or a plastic bonded material. The sink must be of sufficient dimensions to adequately hold a coiled full-length colonoscope without causing the instrument damage. The sink should be supplied with hot and cold running water.
• An area adjacent to this sink where the components of the instrument are removed for cleaning. The 'dirty' bench is then suitable for holding instruments awaiting chemical disinfection.
• An area for disinfection of instruments. In the case of automated disinfectors the dimensions and requirements are determined by the make and model of the machine to be installed. For manual disinfection, a chemical container of sufficient dimensions to hold an instrument without damage to the instrument is required. It is preferable that this container be a fixed sink placed under an appropriate fume extraction system. Otherwise a container especially designed for chemical disinfection of instruments should be available. This must be placed in a fume extraction cupboard.

• Where an automated disinfector is used, rinsing is performed within the machine. Where manual rinsing occurs, a sink designated for rinsing only clean instruments must be available and located within the fume extraction cover.

Reprocessing regimens

Disinfect before and after procedures

Bacteria proliferate rapidly in water. Bacteria may contaminate endoscopes following the disinfection cycle. This contamination may be from unsterile rinsing water including water in AFERS claimed to be bacteria free. Contamination can also occur from the environment. Damaged internal channels may have minute numbers of bacteria remaining after chemical disinfection. A dry environment will prevent proliferation of contaminating bacteria. Conversely a wet environment will result in rapid proliferation to a level where clinical infection during instrument use can occur. Some existing guidelines recommend reprocessing endoscopes before use on the day of use. It would seem that with current drying procedures, gastroscopes and colonoscopes are safe to use within 24 hours post disinfection. Storage cabinets which incorporate heated filtered air perfusing through the channels have been shown to greatly extend the time before repeat disinfection is required. The clinical risk of infection in ERCP, bronchoscopy and cystoscopy from even low levels of contamination is such that instruments used in these procedures should continue to be processed immediately prior to use.

At the end of a list, using 70% isopropyl alcohol to enhance the drying process, the endoscope must be thoroughly forced air dried prior to storage. Methylated spirits is NOT suitable for this process. Drying of endoscopes with alcohol between each use has also been advocated [66–68] but is not widely practised. The current British Society of Gastroenterology guidelines no longer recommend the use of alcohol for drying due to concern about fixation of prion protein matter by the alcohol. They instead require all endoscopes to be reprocessed within 3 hours prior to use to alleviate the risk of microbial proliferation of water borne organisms in the channels. This requirement has prompted the development of cabinets which extend the storage time.

Manual cleaning

The following steps should be performed immediately following a procedure.
1 IMMEDIATELY after each procedure, with the endoscope still attached to the light source, grasp the control head. Using a disposable cloth soaked in detergent solution, wipe the insertion tube from the control head to the distal tip. Discard cloth.

2   Place distal tip in detergent solution. Aspirate through suction channel—depress and release suction button rapidly to promote debris dislodgement.

3   Depress and release the air/water button several times to flush water channel. Occlude the air button to force air through the air channel.

4   Some types of endoscope have an air/water channel cleaning button that should be placed in the air/water valve seat at this point as per manufacturer's instructions to flush both the air and water channels. If there is no such adaptor, remove the water bottle connector from the endoscope, taking care not to contaminate its end. Drain the water channel by occluding the water inlet on the endoscope light guide plug or by positioning of the control lever on the water bottle cap (if present). The endoscope should be removed from the light source, the waterproof cap should be placed over the electrical pins on the light guide plug, and the endoscope taken to the cleaning area. (If, due to local circumstances, there is a delay prior to thorough cleaning, perform the leak test then place the endoscope in a bowl of enzyme solution and soak. However, full processing should occur as soon as possible to avoid microbial proliferation in the cleaning fluid) It is essential that the endoscope is not allowed to dry prior to cleaning as this will allow organic material to dry, making removal from channels difficult or impossible.

5   Remove all valves and control buttons. Leak test the instrument as per manufacturer's instructions. WARNING: It is essential that manufacturer's instructions be followed.

6   Brush and clean valves and buttons, paying particular attention to internal surfaces. Place buttons in an ultrasonic cleaner.

7   Place endoscope in enzymatic/detergent solution and, using appropriate brushes provided by the manufacturer, brush the suction/biopsy channel and the air/water channels if design permits. Particular attention needs to be given to ensuring that all sections of the channels have been accessed. If the brush contains obvious debris it should be cleaned before being withdrawn. Each channel should be brushed until all visible debris is removed. Wash all outer surfaces.

8   Using a soft toothbrush, gently clean the distal tip of the endoscope.

9   Brush control handles and biopsy port. Brush around valve seats.

10   Clean valve seats thoroughly—check that all visible debris has been removed. Use special brushes if provided by manufacturer.

11   Fit cleaning adaptors. Thoroughly flush all channels with enzymatic solution, ensuring all air is removed from channels. Allow solution to remain in contact for time required for the specific product.

12   Rinse outer surfaces. Flush all channels thoroughly with fresh water. It is essential that all detergent be removed prior to disinfection.

13   Purge channels with air to remove rinsing water.

14   Disinfect as follows or machine reprocess as per specific machine instructions.

Manual disinfection

1   After manual cleaning immerse endoscope in disinfectant so that the entire endoscope is submerged. Fill all channels with disinfectant so that all air bubbles are expelled. All channel entrances must be under the surface of the disinfectant during this procedure to ensure that no air enters the channel. Remove the buttons from the ultrasound, rinse, dry, and then immerse buttons and valves in disinfectant or autoclave if applicable. It is preferable to have extra supplies of buttons and valves to ensure that adequate cleaning is performed prior to immersion in disinfectant.
2   Soak instrument for required time in disinfectant of choice. A timer with an alarm is essential to ensure that accurate soak times are achieved. Digital timers are more accurate. A fluid thermometer with digital readout is recommended to constantly monitor temperature of disinfectant solution.
3   Purge disinfectant from all channels with air and remove endoscope, valves, and buttons from disinfectant, taking care to avoid drips and splashes.
4   Rinse exterior of endoscope thoroughly and flush channels with fresh water to remove all traces of chemical. Rinse all valves and buttons thoroughly.
5   Purge all rinsing water from channels.
6   If the instrument is being prepared for reuse, remove the cleaning adaptors. Dry exterior surfaces with a soft cloth, lubricate 'O' rings on buttons, and reassemble endoscope.
If the instrument is to be stored do not remove cleaning adaptors and continue as follows.

At the end of the list

1   Flush all channels with 70% isopropyl alcohol (approximately 2 ml for elevator channels, approximately 20 ml for each other channel). If using a multichannel cleaning adaptor the quantities of alcohol may need to be increased [55].
2   Force air dry all channels. Ensure that the air source has a flow regulator and use lower pressure on fine channels. Use bayonet fittings rather than luer-lock to attach the air tubing to the cleaning adaptors and fit securely but not tightly—if safe pressure is exceeded the bayonet fitting will give way. Use of excessive air pressure may cause damage to the instrument [55].
3   Ensure that all outer surfaces are dry.
4   Check the instrument for any sheath or lens damage. Polish the lens with the cleaner provided by the manufacturer. DO NOT REASSEMBLE ENDOSCOPE.
5   Store endoscope (disassembled) in a well-ventilated storage cupboard, which permits full length hanging on appropriate support structures. Endoscopes

should not be stored in transport cases as these may themselves become contaminated.

6   Store buttons and valves separately (not attached to endoscopes). 'O' rings on buttons and valves should only be lubricated following disinfection prior to use.

Endoscopic accessory equipment

The cleaning and disinfection of reusable endoscopic accessories is equally as important as that of the endoscope. Endoscopic accessories have been implicated in the transmission of infection. As with endoscopes, the cleaning of accessories as a prerequisite to sterilization is mandatory [69].

Cleaning of accessories

1   All equipment should be immersed in enzymatic detergent immediately following use until cleaning can be performed.
2   The equipment should be dismantled as far as possible and all visible soiling removed.
3   Any spiral coil, hinged, or complex structured accessories should be placed in an ultrasonic cleaner and processed according to manufacturers' recommendations. The ultrasound should be used with the lid in place to avoid dispersal of aerosols generated as these may contain biological material.
4   Any fine bore cannula or tubing accessory items will require thorough flushing with enzymatic detergent. Other accessory items, depending on design, will require a combination of flushing and brushing to clean surfaces.
5   Following cleaning by either of these methods, accessory items should be thoroughly rinsed and dried prior to disinfection, autoclaving, or low temperature sterilization.

Disinfection

General accessory equipment used in gastroenterological procedures requires high-level disinfection. Accessories that enter sterile tissue or the vascular system must be sterile. This includes biopsy forceps, injection sclerotherapy needles, and all accessories used for ERCP. Where an alternative exists, all non-autoclavable reusable accessories should be phased out.

1   All autoclavable equipment must be cleaned thoroughly prior to sterilization process.
2   All non-autoclavable equipment should be immersed in disinfectant, ensuring all cavities are flushed with the fluid. The soaking time will depend on whether the accessory item will be required to enter sterile tissue.

Special accessory items

Sclerotherapy needles. Sclerotherapy needles are difficult to clean and repro-cess to a sterile state and may provide an occupational hazard. Therefore it is recommended that only single use sclerotherapy needles be used.

Water bottles and connectors. These accessory items should be autoclaved at the beginning and end of each session as they have been implicated in the trans-mission of infection. All non-autoclavable bottles and connectors should be replaced with those that are fully autoclavable.

Dilators. Dilators are likely to come in contact with tissue that has been abraded or otherwise damaged by the dilation process. They should ideally be sterilized. They must at least have undergone high-level disinfection immedi-ately before the session. Note the operative field will not be sterile as the patient's own microbiological flora will contaminate the area.

Problem areas in endoscope reprocessing

Rinsing water

Poor quality water

The endoscope may well become colonized with significant pathogens after appropriate cleaning and high-level disinfection if the rinsing water itself is con-taminated. *Pseudomonas* spp., atypical mycobacteria, *Legionella* spp., cryp-tosporidia, and a variety of other organisms are frequent contaminants of hospital tap water. The microbiological quality of water varies dramatically from country to country. Surprisingly it may vary widely even within the same city dependent upon a variety of local factors. Municipal water quality varies with the age and condition of water mains. Local hospital factors will include the age and extent of plumbing alterations. 'Dead runs' are particularly import-ant. A temperature of at least 55°C at the point of use is necessary to minimize the growth of organisms in the hot water supply. Contaminants other than microbiological agents may also affect the quality of delivered water. High sediment levels may block filters quickly.

Infections from rinsing water

Organisms introduced into the endoscope by the rinsing water may colonize the instrument and be transferred to patients subsequently examined with the endoscope. The greatest clinical risk has proved to be the transfer of pseudomonas to patients at the time of ERCP. However, many organisms found in the water supply may pose significant clinical hazards to immunocompromised patients. The problem of contamination of AFERs is considered in more detail in that section.

Bacteria free water

Atypical mycobacterial contamination of bronchoscopes has caused epidemics of pseudo-infection with significant clinical consequences to patients [11]. Bronchoscopes and duodenoscopes should therefore be rinsed in bacteria free water. This may be prohibitively expensive for gastroscopes and colonoscopes but substantially bacteria-free water should be used. Unfortunately this is more difficult to achieve than first appears [70–75]. Adequate water filtration is both technically challenging and expensive. A filter bank (usually four) of decreasing mesh size down to a final filter of 0.2 microns is required. There must be a mechanism whereby the filters can be treated to remove microbiological contamination. The way in which this can be achieved will depend on a variety of circumstances including the particular filters, the available water pressure, and the quality of the water both in terms of sediment and microbiological content. In general it is best to have a closed loop arrangement with shut off valves on the input and output side of the filters. Access ports on the filter side of these shut off valves allow circulation of sterilants through the filter bank (note some filters will be damaged by reverse circulation). Agents used to treat the filter bank have included hot water, chlorine releasing agents, and glutaraldehyde. It is important to ensure that the agent used is compatible with the particular filters. Filters should be changed regularly and sent for microbiological examination at the time of replacement when there are problems of machine filter contamination or known high contamination levels of the hospital water supply. It is important not to assume that 0.2 micron filters will be failsafe. Excessive water pressure, excess sediment, gross bacteriological contamination, etc., may all result in bacteria translocating through filter defects. Hospitals with high quality water may not have any problems. Others, presumably with lesser water quality, have reported almost insurmountable difficulties requiring overnight sterilization of filters on a daily basis together with frequent filter replacement.

Water testing

The bacteriological quality of the rinse water available should be tested [73]. Microbiological monitoring should be undertaken in liaison with the local microbiology laboratory. The tap mouth should be flamed to eliminate surface gram negatives (although these in themselves may constitute a significant finding) and a minimum of a litre of tap water collected. Bacteriological quality of tap water should be monitored at least yearly and after any known plumbing alterations at the hospital or unit. More frequent sampling may be appropriate where the tap water has previously been found to be contaminated, where the institution has old plumbing, and in hotter climates.

Recommendations for rinsing water

- Duodenoscopes and bronchoscopes must *always* use sterile or 0.2 micron filtered water for rinsing.
- The bacteriological quality of the unit tap water should be monitored.
- Bacteriological filtering with 0.2 micron final filters is recommended for rinsing when poor water quality exists.
- Filter banks must be serviced and bacteriologically monitored on a regular basis.
- *ALL* endoscopes should have a final alcohol rinse followed by forced air drying at the end of procedure lists.
- Particular problems of AFERs are considered separately.

Variation in cleaning and disinfection regimens depending upon the supposed infective status of the patient

A number of surveys have shown that the practice of varying the cleaning and disinfection regimen according to the supposed infective status of the patient is widespread, with hospitals changing their reprocessing techniques after use in patients with known HIV infection, tuberculosis, or hepatitis [76–79]. There is clear evidence to show that the cleaning and disinfection schedule recommended in this review is adequate to prevent the transmission of infectious disorders including HIV infection, hepatitis, and tuberculosis [9,10,23,24]. There is therefore NO JUSTIFICATION to alter the cleaning and disinfection regimen if patients are known to have these disorders. (The problems associated with prion disease are considered separately)

Compliance with cleaning and disinfection protocols

Investigation of clinical infections related to endoscopic procedures has almost invariably shown that there has been a breach of recommended cleaning and disinfection protocol. In a few cases it has not been possible to determine the reason for the infection. In at least one incident (hepatitis C transmission) the suspicion has fallen on the anesthetic technique [32]. Practice surveys in the past have shown poor compliance with recommended protocols. Raymond [76] in 1990 found that 73% of all units surveyed in France had serious protocol deficiencies. A study in the United States in 1992 showed 40% of units surveyed had unsatisfactory aspects in their reprocessing protocols [77]. Even worse compliance has been reported from a variety of other countries. Fortunately there is evidence of a substantial improvement in recent years. Surveys in the United States in 1998 [78] and 1999 [79] showed major improvements though the World Congress of Gastroenterology survey in 2005 demonstrated deficiencies in practice still remain. Concerns also remain about accessory reprocessing with a small percentage of respondents reprocessing biopsy forceps and other critical items by glutaraldehyde disinfection rather than sterilization [80,81]. Other concerns include rinsing water quality, persisting variation in reprocessing regimens depending on the patient's perceived infective status, and reuse of disposable items.

The investigation of possible endoscopy infection transmission incidents

Investigation may be necessary because of internal recognition of an equipment or protocol failure. Alternatively, a complaint may be initiated by a patient or external agency.

Common causes

Common causes requiring incident investigation include:
• Self-recognition of protocol errors, e.g. failure to recognize and clean jet channels.
• Pump or other mechanical failure on AFERs without adequate alarm systems.
• Bacterial colonization of AFERs.
• Improper use of chemical disinfectants.

Golden rules for investigating potential infection incidents

The golden rules for any unit involved in investigation of a potential infection transmission incident are:
• Inform the appropriate authority immediately.
• Do not try to avoid investigation and do not undertake investigation of patient complaints yourself.
• Do not argue with or suggest alternative possible sources of infection transmission to complainants.
• Ensure that the information listed above is readily available to the investigating authority.
The appropriate regulatory authority should be notified of any incident. Authorities commonly allow in-house investigation of self-recognized low-risk

protocol failures. Investigation of patient complaints, and serious and potentially serious self-recognized incidents, must be conducted at arms length by an appropriate regulatory authority.

The investigation process

The exact process of investigation will depend upon the particular incident but in general the regulatory authority will:
• Inspect the premises to ensure that there is compliance with registration, licensing, and credentialing requirements.
• Ensure that medical and nursing staff are qualified and have acceptable continuing education processes.
• Ensure that endoscopic equipment, endoscope accessories, reprocessing, and safety equipment are appropriate.
• Ensure that internationally accepted endoscope and accessory reprocessing protocols are used [55–61] and protocol compliance is documented.
• Ensure that bacteriological surveillance programs exist.
• Identify involved and at risk patients, endoscopes, accessories, and reprocessing equipment.
• Examine anesthetic procedures.
• Contact affected and at risk patients for serological sampling (e.g. HIV, HCV, HBV) or other appropriate investigations (e.g. sputum samples if tuberculosis transmission is a possibility).

Transmission of viral disease

There is no current evidence that serious viral diseases such as HIV, HBV, or HCV have been transmitted from patient to patient by endoscopy if all aspects of internationally accepted endoscope reprocessing protocols have been followed [55–61].

Automatic flexible endoscope reprocessors (AFERs)

AFERs are widely used in the western world. American surveys in 1998 and 1999 showed around 70% utilization of AFERs [78,79]. These machines certainly reduce unpopular, arduous, repetitive tasks and reduce occupational exposure to irritant chemicals. Unfortunately AFERs have also been responsible for many serious clinical infections including deaths and epidemics of pseudo-infection [8,11,82–85]. The enthusiastic and largely uncritical acceptance of AFERs may owe more to their convenience than to clinical safety. There are numerous AFER models of widely varying quality, durability, and effectiveness.

Perceived advantages of AFERs include:

- Standardization of endoscopic reprocessing.
- Reduced exposure of staff to chemicals.
- Reduction of staff time spent on disinfection.

None of the currently available machines negate the need for thorough manual cleaning as an essential prerequisite to disinfection. Any claim that manual pre-cleaning is unnecessary should be carefully scrutinized and not accepted unless it has been published in respected peer reviewed journals. The US FDA in 2006 approved the marketing of a machine which is claimed to replace manual cleaning with machine processes. The American Society for Gastrointestinal Endoscopy (ASGE) subsequently published a statement urging caution in dispensing with the manual brushing and washing steps that are current practice until the capability of the machine have been confirmed in independent studies and clinical practice. Working parties are currently developing standards for AFERs under the European Committee for Standardization and the International Standards Organization. When completed, parts 1 and 4 of these documents will provide a reasonable international standard for machines.

Machine design and principles

Contamination

AFERs will rarely show contamination when new. Unfortunately this is when most AFERs are trialed. Problems with bacterial contamination rarely become apparent in machines before 6 months of use and become progressively more likely with ongoing use of machines and endoscopes. Increasing wear and age reveal unsuspected defects. Biofilms, valve failure, surface irregularities, fissuring, filter failures, and chemical familiarity all offer colonization opportunities for ever vigilant bacteria.

Water supply

Machines should be plumbed into the water supply rather than be filled manually. Pre-filters are necessary. Filter systems must be regularly serviced and monitored. It is all too easy for filters themselves to become a major source of contamination.

Alarm function

The principal function of AFERs is to pump liquids through endoscope channels. Alarm functions to detect pump failure on all channels are essential.

Self-sterilization

AFERs should have an effective self-sterilization cycle. Most AFERs claim to have one but manydo not stand up to rigorous scrutiny.

Fume containment

The extraction of disinfectant fumes from within the machine should occur prior to completion of the operating cycle and prior to opening the machine. If this is not possible the machine must be contained within a fume extraction hood.

Disinfectant supply

Machines which use a concentrated solution and in-use dilution for a single cycle (e.g. STERIS system) avoid the problem of dilution of the disinfectant with rinsing water. Machines which contain a tank of disinfectant for reuse should be monitored for disinfection concentration to determine appropriate disinfectant change schedules. Machines which require the filling of a disinfectant reservoir must incorporate a pump mechanism to obviate the need for pouring the chemical into the machine.

Reprocessing time

AFERs add significantly to endoscope reprocessing time.

AFERs cannot guarantee to sterilize endoscopes

AFERs cannot guarantee to sterilize endoscopes despite some manufacturers' claims to the contrary. Remember that, unless adequate cleaning has taken place, endoscopes will remain seriously contaminated and have caused serious clinical infections including death, despite being subjected to 'sterilizing processes' including ethylene oxide and peracetic acid exposure.

Cost

AFERs may increase reprocessing costs significantly. Real cost analysis should include the cost of purchase of the machines, extra endoscopes, machine service cost, and filtration costs. With poor quality water supply filtration costs can be extremely high.

Plumbing pathway

Plumbing pathway diagrams must be factual and not schematic. Careful evaluation of plumbing pathways is essential to determine if claimed self-sterilization cycles are to amount to anything more than wishful thinking.

Rinse and dry cycle

AFERs must have a terminal bacteria-free water rinse followed by 70% alcohol and air-drying cycle for use at the end of each list. If such a cycle is not part of the AFER's features it must be carried out manually prior to storage of each endoscope.

Regular bacteriological surveillance

Regular bacteriological surveillance of AFERs is essential. Specimens are usually best collected by pumping not less than 1 litre of water through filters placed in line at the point of endoscope connection and culturing the filters.

Quality control in endoscope reprocessing

Reliable quality control systems are an integral part of any manufacturing or service process. Clinical medicine has been slow to embrace adequate quality control systems and endoscope reprocessing protocols have been particularly deficient. Given the complexity of endoscope construction, the difficulty of ensuring adequate cleaning, and the relatively low safety margin of chemical disinfectants used, formal quality control measures are essential. Automated systems which reduce human error, together with automatic recording of essential parameters and alarm systems are highly desirable.

Unfortunately endoscope cleaning currently remains a manual process. Education and certification of those cleaning endoscopes therefore remains the most practical quality assurance process.

Disinfection, however, lends itself to automation and process monitoring. Regrettably the number of serious clinical infections associated with AFERs shows that current systems remain far from ideal.

Quality control measures

Quality control measures in endoscope reprocessing should include:
1   Appropriate education, examination, and certification of staff reprocessing endoscopes.
2   Proof of compliance with internationally accepted endoscope and accessory reprocessing protocols [55–61].
3   A record system which documents measurable reprocessing parameters. Where manual disinfection is employed this will include disinfection concentration, temperature, immersion time, etc.; for AFERs it will mean documentation of adequate cycle completion. It is essential that the unit has a clear system

which links the particular endoscope with the patient examined, the patient's position on the list, the endoscope cleaner, and the person and/or machine involved in disinfection. A clear and reliable linkage system is essential in investigating possible infection transmission incidents.

4   Accessories which breach sterile surfaces and are difficult to reprocess by a clearly validated sterilizing system should be single use only, e.g. sclerotherapy needles. Accessories which breach sterile surfaces but are not labeled for single use only and can be reprocessed by a validated reliable method such as steam sterilization need not be individually traceable. Accessories which breach sterile surfaces and are labeled 'for single use only' require an institutionally validated reprocessing protocol and must be individually traceable. In some countries, particularly the USA, institutionally validated reprocessing protocols will be extremely onerous [86].

5   A formal system for equipment servicing, maintenance, and replacement. This must include endoscopes and accessories, AFERs, ultrasonic cleaners, and water filtration systems.

6   A regular bacteriological surveillance program of endoscopes, AFERs, and water quality.

7   It is desirable that each unit has some outcome auditing process, which should include at least intermittent infection detection surveys.

Microbiological surveillance in endoscopy

Microbiological surveillance of endoscopes, hospital water supply, water filtration systems, and AFERs is strongly recommended. The area remains controversial because of sampling difficulties, lack of methodological validation, and difficulty interpreting culture results. These criticisms have a degree of validity and highlight the need for supporting methodological evidence. They do not, however, remove the need for bacteriological surveillance, which remains an important indirect validation of reprocessing protocols, provides evidence of internal endoscope damage which may be otherwise undetectable, and allows the early detection of colonization of filtration systems and AFERs [87–92].

Deva *et al.* [25] have shown that the absence of bacterial contamination is an accurate reflection of viral elimination during reprocessing. Thus viral cultures are not performed for surveillance purposes.

Duodenoscopes

There can be little serious argument against bacteriological surveillance of duodenoscopes. Serious clinical infections, usually with *Pseudomonas aeruginosa* or related species, occurred after ERCP in significant numbers in the past and continue to be reported. Endoscopists have frequently failed to recognize the endoscopic causation of these infections. As a result, errors in reprocessing protocols, internal endoscope damage, and colonization of AFERs have all failed early detection.

Bronchoscopes

Failure to detect AFER colonization with pseudomonas and atypical mycobacteria has led to a number of epidemics of infection and pseudo-infection in patients undergoing bronchoscopy [15–20,93].

Recommendations

- Hospital water supply: Endoscopy Unit water supply should be examined on at least a yearly basis, more frequently where there is evidence or recent plumbing alterations.
- Water filters: Water filters should be sent for microbiological examination when there are problems of machine filter contamination or known high contamination levels of the hospital water supply.
- Duodenoscopes and bronchoscopes: These should be monitored at least monthly.
- AFERs: AFERs should be monitored on a monthly basis or more frequently if there have been previous colonization problems.
- Gastroscopes and colonoscopes: These should be monitored 4-monthly depending on instrument age, previous positive culture results, or if other bacteriological surveillance (e.g. AFERs, water filters, etc.) has shown evidence of contamination.

Testing procedures

Assessment should focus on the acceptability of the total number of organisms detected. Detailed taxonomic identification is not indicated except where microbiological failure persists after a rigorous review of compliance with cleaning and disinfection protocols and the structural soundness of the endoscope involved. Cultures should be directed to the detection of common enteric or respiratory organisms and organisms which are known to be associated with AFERs and filter contamination. The most important pathogens include *Pseudomonas* spp., *Klebsiella* spp., *Proteus* spp., *E. coli*, *Salmonella* spp., and atypical *Mycobacterium* spp. Consultation with a clinical microbiologist familiar with the endemic hospital pathogens is essential. Samples should be collected in an aseptic manner. The exact technique may vary with individual microbiological laboratories. In general, the most important sample collection from endoscopes is to fill the biopsy channel with sterile water, and brush it vigorously with a sterile channel cleaning brush which should then be agitated in sterile water in a specimen container. After brush removal, flush some sterile water down the channel. Brushing is not possible for all channels of some endoscopes. It is essential to ensure that specimens reach the laboratory without delay following collection.

Interpretation of cultures

Workplace discussions reveal that one of the common but unvoiced reasons for resistance to bacteriological surveillance is the anxiety engendered by positive culture results. It has to be stressed that the finding of a few bacteria on bacteriological surveillance of an endoscope is not an infection transmission event and does not require patient infection detection protocols to be activated. It is essential to discuss positive culture findings with a clinical microbiologist and to look at the pattern of results from all endoscopes. Some interpretation examples include:

• A light growth of staphylococcus from a single instrument on a single occasion: This is almost certainly an environmental contaminant occurring during sample collection.

• *Any* growth of *Pseudomonas* spp. from a duodenoscope: This is cause for immediate withdrawal of that instrument. Full investigation of the possible source of contamination and activation of patient infection detection protocols for recent patients undergoing ERCP with that instrument.

• Light mixed growth of fecal organisms from different instruments over a period of time: Almost certainly reflects inadequate reprocessing procedures within the unit which need to be traced to either single or multiple staff members and corrective action taken.

• A heavy growth of salmonella from a colonoscope: Either inadequate reprocessing or internal instrument damage. The instrument should be withdrawn and carefully inspected by the manufacturer.

• Moderate growth of atypical mycobacteria from bronchoscope: Likely to be AFER or instrument accessory colonization. Clinicians should be notified that recently bronchoscoped patients may have specimens falsely interpreted as showing atypical mycobacterial infection.

• Growth of *Mycobacterium tuberculosis* from a bronchoscope: Immediate withdrawal of instrument. Full investigation of cause of contamination and activation of infection detection protocols for patients recently bronchoscoped with that instrument.

Microbiological surveillance of AFERs

The method of sample collection for automatic disinfectors will vary depending upon the design of the individual machine. It is therefore appropriate to seek advice from the manufacturer and/or consult with the hospital clinical microbiologist. Common sense would suggest that the most appropriate point for machine sampling is the attachment of the machine to the endoscope. For machines with a single point of attachment (e.g. Medivator) this is relatively simple. Where there are multiple endoscope connections the process becomes more complicated. It is essential to know the design of the machine to determine which is the optimum part of the cycle in which to collect samples. In most cases this will be in the rinsing cycle.

Early detection of machine contamination is best effected by a concentration process. A sterile sealed filter (e.g. Millipore filter) is connected to the outlet of the machine where it normally attaches to the endoscope and a minimum of 200 ml of fluid is cycled through the filter in the rinse cycle mode. The disc can then be removed and plated directly. Since the principal contaminants of automatic disinfectors are *Pseudomonas* and related species and various forms of atypical mycobacteria, cultures should be particularly directed towards these organisms.

Outstanding issues and future trends

Serious infections associated with endoscopy are almost invariably due to failure to follow recognized guidelines for endoscope reprocessing or prophylactic antibiotic administration. Even minor deviations from accepted cleaning protocols results in persistent microbiological contamination of endoscopes after attempted high-level disinfection or sterilization. Present reprocessing techniques therefore have a lower margin of safety than is desirable. In the short term the emphasis must be to ensure that all staff involved in endoscope reprocessing have been adequately trained and assessed. Quality control systems must be fully implemented, including microbiological surveillance of all endoscopes. Endoscopes and AFER manufacturers and distributors must develop more responsible attitudes. There is a growing concern that companies fail to disseminate information on real or potential product defects. Restricting product warnings to known purchasers of individual instruments is quite inadequate, not least because such devices may have been on-sold or transferred to other hospitals with health care networks.

Currently there is widespread lack of recognition of the difficulties in providing rinse water of adequate quality. More effective education about the problems of biofilms and filter difficulties is urgently required.

AFER design and function continue to rapidly improve. However, few if any current machines can claim to have adequate self-sterilization cycles which involve all necessary parts of the machine, individual flow alarms on all channels, and reliable sterile water for rinsing cycles. Manufacturers clearly have ample scope for further improvement. The AFER manufacturer who can develop a machine with the above qualities combined with an automated adequate and reliable cleaning system will have instant command of the market.

The inherent complexity of endoscope design, together with the clinical requirements for flexibility, are often inadequately understood. The aim must be to develop endoscopes and accessories whose sterility can be guaranteed. Despite claims to the contrary we are still a long way from this goal.

References

1 Favero MS, Bond WW. (1991) Chemical disinfection of medical and surgical materials, In: *Disinfection, Sterilization and Preservation*, 4th edn, (ed. Block, S. S.) pp. 617–41. Lea & Febiger, Philadelphia.
2 Favero MS. Sterility assurance: concepts for patient safety, In: *Disinfection, Sterilization and Antisepsis: Principles and Practices in Healthcare Facilities* 2001, (ed. W. A. Rutla). pp. 16–27. APIC, Washington.
3 Rutala WA. APIC guidelines for selection and use of disinfectants. *Am J Infect Control* 1996; 24: 313–42.
4 Bond WW. Overview infection control problems. *Gastroenterol Clin North Am* 2000; 10 (2): 199–213.
5 Webb SF, Vall-Spinosa A. Outbreak of *Serratia marcescens* associated with the flexible fiberbronchoscope. *Chest* 1975; 68: 703–8.
6 Nicholson G, Hudson RA, Chadwick MV, Gaya H. The efficacy of the disinfection of bronchoscopes contaminated in vitro with *Mycobacterium tuberculosis* and *Mycobacterium avium-intracellulare* in sputum: a comparison of Sactimed-I-Sinald and glutaraldehyde. *J Hosp Infect* 1995; 29: 257–64.
7 Beecham HJ, Cohen ML, Parkin WE. *Salmonella typhimurium*: transmission by fiberoptic upper gastrointestinal endoscopy. *JAMA* 1979; 241: 1013–15.
8 Wenzor RP, Edmond MB. Tuberculosis infection after bronchoscopy. *JAMA* 1997; 278 (13): 1111.
9 Ramsey AH. An outbreak of bronchoscopy-related *Mycobacterium tuberculosis* infection due to lack of bronchoscope leak testing. *Chest* 2002; 121: 976–81.
10 Hanson PJV, Chadwick MV, Gaya H, Collins JV. A study of glutaraldehyde disinfection of fibreoptic bronchoscopes experimentally contaminated with *Mycobacterium tuberculosis*. *J Hosp Infect* 1992; 22: 137–42.
11 Gubler JG, Salfinger M, von Graevenitz A. Pseudoepidemic of nontuberculosis mycobacteria due to a contaminated bronchoscope machine. *Chest* 1992; 101 (5): 1245–9.
12 Langenberg W, Rauws EA, Oudbier JH, Tytgat GN. Patient-to-patient transmission of *Campylobacter pylori* infection by fibreoptic gastro-duodenoscopy and biopsy. *J Infect Dis* 1990; 161: 507–11.
13 Classen DC, Jacobson JA, Burke JP, Jacobson JT, Scott Evans R. Serious pseudomonas infections associated with endoscopic retrograde cholangiopancreatography. *Am J Med* 1988; 84: 590–6.
14 Seigman-Igra Y, Isakov A, Inbar G, Cahaner J. *Pseudomonas aeruginosa* septicemia following endoscopic retrograde cholangiopancreatography with a contaminated endoscope. *Scand J Infect Dis* 1987; 19: 527–30.

15 Kovacs BJ, Aprecio R, Kettering JD *et al*. Efficacy of various disinfectants in killing a resistant strain of *Pseudomonas Aeruginosa* by comparing zones of inhibition: implications for endoscopic equipment reprocessing. *Am J Gastroenterol* 1998; 93: 2057–9.

16 Srinivasan A, Wolfenden LL, Song X, Mackie K, Hartsell T, Jones H *et al*. An outbreak of Pseudomonas aeruginosa infections associated with flexible bronchoscopes. *New Engl J Med* 2003; 348: 221–7.

17 Corne, P, Godreuil, S, Jena-Pierre, H, Jonquet, O, Campos, J, Jumas-Bilak, E, Parer, S, Marchandin, H. Unusual implication of biopsy forceps in outbreaks of Pseudomonas aeruginosa infections and pseudo-infections related to bronchoscopy. *J Hosp Infect* 2005; 61: 20–6.

18 Kirschke DJ, Jones TJ, Craig AS, Chu PS, Mayernick GG, Patel JA, Schaffner W. Pseudomonas aeruginosa and Serratia marcescens contamination associated with a manufacturing defect in bronchoscopes. *New Engl J Med* 2003; 348: 214–19.

19 Sorin M, Segal-Maurer S, Mariano N, *et al*. Nosocomial transmission of imipenem-resistant Pseudomonas aeruginosa following bronchoscopy associated wih improper connection to the Steris System 1 processor. *Infect Control Hosp Epidemiol* 2001; 22: 409–13.

20 Blanc DS, Parret T, Janin B, Raselli P, Francioli P. Nosocomial infections and pseudoinfections from contaminated bronchoscopes: two-year follow up using molecular markers. *Infect Control Hosp Epidemiol*. 1997; 18: 134–6.

21 Cetre JC, Nicolle MC, Salord H *et al*. Outbreaks of contaminated broncho-aveolar lavage related to intrinisically defective bronchoscopes. *J Hosp Infect* 2005; 61: 39–45.

22 Hanson PJV, Gor D, Jeffries DJ, Collins JV. Chemical inactivation of HIV on surfaces. *Br Med J* 1989; 298: 862–4.

23 Hanson PJV, Gor D, Clarke JR *et al*. Contamination of endoscopes used in AIDS patients. *Lancet* 1989; 2: 86–8.

24 Hanson PJV, Gor D, Jeffries DJ, Collins JV. Elimination of high titre HIV from fibreoptic endoscopes. *Gut* 1990; 31: 657–9.

25 Deva AK, Vickery K, Zou J, West RH, Harris JP, Cossart YE. Establishment of an in use testing method for evaluating disinfection of surgical instruments using duck Hepatitis B model. *J Hosp Infect* 1996; 33: 119–30.

26 Birnie GG, Quigley EM, Clements GB, Follet EAC, Watkinson G. Endoscopic transmission of hepatitis B virus. *Gut* 1983; 24: 171–4.

27 Lok ASF, Lai C-L, Hui W-M *et al*. Absence of transmission of hepatitis B by fibreoptic upper gastrointestinal endoscopy. *J Gastroenterol Hepatol* 1987; 2: 175–80.

28 Tennenbaum R, Colardelle P, Chochon M *et al*. Hepatite C apres cholangiographic retrograde. *Gastroenterol Clin Biol* 1993; 17: 763–4.

29 Bronowicki JP, Venard V, Botte C *et al*. Patient-to-patient transmission of Hepatitis C virus during colonoscopy. *New Engl J Med* 1997; 337 (4): 237–40.

30 Crenn P, Gigou M, Passeron J *et al*. Patient to patient transmission of Hepatitis C virus during gastroscopy on neuroleptanalgesia. *Gastroenterology* 1988; 114: 4, A1229.

31 Muscarella LF. Recommendations for preventing Hepatitis C virus infection: analyses of a Brooklyn endoscopy clinic outbreak. *Infect Control Hosp Epidemiol* 2001; 22 (11): 669.

32 Comstock RD, Mallonee S, Fox JL *et al*. A large nosocomial outbreak of hepatitis C and hepatitis B among patients receiving pain remediation treatments. *Infect Control Hosp Epidemiol* 2004; 25 (7): 576–83.

33 Brown P, Preece M, Brandel JP *et al*. Iatrogenic Creutzfeldt-Jakob disease at the millennium. *Neurology* 2000; 55: 1075–81.

34 Brown P, Gibbs C, Rodgers-Johnson P *et al*. Human spongiform encephalopathy: the National Institutes of Health series of 300 cases of experimentally transmitted disease. *Ann Neurol* 1994; 35: 513–29.

35 Rutala WA, Weber DJ. Creutzfeldt-Jakob disease: recommendations for disinfection and sterilization. *Healthcare Epidemiol CID* 2001; 32: 1348–56.

36 Bruce ME, Will RG, Ironside JW *et al*. Transmission to mice indicates that 'new variant' CJD is caused by the BSE agent. *Nature* 1997; 389: 498–501.

37 Bruce ME, McConnell I, Will RG, Ironside JW. Detection of variant Creutzfeldt-Jakob disease infectivity in extraneural tissues. *Lancet* 2001; 358 (9277): 208–9.

38 Wadsworth JD, Joiner S *et al.* Tissue distribution of protease resistant prion protein in variant Creutzfeldt-Jakob disease using a highly sensitive immunoblotting assay. *Lancet* 2001; 358 (9277): 171–80.

39 The National Creutzeldt-Jacob Disease Surveillance Unit. www.cjd.ed.ac.uk.

40 Endoscopy equipment guidance revised. www.healthstatejournal.com/story.

41 La Scolla B, Rolain JM, Maurin M, Raoult D. Can Whipple's disease be transmitted by gastroscopes? *Infect Control Hosp Epidemiol* 2003; 24(3): 191–4.

42 Stephenson PM, Dorrington L, Harris Od Rao A. Bacteremia following oesophageal dilation and oesophago-gastroscopy. *Aust N Z J Med* 1977; 7: 32–5.

43 Cohen FL, Koerner RS, Taub SJ. Solitary brain abscess following endoscopic injection sclerosis of oesophageal varices. *Gastrointest Endosc* 1985; 31: 331–3.

44 Tseng C-C, Green RM, Burke SK *et al.* Bacteremia after endoscopic band ligation of oesophageal varices. *Gastrointest Endosc* 1992; 38: 336.

45 Struelens MJ, Rost F, Deplano A *et al. Pseudomonas aeruginosa and Enterobacteriaceae* bacteremia after biliary endoscopy: an outbreak investigation using DNA macrorestriction analysis. *Am J Med* 1993; 95: 489.

46 Bass DH, Oliver S. Bornman PC. Pseudomonas septicemia after endoscopic retrograde cholangiopancreatography: an unresolved problem. *S Afr Med J* 1990; 77: 509.

47 Gossner L, Keymling J, Hahn EG, Ell C. Antibiotic prophylaxis in percutaneous endoscopic gastrostomy (PEG): a prospective randomised clinical trial. *Endoscopy* 1999; 31 (2): 119–24.

48 Dajani AS, Taubert KA, Wilson W *et al.* Prevention of bacterial endocarditis: recommendations by the American Heart Association. *Clin Infect Dis* 1997; 25 (6): 1448–58.

49 British Society of Gastrointestinal Endoscopy. Antibiotic prophylaxis in gastrointestinal endoscopy. A report by a Working Party for the BSG. (2001). *BSG Guidelines in Gastroenterology*, pp. 1–10.

50 Wilson W, Taubert KA, Gewitz M *et al.* Prevention of infective endocarditis. *Circulation* 2007 Apr 19; (Epub ahead of print).

51 Harris A, Chan ACH, Torres-Viera C *et al.* Meta-analysis of antibiotic prophylaxis in endoscopic retrograde cholangiopancreatography (ERCP). *Endoscopy* 1999; 31 (9): 718–24.

52 Zuhisdorf B, Martiny H. Intralaboratory reproducibility of the German test method of prEN ISO 15883-1 for determination of the cleaning efficacy of washer-disinfectors for flexible endoscopes. *J Hosp Infect* 2005; 59: 286–91.

53 Martiny H, Floss H, Zuhlsdorf B. The importance of cleaning for the overall results of processing endoscopes. *J Hosp Infect* 2004; 56(Suppl 2): S16–22.

54 Heeg P. Reprocessing endoscopes: national recommendations with a special emphasis on cleaning—the German perspective. *J Hosp Infect* 2004; 56(Suppl 2): S23–6.

55 Cowen AE, Jones D, Wardle E. (2003) *Infection Control in Endoscopy*, 2nd edn. Gastroenterological Society of Australia, Sydney.

56 Alvarado CJ, Reichelderfer M. APIC guideline for infection prevention and control in flexible endoscopy. *Am J Infect Control* 2000; 28: 138–55.

57 Guidelines for Decontamination of Equipment for Gastrointestinal Endoscopy. BSG Working Party Report 2003 (Updated 2005) The Report of a Working Party of the British Society of Gastroenterology Endoscopy Committee. www.bsg.org.uk

58 European Society of Gastrointestinal Endoscopy and European Society of Gastrointestinal Endoscopy Nurses and Associates. (2003) Technical Note on Cleaning and Disinfection Endoscopy. www.esge.com/downloads/pdfs/guidelines.

59 Nelson DB, Jarvis WR, Rutala WA *et al.* Multi-society guideline for reprocessing flexible gastrointestinal endoscopes. *Infect Control Hosp Epidemiol* 2003, 24(7): 532–7.

60 American Society for Testing and Materials (2000). *Standard Practice for Cleaning and Disinfection of Flexible Fibreoptic and Video Endoscopes Used in the Examination of the Hollow Viscera.* F1518-00. ASTM, West Conshohocken, PA.

61 Association of PeriOperative Registered Nurses. Recommended practices for cleaning and processing endoscopes and endoscope accessories. *AORN J* 2003, 77(2): 434–8, 441–2.

62 Obee PC, Griffith CJ, Cooper RA, Cooke RP, Bennion NE, Lewis M. Real-time monitoring in managing the decontamination of flexible gastrointestinal endoscopes. *Am J Infect Control* 2005; 33: 202–6.

63 Cheetham NWH, Berentsveig V. Relative efficacy and activity of medical instrument cleaning agents. *Aust Infect Control* 2002, 7 (3): 105–11.

64 Vickery K, Pajkos A, Cossart Y. Removal of biofilm from endoscopes: evaluation of detergents efficiency. *Am J Infect Control* 2004, 32 (3): 170–6.

65 Hutchisson B, LeBlanc C. The truth and consequences of enzymatic detergents. *Gastroenterol Nurs* 2005; 28: 372–6.

66 Muscarella L. Leading a horse to water: are crucial lessons in endoscopy and outbreak investigations being learned? *Infect Control Hosp Epidemiol* 2002, 23 (7): 358–60.

67 Muscarella, L. To dry or not to dry the endoscope? *Healthcare Purchasing News* 2003, 27 (10): 62–5.

68 Society of Gastroenterology Nurses and Associates. Frequently asked questions. *SGNA News* 2004, Jan-Feb: 7.

69 European Society of Gastrointestinal Endoscopy and European Society of Gastrointestinal Endoscopy Nurses and Associates. (1999)Protocols for Reprocessing Endoscopy Accessories. www.esge.com/downloads/pdfs/guidelines/reprocesingendoacc.pdf

70 Muscarella, L. Déjà vu … all over again? The importance of instrument drying. Letter to Editor. Custom Ultrasonics Inc, Ivyland, Pennsylvania. *Infect Control Hosp Epidemiol* 2000, 21 (10): 628–9.

71 Cooke RPD, Whymant-Morris A, Umasankar RS, Goddard SV. Bacteria-free water for automatic washer-disinfectors: an impossible dream? *J Hospital Infect* 1998; 39 (1): 63–5.

72 Working Party Report. Rinse water for heat labile endoscopy equipment. *J Hosp Infect* 2002; 51: 7–16.

73 Willis C. Bacteria-free endoscopy rinse water—a realistic aim? *Epidemiol Infect* 2006; 134: 279–84.

74 Pang J, Perry P, Ross A *et al*. Bacteria-free rinse water for endoscope disinfection. *Gastrointest Endosc* 2002; 56: 402–6.

75 Mackay WG, Leanord AT, Williams CL. Water, water everywhere nor a sterile drop to rinse your endoscope. *J Hosp Infect* 2002; 51: 256–61.

76 Raymond JM *et al*. Evaluation des procédures de décontamination utilisées dans les centres d'endoscopie digestive de Gironde. *Gastroenterol Clin Biol* 1990; 14: 134–9.

77 Reynolds CD, Rhinehart E, Dreyer P, Goldman DA. Variability in reprocessing policies and procedures for flexible fiberoptic endoscopes in Massachusetts hospitals. *Am J Infect Control* 1992; 20: 283–90.

78 Cheung RJ, Oritz D, DiMarino AJ Jr. GI endoscopic reprocessing practices in the United States. *Gastrointest Endosc* 1999; 50 (3): 362–8.

79 Muscarella LF. Current instrument reprocessing practices: results of a national survey. *Gastroenterol Nurs* 2001; 24 (5): 253–60.

80 Rateb G, Sabbagh L, Rainoldi J *et al*. Reprocessing of endoscopes: results of an OMED-OMGE survey. *The Canadian J Gastroenterol* www.pulsus.com/WCOG/abs/DR.1054

81 Moses FM, Lee JS. Current GI endoscope disinfection and QA practices. *Dig Dis Sci* 2004; 49: 1791–7.

82 Fraser VJ, Jones M, Murray PR *et al*. Contamination of flexible fiberoptic bronchoscopes with *Mycobacterium chelonae* linked to an automated bronchoscope disinfection machine. *Am Rev Respir Dis* 1992; 145: 853.

83 Nosocomial infection and pseudoinfection from contaminated endoscopes and bronchoscopes – Wisconsin and Missouri. *JAMA* 1991; 266: 2197.

84 Alvarado CJ, Stolz SM, Maki DC. Nosocomial infections from contaminated endoscopes: a flawed automated endoscope washer. An investigation using molecular epidemiology. *Am J Med* 1991; 91 (Suppl. 3B): 272S–280S.

85 Reichert M. Automatic washers/disinfectors for flexible endoscopes. *Infect Control Hosp Epidemiol* 1991; 12: 497–9.

86 Ulatowski TA. (2001) Re-use of single use devices. In: *Disinfection, Sterilization and Antisepsis: Principles and Practices in Healthcare Facilities*. (ed. W. A. Rutala). pp. 16–27 APIC, Washington.

87 Tunuguntla A, Sullivan MJ. Monitoring quality of flexible endoscope disinfection by microbiologic surveillance cultures. *Tenn Med* 2004; 97: 453–6.

88 Muscarella LF. Application of environmental sampling to flexible endoscope reprocessing: the importance of monitoring the rinse water. *Infect Control Hosp Epidemiol* 2002; 23: 285–9.

89 Nelson DB. Recent advances in epidemiology and prevention of gastrointestinal endoscopy related infections. *Curr Opin Infect Dis* 2005; 18: 326–30.

90 Standards New Zealand. (2002) *Microbiological Surveillance of Flexible Hollow Endoscopes* SNZ HB 8149:2001.

91 Merighi A. Quality improvement in gastrointestinal endoscopy: microbiologic surveillance of disinfection. *Gastrointest Endosc* 1996; 43: 457–62.

92 WGO-OMGE/OMED. (2006) Practice Guideline. Endoscope Disinfection. www.worldgastroenterology.org /global guidelines /guide14.

93 Srinivasan A, Wolfenden LL, Song X, Perl TM, Haponik EF. Bronchoscope reprocessing and infection prevention and control: bronchoscopy-specific guidelines are needed. *Chest* 2004; 125: 307–14.

CHAPTER 8

Risks, prevention, and management

PETER B. COTTON

Synopsis

This review emphasizes key issues for reducing the burden of risk inherently involved in all interventional procedures, and the need to ensure that patients are informed sufficiently to be able to participate in decisions about their care. Whilst each patient and each procedure may be unique, the principles of risk minimization and management are universal. Procedures must be done for appropriate indications, by well-trained endoscopists, assisted by expert staff, using the correct equipment. Known risk factors should be reviewed before-hand, and steps taken to accommodate them whenever necessary and possible. Patient consent exists only when there has been a meaningful educational process, adjusted appropriately to the individual patient and clinical situation. Unplanned events should be defined carefully and their occurrence monitored, so that standard methods for continuous quality improvement can be applied.

Introduction

Endoscopy ('looking inside') is invasive by definition, and therefore potentially hazardous. Therapeutic interventions add to the risk. The goal of everybody involved in an endoscopy procedure, not least the patient, is to maximize the benefits and to minimize the risks.

This contribution focuses on the potential risks of endoscopy in general. Specific risks of individual procedures (such as ERCP, and various therapeutic manoeuvres) are addressed in the relevant sections. However, the principles are the same. Endoscopists must understand the risks, the factors which affect them, the ways to reduce them, and how best to educate our patients about them. There have been many reviews of this topic [1–23].

The contract with the patient; informed consent

Endoscopy is normally conducted as part of a comprehensive evaluation by a gastroenterologist or by another digestive specialist. It is used mostly electively in the practice environment, or hospital outpatient clinic, but may sometimes be needed elsewhere (e.g. emergency room, intensive care unit). Sometimes, endoscopists offer an 'open access service' where the initial clinical assessment and continuing care is performed by another physician.

Responsibility

In all of these situations it is the responsibility of endoscopists to assure themselves that the potential benefits of the proposed procedure exceed the potential risks, and to convey that information clearly to their patients. Truly informed consent means that the patient really does understand the potential risks and benefits, as well as the possible limitations and any available alternative approaches [24]. That is our contract with the patient. Signing an 'informed consent form' is a medico-legal requirement in many institutions, but it is nothing more than confirmation of the education process.

Educational materials

Nothing can replace a detailed discussion between the endoscopist and the patient (and any accompanying persons), but this process can be enhanced with written, video-, or web-based educational materials. Suitable brochures are available from national organizations, and on many websites (e.g. www.ddc. musc.edu). They can be adapted for local conditions. Whatever the details of the education process, patients must be given the opportunity to ask questions of their endoscopist (and support staff) immediately before the procedure. The process of informed consent must be clearly documented, and preferably witnessed.

Humanity

It is appropriate here to emphasize also the importance of simple courtesies and common humanity in dealing with our customers. What is familiar and routine to the endoscopist and staff may be viewed by patients as a major ordeal—especially by those unfortunate enough to experience a significant adverse event.

What are 'risks' and 'complications'?

Definitions

Risks cannot be described, discussed, measured or monitored unless there is agreement about their definition. This has proved to be a challenge [25,26]. The word 'complication' has unfortunate medico-legal connotations. It suggests that something has 'gone wrong'. It seems preferable to use a more neutral term, like 'unplanned event', which simply indicates that the procedure has not gone completely 'according to plan', a subtle but important difference in emphasis. Some use the term 'adverse events' instead of complications. However, not all unplanned events are actually adverse; occasionally, things may go better than expected. The logic of using 'unplanned event' is that it ties directly in with the informed consent process. The truly informed patient knows what the plan is, and has specific expectations about what will happen before, during, and after the procedure, as well as the likely outcomes, both positive and negative.

Threshold for 'a complication'

Some unplanned events are relatively trivial, e.g. the need for sedation reversal during or after a procedure, or self-limited bleeding at the site of an endoscopic incision. These events should be adequately documented, so that the causes can be explored and quality improvement processes can be applied, but they are not significant enough clinically to be called complications. Mostly, patients are unaware of such events. However, there is a level of severity at which an 'unplanned event' does become clinically important, and where 'complication' is a legitimate descriptor. The question is where to place the threshold, i.e. at what level of severity does an unplanned event become a complication? We attempted to define that threshold in 1991 at a consensus conference discussing outcomes of ERCP [27]. We stated that 'a complication is an unplanned event, related to the procedure, that requires the patient to be admitted to hospital, or to stay in hospital longer than expected, or to undergo other unplanned interventions'. By this definition, we do not count in our statistics of 'complications' any deviation that occurs during a procedure but which is not obvious to the patient afterwards (e.g. transient bleeding), or one which can be treated on an outpatient basis (e.g. localized thrombophlebitis at an infusion site). This definition is not an attempt to hide such events, merely an effort to provide a common language. This is essential if we are to collect data, for, without data, we cannot study our outcomes or improve them.

Severity

A complication is an unplanned event that reaches a certain level of severity. But not all complications are of equal importance. They vary from relatively minor episodes (e.g. one day of pancreatitis after ERCP) to those which are life threatening (e.g. perforation). It seems reasonable to stratify the severity of complications by the extent of the disturbance which they cause to the patient. The consensus conference settled on the following stratification of severity:

- Mild; unplanned events requiring hospitalization of 1–3 days.
- Moderate; needing 4–9 days in hospital.
- Severe; more than 10 days in hospital, or needing surgery, or intensive care.
- Fatal; death attributable to the procedure.

Attribution

Use of the terms 'attributable' and 'related to the procedure' (in the earlier general definition) introduces a regrettable element of subjectivity, with the potential for reporting bias. That could be avoided by counting everything adverse that occurs within a certain period (say 30 days, as used to be the case after surgery). However, this would not be appropriate. No one would causally connect a simple diagnostic endoscopy with a myocardial infarction which occurred 29 days afterwards, in an elderly patient with known heart disease, especially if they had undergone multiple other medical interventions in the meantime. However, attribution would seem reasonable if the same event had occurred only two days after the endoscopy, especially if aspirin had been discontinued, or if the patient had experienced transient hypotension or hypoxia. Other issues with unplanned events and complications are whether they cause the procedure to be interrupted or aborted, and whether they leave any permanent sequelae.

Timing of unplanned events

Most unplanned events occur during or immediately after the procedures. However, they can happen even before the endoscope is introduced (e.g. a reaction to prophylactic antibiotics or other preparation), during the procedure (e.g. transient bradycardia or hypoxia), immediately afterwards (e.g. pain due to perforation), a few hours later (e.g. pancreatitis after ERCP), or can be delayed for several days or weeks (e.g. aspiration pneumonia or delayed bleeding). Some events (e.g. viral transmission) may be so far delayed that the connection is difficult to make, or is missed completely. Keeping track of unplanned events which occur after patients leave the procedure unit is a challenge. Making routine follow-up phone calls is time-consuming, and not completely reliable. Perhaps automatic, computer-generated phone calls or e-mail will be useful in the future.

Direct and indirect events

When considering complications, most endoscopists think first about the obviously related *direct* events (such as bleeding and perforation) that occur in organs which are being traversed or treated. However, there are also many *indirect* events, which occur outside the digestive tract. Cardiopulmonary complications (often related to sedation) are probably the commonest of the unplanned events. Renal, neurological, and musculoskeletal complications have all occurred. Indirect events are more likely to occur after the patient leaves the procedure unit, and are thus more often overlooked and under-reported.

Data set for unplanned events

A proposed data set for documentation of unplanned events, their consequences, and their severity is shown in Table 8.1 [28].

General issues of causation and management

The issues impacting each specific type of event are discussed in detail below. However, there are some general risk factors, and important points to be made about the recognition and management of unplanned events.

Unplanned events may occur because of:
- Poor technical or cognitive performance by the endoscopist or staff.
- Patients' 'fitness' or, really, 'unfitness'. This is a combination of, and interaction between the complexity/severity of the presenting complaint and the patients' comorbidities (including allergies).
- Non-compliance by patients and their helpers.

Technical and cognitive performance

The skill of the endoscopist (both clinical and technical) is probably the most important single factor determining the likelihood of unplanned events. As for certain surgeries, there is now good evidence that better-trained and more experienced endoscopists have higher success rates and fewer complications [29]. This raises the important and controversial issues of training, assessment of competence, report cards, recredentialing, and regionalization of specialist services [30]. However, endoscopists do not work on their own. Their specialist nursing and technical associates have much responsibility for many aspects of patient safety. The most important areas for them are the preparation of the patient, and the equipment, sedation, and monitoring of patients during and after the procedures.

Fitness for procedures

Defining a patient's 'fitness' for a procedure is a complex issue. Their 'unfitness', or degree of 'illness' is a combination of the presenting disease and any existing comorbidities (and their possible interactions, which are sometimes complex).

Table 8.1 Unplanned events

1 Nature
   Medication/sedation/anesthesia
   ☐ Allergic reaction (antibiotic; contrast-related; other ……………................)
   ☐ Hypoxia (transient; prolonged)
   ☐ Hypotension
   ☐ Hypertension
   ☐ Drug interaction (Details: …………………………………………….........)
   ☐ Neuropsychiatric reaction
   ☐ IV site problems
   ☐ Other (State: …………………………………………………...................)

   Direct GI events
   ☐ Endoscopic perforation
   ☐ Snare/diathermy perforation
   ☐ Dilator perforation
   ☐ Bleeding
   ☐ Infection
   ☐ Peritonitis
   ☐ Other (State: ……………………………………………………..........)
   ☐ Sphincterotomy perforation*
   ☐ Duct penetration/dissection*
   ☐ Hemobilia*
   ☐ Pancreatitis*
   ☐ Biliary infection*
   ☐ Cholecystitis*
   ☐ Pseudocyst infection*
   ☐ Basket impaction*

   * = ERCP only

   Indirect (non-GI) events
   ☐ Pulmonary (aspiration; pneumonia; wheezing)
   ☐ Cardiac (ischemia; dysrhythmia)
   ☐ Renal impairment
   ☐ Neurological
   ☐ Musculoskeletal
   ☐ Pregnancy-related
   ☐ Pain, cause unclear
   ☐ Fever, cause unclear
   ☐ Other (State: ………………………………………………………..)

   Equipment malfunction
   ☐ Endoscope
   ☐ Radiology equipment
   ☐ Accessories
   ☐ Diathermy
   ☐ Implanted devices

Continued p. 179

Table 8.1 (*cont'd*)

2 Timing (of onset)
- ☐ Preprocedure (from starting prep to entering endoscopy room)
- ☐ Procedure (in room)
- ☐ Early recovery (< 4 h)
- ☐ Late recovery (4–24 h)
- ☐ Delayed (1–30 days)
- ☐ Late (> 30 days)

3 Procedure
- ☐ Not started; Stopped prematurely; Completed

4 Changes in care plan
- ☐ None
- ☐ Extra consultation (Details: ....)
- ☐ Unplanned admission (....... days)
- ☐ Prolonged admission (....... days)
- ☐ ICU admission (....... days)

5 Treatment needed
- ☐ Medications (naloxone, flumazenil, atropine, oxygen)
- ☐ Transfusion (type, units ....)
- ☐ Ventilation assistance
- ☐ Intubation
- ☐ Emergency code called
- ☐ Endoscopy (Details: ....)
- ☐ Radiology intervention (Details: ....)
- ☐ Surgery (Details: ....)
- ☐ Other intervention (Details: ....)

6 Outcome
- ☐ Full recovery
- ☐ Permanent disability/loss of function (Details: ....)
- Death (Date .... ; Days after procedure ....)

7 Attribution (event related to endoscopy?)
- ☐ Yes; Probably; No; Uncertain

8 Detail of events:

....

....

As yet, there is no agreed and relatively simple score that can be used to compare the acuity of different patients and populations of patients undergoing endoscopic and related procedures.

ASA score

The American Society of Anaesthesiology grading system is well validated for operative procedures requiring anaesthesia [31]. It has some correlation with the cardiopulmonary responses to sedation during endoscopy, but other specific issues are more important.

Other risk indices

Many other risk indices are in use in other areas, e.g. APACHE, POSSUM, Charlson, but none measure the likely risk of endoscopic procedures [32–34]. Developing an overall (and procedure specific) risk score can be done only by collecting the data on large numbers of patients and procedures, and analysing the outcomes. This has been done in certain contexts, e.g. ERCP and sphincterotomy [28,35].

Prompt recognition and management

The keys to effective management of complications are early recognition and prompt focused action. Delay is dangerous both medically and legally [36]. Patients in pain and distress after procedures should always be examined carefully, and never simply 'reassured' without careful evaluation.

Communication

Poor communication is the basis for much unhappiness, and many lawsuits. Remember that the truly informed patient (and relatives) have been told already that complications can happen. This is an integral, important part of the consent process. So it is appropriate and correct to address suspected complications in that spirit. 'It looks as if we have a perforation here. We discussed that as a remote possibility beforehand, and I am sorry that it has occurred. Here is what I think we should do.'

Distress

Your distress is understandable and worthy, and it is important to be sympathetic, but equally important to be professional and matter of fact. Excessive apologies may give the impression that some avoidable mishap has occurred. Never, never, attempt to cover up the facts.

Document

Document what has happened and communicate widely, with the patient, interested relatives, referring physicians, supervisors, and your Risk Management advisors.

Act promptly

Get appropriate laboratory studies and radiographs, and consult other experts in the relevant fields, including a surgeon for anything that might remotely require surgical intervention. Sometimes it may be wise to offer to transfer the patient's care to a specialty colleague, or to a larger medical centre, but if this happens, try to keep in touch, and to show continuing interest and concern. Apparent abandonment alienates patients and their relatives, and may lead to initiation of legal action.

Specific unplanned events

Whilst cardiopulmonary events related to sedation are probably the commonest unplanned events, medico-legal claims arise more often from failure to diagnose and from perforation (and pancreatitis after ERCP) [37]. It is therefore smart to emphasize both of these risks in the informed consent process.

Failure to diagnose

Missing, or apparently missing, cancer and precursors is a particular risk in colonoscopy, but can occur in other organs [38]. Endoscopists have been faulted for failing to follow suspicious lesions (e.g. gastric ulcers), even when poor compliance of the patient has been the main issue.

Perforation

Perforation is the most feared complication of endoscopic procedures, because the consequences may be severe, and because its occurrence suggests (but does not prove) imperfect practice [39–43]. It can occur anywhere that endoscopes travel. It may be caused by the endoscope tip, or by pressure from the shaft in a tight loop, or by therapeutic dilatation or incision.

Risk factors. The risk of esophageal perforation is greater in the elderly, particularly in the presence of a Zenker's diverticulum. It is also markedly increased during esophageal dilatation, especially in patients with malignancy or achalasia [44]. Perforation of the stomach or duodenum is very unusual in patients without major focal pathology. Retroperitoneal perforation occurs after endoscopic sphincterotomy, particularly when the needle-knife or precut technique is used by inexperienced operators. Perforation of the afferent loop is a possibility during manipulations after Billroth II gastrectomy, and other surgical diversions. Colonic perforation is the most severe complication of colonoscopy. The risk may be increased by focal disease, such as diverticula or tumours.

Recognition. Early recognition of perforation is essential. The endoscopic view may leave no room for doubt. Pain and distress are the hallmark symptoms. Patients with esophageal perforation may develop subcutaneous emphysema. Perforation at colonoscopy is often associated with dramatic abdominal distension. Tachycardia is common. Steps should be taken immediately to clarify the situation. Plain radiographs usually are diagnostic, but CT scanning is more sensitive and should be carried out quickly if perforation is suspected and standard radiographs are negative or equivocal. The retroperitoneal nature of perforation after endoscopic sphincterotomy may delay recognition and has few specific signs. The patient may appear to have pancreatitis. Severe pain without impressive elevation of serum amylase or lipase is suggestive of perforation, and early CT scan is advised.

Treatment. Treatment of perforation is sometimes controversial. Careful assessment, review of the available literature, and surgical advice are essential. Whilst prompt surgical intervention might seem to be the obvious solution (especially to surgeons), it is not always necessary. Intra-abdominal perforations are almost always treated surgically, although a few selected cases have been managed conservatively, and by endoscopic clipping or sewing. Many esophageal and most sphincterotomy perforations have been treated conservatively (nil by mouth, intravenous fluids, antibiotics, and sometimes with targeted drainage tubes). Collaborative management with specialist (surgical) colleagues is strongly recommended whatever strategy is proposed, with frequent review —and much communication with the patient and anxious relatives.

Bleeding

Bleeding may occur due to endoscopic manipulations (e.g. biopsy, polypectomy, or sphincterotomy), or can arise during procedures from existing lesions (e.g. an ulcer with a visible vessel), or occasionally due to retching (Mallory Weiss tear). The risk of bleeding is a balance between the technique of the endoscopist, the specific clinical lesion carried by the patient, and by the coagulation status.

Risk factors. Patients with poor coagulation and/or portal hypertension are clearly at increased risk. Coagulopathy should be normalized or improved wherever possible, preferably to achieve coagulation parameters like those usually accepted for percutaneous liver biopsy. Anticoagulation should be stopped ahead of time, and (if clinically necessary) replaced temporarily by intravenous heparin for the procedure, and during the phase of early recovery. The use of antiplatelet drugs also increases the risk of bleeding, although the extent is difficult to determine [45]. There is little evidence to support the widely held belief that aspirin and non-steroidal anti-inflammatory drugs (NSAIDS) increase the risk, but many endoscopy units recommend that these agents be discontinued for five days or more before endoscopy (and for a week or so afterwards). It used to be common practice to measure coagulation parameters in all patients scheduled for therapeutic endoscopy. However, this practice is not supported by data, nor by the recent guidelines from the ASGE. A careful personal and family history of bleeding problems is more discriminating [46].

Endoscopic incisions (e.g. for polypectomy or sphincterotomy) should be performed in a controlled manner, to provide sufficient coagulation of local vessels. The addition of epinephrine to a 'saline cushion' may be helpful when resecting sessile polyps. Polyps with large stalks often have large vessels. The risk of bleeding may be reduced by injecting epinephrine or sclerosant into the stalk, or by deploying a detachable loop. The risk of inducing immediate or delayed bleeding from lesions which have themselves recently bled (e.g. ulcers or varices) depends on the size of the vessel and the pressure within it, and on the precise endoscopic technique. Endoscopic ultrasound and Doppler techniques have been used to detect significant submucosal vessels.

Recognition. Recognition of bleeding is usually obvious, during or after endoscopy. Occasional patients may present later only with anaemia. Delayed bleeding should not be attributed to the treated area without endoscopic confirmation.

Treatment. Most endoscopically induced bleeding can be treated by standard medical means, with repeat endoscopic assessment and treatment when bleeding is persistent or severe. Expert angiographic investigation and treatment has been used successfully. Surgery is needed very rarely.

Cardiopulmonary and sedation complications

Cardiopulmonary problems and adverse reactions to sedation are the commonest cause of significant unplanned events attributable to endoscopy [47–66].

The stress of the procedures (and the presence of the tube itself) may provoke dysrhythmias or induce hypotension or hypoxia, especially in patients with established cardiac or pulmonary disease, and in the morbidly obese. Aggressive sedation (with inadequate monitoring) can be disastrous. The cardiopulmonary status of potential patients should be assessed carefully (and improved if possible), and the approach to sedation/anaesthesia should be cautious and intelligent. A history of toleration of past procedures may be helpful. Some patients can accept simple endoscopy procedures without any sedation or analgesia. Others with significant comorbidities, and predictable airway difficulties, are best managed by anaesthesiologists. Endoscopists and staff should be fully trained in sedation, monitoring, and resuscitation, with ready access to all necessary equipment. Cardiological consultation may be appropriate in patients with unusual rhythms (or medications), pacemakers and implantable defibrillators.

Infection

Endocarditis. Endoscopy can provoke bacteremia, especially during therapeutic procedures such as dilatation. This may be dangerous in a very small number of patients who are immunocompromised, or who have important cardiovascular lesions. Endoscopy-induced endocarditis is extremely rare (and therefore difficult to study). Hard facts are scarce, and there is certainly room for disagreements in practice [67]. Guidelines concerning the use of antibiotic prophylaxis have been developed by many cardiological and endoscopic authorities [68–70]. Most recommend giving antibiotics to certain 'high risk' patients undergoing the higher risk procedures, but leave much leeway for individual judgement. The American Heart Association has recently concluded that administration of antibiotics solely to prevent endocarditis is not recommended for patients undergoing a gastrointestinal tract procedure [71]. This change of heart will no doubt be debated and eventually digested by GI organizations.

Infections. Infections can be transmitted in the endoscopy unit [72]. Outbreaks of salmonella, shigella, pseudomonas, hepatitis and other infections have been reported [73]. Such patient-to-patient transmission should be prevented by assiduous attention to cleaning and disinfection regimes, and appropriate management of accessories, tissues, and fluids. Patient-to-staff transmission (e.g. of *H. pylori*) has probably occurred, when staff protection precautions are inadequate. Transmission of tuberculosis, and of prion diseases, is a cause for concern [73,75]. Staff-to-patient transmission is theoretically possible. Prevention of infection in the endoscopy unit clearly requires a comprehensive approach, involving appropriate 'universal precautions', assiduous cleaning and disinfection practice, and continuous monitoring. Selective immunization of staff is relevant.

Instrumentation. Instrumentation can stir up dormant colonization, e.g. when contrast is injected under pressure into a contaminated biliary tree. The same is theoretically true when endoscopy manipulates other infected areas, such as a small peri-diverticular abscess.

Allergic reactions

Certain patients may react adversely to medications used during endoscopy procedures. Local anaesthetic agents, antibiotics, and iodine-containing contrast materials are most commonly cited. What to do about suspected iodine allergy before ERCP is controversial [76]. Some patients are allergic to latex rubber. Staff can become sensitized to gluteraldehyde. Obviously, a careful history of drug use and allergies is mandatory.

IV site issues

Blemishes and local phlebitis are common. Spreading infection is very rare.

Miscellaneous and rare events

There are many other theoretical and rare unplanned events. Patients may sustain injuries during sedation, by falling, or by pressure on nerves. Teeth have been damaged or lost, and more than one shoulder has been dislocated. Electrical injury can occur during diathermy, and there have been colonic explosions. Very rarely, endoscopes have become impacted, e.g. by retroversion up the esophagus, or have caused serious damage to adjacent structures, e.g. avulsion of the spleen.

Risk reduction and management

The responsibility for safety (and any unplanned event) falls ultimately on the endoscopist, and there are very important issues of training, competence, and credentialing. The recent emphasis on monitoring quality with defined metrics, report cards and benchmarking is a major step forward in protecting patients from inadequately trained practitioners [77,78]. However, it is equally clear that the professionalism of nurses and other staff is crucial. Electronic monitoring of some aspects is helpful, but the personal involvement of educated staff is even more so. Emergency equipment must be readily available. Endoscopists should be trained in advanced cardiac life support techniques.

Endoscopy can never be completely safe. Keeping unplanned events to a minimum should be of the highest priority for the endoscopy team, and for the patient. Understanding the risks and risk factors is fundamental. Careful pro-spective monitoring of defined events allows continuous quality improvement.

Studying the genesis of medico-legal complaints can help to minimise them [79,80]. Practicing within established standards of care, and ensuring good communications are key factors.

Outstanding issues and future trends

Reducing the burden of unplanned events in the future will involve progress in many different areas, including:

- Reducing the use of endoscopy for purely diagnostic purposes, using better patient selection (e.g. by genetic markers or fecal DNA testing), and alternative non-invasive methods (e.g. CT colonography).
- Refining methods for therapeutic endoscopy.
- Improving the training of endoscopists and support staff, with objective testing of competence for credentialing, and recredentialing.
- Continuous quality improvement, through structured documentation of outcomes, and appropriate feedback.
- Making endoscopes easier to clean and disinfect, even sterilize.
- Fostering patient empowerment, through meaningful education and the widespread use of report cards.

References

1 Arrowsmith JB, Gerstman BB, Fleische DE, Benjamin SR. Results from the American Society for Gastrointestinal Endoscopy/U.S. Food and Drug Administration collaborative study on complication rates and drug use during gastrointestinal endoscopy. *Gastrointest Endosc* 1991; 37 (4): 421–7.

2 Carey WD. (1987) Indications, contraindications, and complications of upper gastrointestinal endoscopy. In: *Gastrointestinal Endoscopy* (eds. MV Sivak). p. 301. W.B. Saunders, Philadelphia.

3 Chan MF. Complications of upper gastrointestinal endoscopy. *Gastrointest Endosc Clin N Am* 1996; 6 (2): 287–303.

4 Cooper GS, Blades EW. (2000) Indications, Contraindications, and Complications of Upper Gastrointestinal Endoscopy, in Gastroenterologic Endoscopy. In: *Gastrointestinal Endoscopy Vol 1* (eds. MV Sivak). pp. 438–54. W.B. Saunders, Philadelphia.

5 Delvaux M. The complications of digestive endoscopy. *Gastroenterol Clin Biol* 1995; 19: B23–32.

6 Eimiller A. Complication in endoscopy. *Endoscopy* 1992; 24 (1–2): 176–84.

7 Eisen GM, Baron TH, Dominitz JA, Faigel DO, Goldstein JL, Johanson JF *et al.* Complications in Upper GI Endoscopy. *Gastrointest Endosc* 2002; 55 (7): 784–93.

8 Freeman ML, Nelson DB, Sherman S, Haber GB, Herman ME, Dorsher PJ *et al.* Complications of endoscopic biliary sphincterotomy. *N Engl J Med* 1996; 335: 909–18.

9 Froehlich F, Gonvers JJ, Vader JP, Dubois RW, Burnand B. Appropriateness of gastrointestinal endoscopy: risk of complications. *Endoscopy* 1999; 31 (8): 684–6.

10 Hart R, Classen M. Complications of diagnostic gastrointestinal endoscopy. *Endoscopy* 1990; 22: 229–33.

11 Kavic SM, Basson MD. Complications of endoscopy. *Am J Surg* 2001; 181 (4): 319–32.

12 Keeffe EB. (1991) Endoscopic procedural safety. In: *Quality Control in Endoscopy* (ed. R. Mccloy) pp. 33–45. Springer-Verlag, Berlin.

13 Muhldorfer SM, Kekos G, Hahn G, Ell C. Complications of therapeutic gastrointestinal endoscopy. *Endoscopy* 1992; 24: 276–83.

14 Newcomer MK, Brazer SR. Complications of upper gastrointestinal endoscopy and their management. *Gastrointest Endosc Clin North Am* 1994; 4 (3): 551–70.

15 Quine MA, Bell GD, McCloy RF, Charlton JE, Devlin HB, Hopkins A. A prospective audit of upper gastrointestinal endoscopy in two regions of England: safety, staffing and sedation methods. *Gut* 1995; 36: 462–7.

16 Rankin GB, Sivak MV. (2000) Indications, contraindications, and complications of colonoscopy. In: *Gastroenterologic Endoscopy, Vol. 2* (eds. MV Sivak). pp. 1222–52. W. B. Saunders, Philadelphia.

17 Reiertsen O, Skjoto J, Jacobsen CD, Rosseland AR. Complications of fiberoptic gastrointestinal endoscopy—five years' experience in a central hospital. *Endoscopy* 1987; 19 (1): 1–6.

18 Rothbaum RJ. Complications of pediatric endoscopy. *Gastrointest Endosc Clin N Am* 1996; 6 (2): 445–59.

19 Schauer PR, Schwesinger WH, Page CP, Stewart RM, Levine BA, Sirinek KR. Complications of surgical endoscopy. A decade of experience from a surgical residency training program. *Surg Endosc* 1997; 11 (1): 8–11.

20 Schmitt CM. Procedure-specific outcomes assessment for esophagogastroduodenoscopy. *Gastrointest Endosc Clin N Am* 1999; 9 (4): 609–24, vi–vii.

21 Silvis SE, Nebel O, Rogers G, Sugawa C, Mandelstam P. Endoscopic complications. Results of the 1974 American Society for Gastrointestinal Endoscopy Survey. *JAMA* 1976; 235 (9): 928–30.

22 Taylor MB. (1992) Complications of upper endoscopy and colonoscopy. In: *Gastrointestinal Emergencies* (eds. MB Taylor). pp. 551–6. Williams & Wilkins, Baltimore.

23 Zubarik R, Eisen G, Mastropietro C, Lopez J, Carroll J, Benjamin S, Fleischer DE. Prospective analysis of complications 30 days after outpatient upper endoscopy. *Am J Gastroenterol* 1999; 94 (6): 1539–80.

24 Plumeri PA. Informed consent for upper gastrointestinal endoscopy. *Gastrointest Endosc Clin North Am* 1994; 4 (3): 455–62.

25 Cotton PB. Outcomes of endoscopy procedures: struggling towards definitions. *Gastrointest Endosc* 1994; 40: 514–18.

26 Fleischer DE. Better definition of endoscopic complications and other negative outcomes. *Gastrointest Endosc* 1994; 40: 511–14.

27 Cotton PB, Lehman G, Vennes J, Geenen JE *et al.* Endoscopic sphincterotomy complications and their management: an attempt at consensus. *Gastrointest Endosc* 1991; 37: 383–93.

28 Cotton PB. Income and outcome metrics for the objective evaluation of ERCP and alternative methods. *Gastrointest Endosc* 2002; 56 (6): S283–90.

29 Freeman ML. Training and competence in gastrointestinal endoscopy. *Rev Gastroenterol Disord* 2001; 1 (2): 73–86.

30 Cotton PB. How many times have you done this procedure, Doctor? *Am J Gastroenterol* 2002; 97: 522–3.

31 Keat AS. The ASA classification of physical status: a recapitulation. *Anesthesiology* 1978; 49: 233–7.

32 Knaus WA, Wagner DP, Draper EA, Zimmerman JE, Bergner M, Bastos PG *et al.* The APACHE III prognostic system: risk prediction of hospital mortality for critically ill hospitalized adults. *Chest* 1991; 100: 1619–36.

33 Charlson ME, Pompei P, Ales KL, Mackenzie CR. A new method of classifying prognostic comorbidity in longitudinal studies: development and validation. *J Chron Dis* 1987; 40: 373–83.

34 Prytherch DR, Whiteley MS, Higgins B, Weaver PC, Prout WG, Powell SJ. POSSUM and Portsmouth POSSUM for predicting mortality. *Br J Surg* 1998; 85: 1217–20.

35 Freeman ML, DiSario JA, Nelson DB, Fennerty MB, Lee JG, Bjorkman DJ *et al.* Risk factors for post-ERCP pancreatitis: a prospective, multicenter study. *Gastrointest Endosc* 2001; 54: 425–34.

36 American Society for Gastrointestinal Endoscopy ad hoc Risk Management Committee. (2001). *Risk management for the GI endoscopist.*

37 Gerstenberger PD, Plumeri PA. Malpractice claims in gastrointestinal endoscopy: analysis of an insurance industry data base. *Gastrointest Endosc* 1993; 39: 132–8.

38 Plumeri PA. The failure to diagnose colon cancer. A potential medical-legal disaster. *Gastrointest Endosc Clin North Am* 1993; 3 (4): 749–61.

39 Adamek HE, Jakobs R, Dorlars D, Martin WR, Kromer MU, Riemann JF. Management of esophageal perforations after therapeutic upper gastrointestinal endoscopy. *Scand J Gastroenterol* 1997; 32: 411–14.

40 Fernandez FF, Richter A, Freudenberg S, Wendt K, Manegold BC. Treatment of endoscopic esophageal perforation. *Surg Endosc* 1999; 13: 962–6.

41 Enns R, Branch MS. Management of esophageal perforation after therapeutic upper gastrointestinal endoscopy. *Gastrointest Endosc* 1998; 47 (3): 318–20.

42 Moghissi K. Instrumental perforations of the oesophagus. *Br J Hosp Med* 1988; 39 (3): 231–6.

43 Quine MA, Bell GD, McCloy RF, Matthews HR. Prospective audit of perforation rates following upper gastrointestinal endoscopy in two regions of England. *Br J Surg* 1995; 82: 530–3.

44 Clouse RE. Complications of endoscopic gastrointestinal dilation techniques. *Gastrointest Endosc Clin N Am* 1996; 6 (2): 323–41.

45 Miller AM, McGill D, Bassett ML. Anticoagulant therapy, anti-platelet agents and gastrointestinal endoscopy. *J Gastroenterol Hepatol* 1999; 14: 109–13.

46 Eisen GM, Baron TH, Dominitz JA, Faigel DO, Goldstein JL, Johanson JF *et al.* Guideline on the management of anticoagulation and antiplatelet therapy for endoscopic procedures. *Gastrointest Endosc* 2002; 55 (7): 775–9.

47 Lipper B, Simon D, Cerrone F. Pulmonary aspiration during emergency endoscopy in patients with upper gastrointestinal haemorrhage. *Crit Care Med* 1991; 19: 330–3.

48 Benjamin SB. Complications of conscious sedation. *Gastrointest Endosc Clin N Am* 1996; 6 (2): 277–86.

49 Daneshmend TK, Bell GD, Logan RFA. Sedation for upper gastrointestinal endoscopy: results of a nationwide survey. *Gut* 1991; 32: 12–15.

50 Eckardt VF, Kanzler G, Schmitt T, Eckardt AJ, Bernhard G. Complications and adverse effects of colonoscopy with selective sedation. *Gastrointest Endosc* 1999; 49 (5): 560–5.

51 Freeman ML. Sedation and monitoring for gastrointestinal endoscopy. *Gastrointest Endosc Clin N Am* 1994; 4 (3): 475–99.

52 Froehlich F, Gonvers JJ, Fried M. Conscious sedation, clinically relevant complications and monitoring of endoscopy: results of a nationwide survey in Switzerland. *Endoscopy* 1994; 26 (2): 231–4.

53 Holm C, Rosenberg J. Pulse oximetry and supplemental oxygen during gastrointestinal endoscopy: a critical review. *Endoscopy* 1996; 28 (8): 703–11.

54 Keeffe EB, O'Connor KW 1989 A/S/G/E survey of endoscopic sedation and monitoring practices. *Gastrointest Endosc* 1990; 36: S13–18.

55 Lazzaroni M, Porro GB. *Preparation, Premedication, Surveillance Endoscopy* 2001; 33 (2): 103–8.

56 McCloy R. (1997) Safety, sedation and emergencies in endoscopy. In: *Practical Endoscopy* (eds. M Shephard and J Mason). p. 139. Chapman & Hall, London.

57 American Society for Gastrointestinal Endoscopy. Sedation and monitoring of patients undergoing gastrointestinal endoscopic procedures. *Gastrointest Endosc* 1995; 42 (6): 626–9.

58 Sieg A, Hachmoeller-Eisenbach U, Heisenbach T. How safe is premedication in ambulatory endoscopy in Germany? A prospective study in gastroenterology specialty practices. *Dtsch Med Wochenschr* 2000; 125 (43): 1288–93.

59 The American Society for Gastrointestinal Endoscopy. Preparation of patients for gastrointestinal endoscopy. *Gastrointest Endosc* 1998; 48: 691–4.

60 Wong RC. The menu of endoscopic sedation: all-you-can-eat, combination set, a la carte, alternative cuisine, or go hungry. *Gastrointest Endosc* 2001; 54 (1): 122–6.

61 Zuccaro G Jr. Sedation and sedationless endoscopy. *Gastrointest Endosc Clin N Am* 2000; 10 (1): 1–20.

62 Banks MR, Kumar PJ, Mulcahy HE. Pulse oximetry saturation levels during routine unsedated diagnostic upper gastrointestinal endoscopy. *Scand J Gastroenterol* 2001; 36: 105–9.

63 Bell GD. Premedication, preparation and surveillance. *Endoscopy* 2000; 32: 92–100.

64 Bell GD, Jones JG. Routine use of pulse oximetry and supplemental oxygen during endoscopic procedures under conscious sedation: British beef or common sense? *Endoscopy* 1996; 28 (8): 718–21.

65 Charlton JE. Monitoring and supplemental oxygen during endoscopy. *Br Med J* 1995; 310: 886–7.

66 Sandlin D. Capnography for nonintubated patients: the wave of the future for routine monitoring of procedural sedation patients. *J Perianesth Nurs* 2002; 17 (4): 277–81.

67 Roduit J, Jornod P, Dorta N, Blum AL, Dorta G. Antibiotic prophylaxis of infective endocarditis during digestive endoscopy: over- and underuse in Switzerland despite professed adherence to guidelines. *Endoscopy* 2002; 34 (4): 322–4.

68 Antibiotic prophylaxis in gastrointestinal endoscopy. http://www.bsg.org.uk

69 Dajani AS, Taubert KA, Wilson W, Bolger AF, Bayer A, Ferrieri P *et al*. Prevention of bacterial endocarditis. Recommendations by the American Heart Association. *Circulation* 1997; 96: 358–66.

70 Antibiotic prophylaxis for gastrointestinal endoscopy. http://www.asge.org

71 Wilson W, Taubert KA, Gewitz M *et al*. Prevention of infective endocarditis. *Circulation* 2007 Apr 19; (Epub ahead of print).

72 Nelson DB. Infection control during gastrointestinal endoscopy. *J Laboratory Clin Med* 2003; 141: 159–67.

73 Ponchon T. Transmission of hepatitis C and prion diseases through digestive endoscopy: evaluation of risk and recommended practices. *Endoscopy* 1997; 29: 199–202.

74 Ramakrishna B. Safety of technology: infection control standards in endoscopy. *J Gastroenterol Hepatol* 2002; 17: 361–8.

75 Working Party for E/S/G/E. ESGE guidelines for the prevention of endoscopic transmission of type C hepatitis and update in Creutzfeldt–Jakob disease. *Endoscopy* 1997; 29: 203–4.

76 Draganov P, Cotton PB. Iodinated contrast sensitivity in ERCP. *Am J Gastroenterol* 2000; 95 (6): 1398–401.

77 Bjorkman DJ. Popp JW. Measuring the quality of endoscopy. *Am J Gastro* 2006: 101: 864–5 (and subsequent articles).

78 Cotton PB, Hawes RH, Barkun A *et al*. Excellence in endoscopy; toward practical metrics. *Gastrointest Endosc.* 2006 63 286–291.

79 Neale G. Reducing risks in gastroenterological practice. *Gut* 1998; 42 (1): 139–42.

80 Cotton PB. Learning from lawsuits. *Gastointest Endosc* 2006.

CHAPTER 9

Pathology

DAVID N. LEWIN

Synopsis

A gastroenterologist need not be an expert histopathologist or cytopathologist (hopefully they have one in their local pathology department); however, they should understand the importance of gastroenterologist–pathologist communication [1], specimen handling, and interpretation issues, and the relative efficacy of endoscopic sampling methods for a particular clinical situation. Attention to quality of endoscopic biopsy plays a crucial role in maximizing the effectiveness of this diagnostic technique.

Introduction

Histopathological and cytological examination of the gastrointestinal tract is reviewed. This chapter is not intended to be a comprehensive review of all gastrointestinal pathology; however, a number of general concepts are examined and the major gastrointestinal lesions are illustrated. The chapter has been divided into endoscopic biopsy specimens (histology), exfoliative and fine-needle aspiration specimens (cytology), and an overview of the major conditions in each organ system. Additionally, general comments pertaining to communication, special stains, and future trends are all presented.

Gastroenterologist–pathologist communication

Effective gastroenterologist–pathologist communication drives the ability to make accurate diagnoses. Communication can take many forms, from a written request to a verbal consultation. Communication clearly is a 'two-way street', with information communicated from the gastroenterologist to the pathologist and vice versa. There are two critical parts of this communication:
1 Communicating adequate, concise information.
2 Using a common terminology.

Endoscopist communication responsibility

The pathologist needs the typical important patient information, including relevant clinical history, bowel preparation (for colonic specimens), and current medications. Additionally, the endoscopist assumes the responsibility for two tasks normally completed by the pathologist in autopsy and 'traditional' surgical pathology: doing the gross examination, via the endoscope, and taking adequate representative samples. Thus the endoscopist needs to communicate the results of the gross (endoscopic) examination and where the biopsies were taken from. More information about each organ system will be discussed later.

Pathologist communication responsibility

The pathologist should provide feedback regarding the artefacts and adequacy of a specimen for interpretation. The pathologist must also resist the urge to find an abnormality, no matter how subtle, in every biopsy specimen.

Question-orientated approach

One method is to use a question-orientated approach. This will ensure that specific information is included in the pathology report and that the endoscopists receive the answers to the specific question for which they are performing the endoscopy. The clinician can provide simple focused questions for the pathologist to answer. For example, in a patient with long-standing ulcerative colitis undergoing surveillance colonoscopy, the primary question is whether or not there is dysplasia present and not to make a diagnosis of inflammatory bowel disease. The pathologist may agonize over trying to make a diagnosis of inflammatory bowel disease, and not address the question of dysplasia if not asked.

Common terminology

Probably the most crucial aspect of communication is using a common terminology, the implications of which are understood by all parties. While there have been a number of attempts to create standardized terminology for both endoscopy and pathology [2–4], these are not used universally. Terminology may be different in various parts of the United States and is clearly different between different countries [5]. For the endoscopist this means describing the endoscopic exam using simple, descriptive terms. Jargon should be avoided. For example, the term 'gastritis' can imply anything from colour changes to erosions. Endoscopic photographs of lesions for the pathologist can potentially help mitigate this problem. For the pathologist this means using accepted pathological diagnoses. Non-standard diagnoses should be avoided or at least explained with a comment. For example, in a study of inflammatory bowel disease [6] non-specific inflammation was used by various pathologists to mean the following:

1 Confident of IBD or irradiation colitis, but cannot discriminate.
2 Cannot discriminate between ulcerative colitis and Crohn's disease.
3 Probably Crohn's disease.
4 No histological evidence of inflammatory bowel disease.

Terms such as atypia need to be qualified, usually with a reassuring qualifier term such as 'reactive' or 'inflammatory', as for many clinicians this term is often synonymous with dysplasia, which is not typically true in the United States (however it is true in Japan [5]). Similar to endoscopic photographs, histologic images of pertinent findings on reports can be helpful adjuncts to the communication.

Endoscopic biopsy specimens

Endoscopic specimens comprise the majority of the pathology specimens received from gastroenterologists. Most are obtained with pinch biopsy forceps and contain mucosa (epithelium and the lamina propria) down to the muscularis mucosa. Endoscopic biopsy is a very good technique for diagnosing mucosal abnormalities; however, it is very poor for submucosal (and deeper) lesions [7]. Polypectomy and endoscopic mucosal resections will be discussed subsequently. There will be a brief overview of specimen handling and interpretation issues, followed by major conditions in each organ site.

Specimen handling and interpretation issues

The handling of the specimens, in the endoscopy suite and the pathology laboratory, plays a large role in the ability of the pathologist to render an accurate diagnosis. Some of the major issues: orientation of the specimen, fixation, number of biopsies per container, tissue processing, crush artifact, burn/cautery artifact, are discussed. Many of the interpretation discrepancies between pathologists occur secondary to poor qualityspecimens.

Orientation

Orientation of mucosal biopsy is crucial for the pathologist. Ideally the pathologist would like to see the full thickness of the mucosa (from surface epithelium to the muscularis mucosa below) (Fig. 9.1) [8]. Tangential sections (Fig. 9.2) are

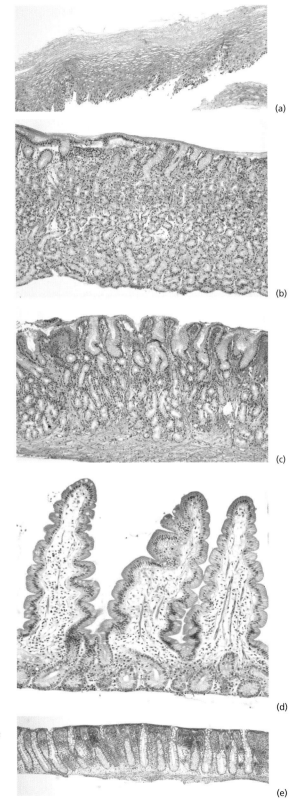

Fig. 9.1 Histological sections of well-oriented biopsies from various areas of the gastrointestinal tract. All reveal mucosa to the muscularis mucosa (at the lower portion of the photomicrograph). (a) Esophageal (squamous mucosa). (b) Gastric fundic (or oxyntic) type mucosa with a central parietal (pink cells) zone. (c) Gastric antral type mucosa with the basal mucous gland. (d) Small bowel mucosa with finger-like villi; the gland-to-villus ratio should be at least 3 : 1. (e) Colon with a parallel 'test-tube' arrangement of the crypts.

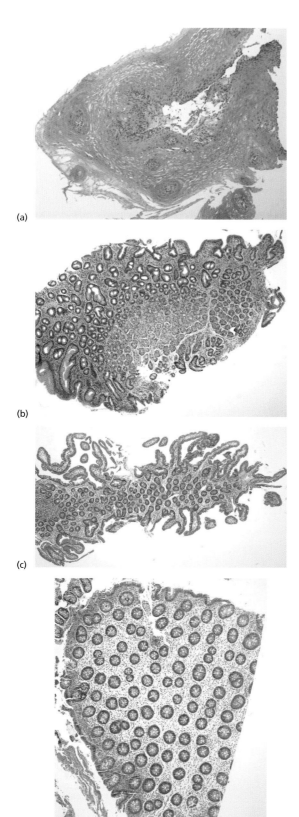

(a)

(b)

(c)

(d)

Fig. 9.2 Histological sections of tangentially oriented normal mucosa from various areas of the gastrointestinal tract. (a) Esophageal (squamous mucosa) with relative increased amount of basal cells (center) due to orientation. (b) Gastric fundic (or oxyntic) type mucosa with increased amount of foveolar tissue due to poor orientation. (c) Small bowel mucosa in which it is very difficult to assess the villus-to-crypt ratio. (d) Colonic mucosa with loss of the 'test-tube' arrangement and instead numerous small cross-sections of each crypt.

much more difficult to interpret [9]. This is especially the case in those instances of dysplasia in Barrett esophagus, where one of the major criteria is nuclear atypia that extends to the surface epithelium. Well-orientated specimens will do wonders for your pathologist's ability to make accurate diagnoses.

Orientation of the biopsy can be accomplished in the endoscopy unit [10]. This requires the endoscopy assistants to orientate and mount biopsies mucosal side up on some sort of mounting media. This is done by relatively few centers and is probably not necessary. It can cause problems if done by untrained individuals. The biopsies are very easy to crush and the surface epithelium can be dislodged easily. If this is being considered, one needs good communication with the pathology laboratory to choose a mounting media and get continual quality control feedback. Well-trained histotechnologists in the pathology laboratory can orientate most biopsies, assuming they are adequate (do not put puny specimens into the fixative). Biopsies should be transferred from the forceps by using a needle (or toothpick) to push the biopsy out of the forceps into the fixative. Shaking the biopsy off the forceps into the fixative can cause trauma to the tissue. The surface epithelium can be lost.

Fixation

Fixation of the biopsy is very important. Biopsies should be transferred to the fixative immediately. This will prevent air drying artifacts, which can be very difficult to interpret. There are a number of different fixatives used by pathology laboratories and each has its advantages and disadvantages. In general, your pathologist will have their standard fixative and it is best to stick with that. Every fixative has its own artefacts and changes the histology slightly. The most common fixative is formalin; however, many labs prefer to use Bouin's or Hollande's (a modification of Bouin's solution). Bouin's creates less shrinkage artefact and gives better nuclear detail; however, it does leach out granules of eosinophils and disposal is more difficult.

Number of biopsies per container

There is a great temptation to put numerous biopsies in a single specimen container, primarily because most pathology laboratory's charge based on the number of containers. I have received ulcerative colitis surveillance cases with 20 biopsies in a single container. There are a number of problems with this approach. (1) It is really not possible to line up more than four biopsies in a tissue block (Fig. 9.3) and an attempt to put more biopsies in a tissue block will result in many of the biopsies being uninterpretable (Fig. 9.4). (2) An additional problem is that there is no way of identifying where the biopsy came from if it is

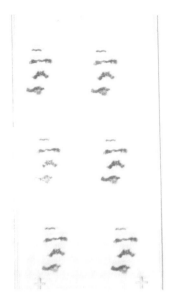

Fig. 9.3 Slide view of serial sections of four well-oriented biopsies in parallel.

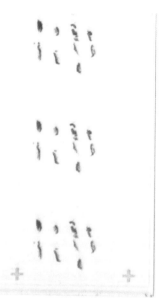

Fig. 9.4 Slide view of numerous (greater than 10) biopsies placed in a single container. A few of the biopsies are of reasonable size; however, some are not well represented.

not separately labelled. If 1 of 20 biopsies has dysplasia, without the proper label there is no way to go back and take additional biopsies if needed. One approach we have taken in our institution is to make multiple blocks from a single container if it contains more than four biopsies. There is an increased technical charge from the lab, but not an increased professional charge.

Tissue processing

Tissue processing is a component of the pathology laboratory and typically not under the purview of the endoscopist. This also plays a crucial role in the ability of the pathologist to make an accurate diagnosis. There are a number of technical flaws that are readily preventable. Problems that can be seen include misorientation of the biopsy specimen, sections that are too thick, folding of the tissue (Fig. 9.5), and shattering of the tissue (Fig. 9.6) by either dull blades or over-cooling of the tissue block. The sections should include multiple ribbons (Fig. 9.7) through the core of the tissue biopsy to allow adequate appraisal of the tissue.

Prep-induced artefact. Different bowel preparation solutions have been reported to cause histological changes in colonic mucosa. Oral sodium phosphate bowel preparation can cause aphthoid ulcers, focal active colitis [11,12], and rare reports of ischemic colitis [13]. It also appears to induce colorectal crypt proliferation. Sodium phosphate enema has been reported to cause sloughing of the surface epithelium. Magnesium citrate and 'X-prep' senna derivative appears

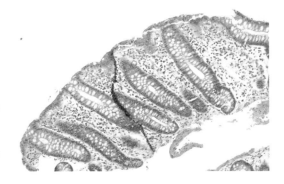

Fig. 9.5 Section of colonic tissue with central fold (irregular dark line through the center of the biopsy). This artifact, if pronounced, can make areas of the biopsy impossible to evaluate.

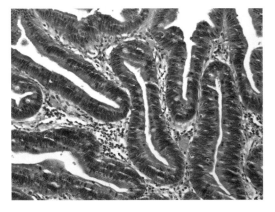

Fig. 9.6 Medium-power view of a tubular adenoma with a subtle shattering of the tissue. This is caused in the histology laboratory by a dull microtome blade and causes linear lines through the tissue. This can cause interpretation problems.

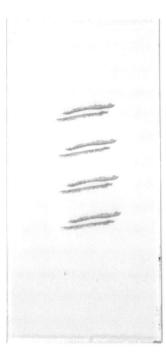

Fig. 9.7 Slide view of a single well-oriented biopsy with multiple ribbons (sections) of the tissue on a single slide. This allows the pathologist to follow suspicious areas through the depth of the tissue. This can be especially important when trying to identify granulomas for the diagnosis of Crohn's disease.

to flatten the surface epithelial cells, cause mucin depletion, and increase lamina propria edema [14]. Anthraquinone glycoside [15] preparations appear to cause epithelial proliferation. Bisacodyl [16–19] has been reported to cause sloughing of the surface epithelium. Information given to the pathologist about the type of colon preparation can be very helpful in interpreting the histological changes identified.

Endoscopy-induced artifacts

Endoscopic trauma can also induce artifacts seen on histology. Typically these are mild and difficult to differentiate from prep-induced artifacts. They consist of edema and hemorrhage in the lamina propria.

Biopsy-induced artifacts

Crush artifact. Every endoscopic biopsy has some crush artifact, typically at the periphery of the biopsy (Fig. 9.8) [18,19]). One would like to minimize that amount of tissue crush by minimizing the handling of the specimen (except in those institutions that mount the tissue biopsy), not shaking the biopsy off the forceps or pushing the biopsy out of the cup from the top.

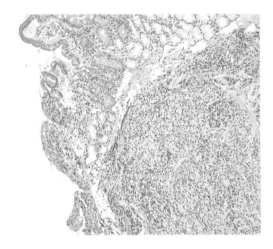

Fig. 9.8 Crush artifact: a medium-power view of the edge of a duodenal biopsy with a carcinoid tumor. Crush is present in virtually all biopsies to some degree. Lymphocytes and endocrine cells (as in this biopsy) are often most affected by the crush. The cells lose their usual rounded appearance and become dark, elongated, and uninterpretable.

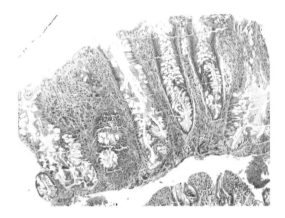

Fig. 9.9 Burn/cautery artifact: a medium-power view of a colonic biopsy with moderate cautery artifact. The cells and nuclei elongate and the architecture of the lesion is distorted. Architecturally this polyp appears to be a hyperplastic polyp; however, differentiation from a tubular adenoma or serrated adenoma due to the nuclear enlargement is impossible.

Burn/cautery artifact. Endoscopic biopsies taken with electrocautery current (hot biopsies and polypectomies) will show cautery artefact (Fig. 9.9). This can be useful in identifying the margin of resection for polypectomy specimen; however, depending on the amount and type of cautery used it can make the tissue uninterpretable. Typically the cells and nuclei elongate (Fig. 9.10) with electrocautery and the differentiation between dysplastic adenomatous epithelium and hyperplastic epithelium becomes impossible.

Polypectomy

Identification of the polyp stalk (Fig. 9.11) is an important aspect of interpreting these specimens. (Fig. 9.12) [20–22]. After polypectomy and with fixation, the stalk retracts and can 'disappear' by the time it is received in the pathology laboratory. Ideally the specimen should be bisected or trisected by the

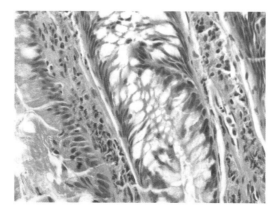

Fig. 9.10 Burn/cautery artifact: a high-power view of a colonic polyp to illustrate the elongation of the nuclei. The artifact gives the suggestion of dysplastic nuclei; however, it is unclear if this represents an adenoma or not.

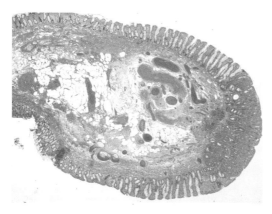

Fig. 9.11 Low-power view of a polypectomy specimen. The adenoma and focal invasive carcinoma are present in the tip at the lower right portion of the specimen. The stalk is covered by normal colonic mucosa and has a loose (pale) fibrovascular core. The margin is present at the other end.

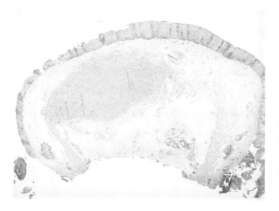

Fig. 9.12 Low-power view of an endoscopic mucosal resection of a granular cell tumor of the esophagus. The surface (*top of picture*) is covered with squamous mucosa. There is a pink cellular lesion (granular cell tumor) in the center and the deep portion represents the cauterized submucosal margin.

pathologist through the stalk; however, if they cannot identify the stalk, this may not be done. There are a couple ways of identifying the stalk for the pathologist. One is to impale the polyp with a short 25-gauge needle, while a second is to put a drop of india ink on the polyp stalk after removal. I prefer the second method, for reasons of safety in the pathology laboratory. With the needle in

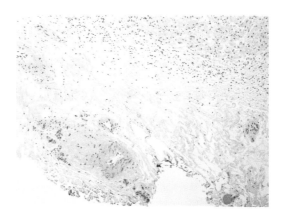

Fig. 9.13 High-power view of an EMR of a granular cell tumor. The deep surgical margin (*inferior portion of picture*) has been inked with black ink. There is an adjacent artery. The tumor is in the top right hand portion of the image.

the specimen there is always the risk of the pathologist blindly sticking themselves with the needle while handling the specimen.

Endoscopic mucosal resection

Similar to polypectomy specimens, the margins of endoscopic mucosal resections (Fig. 9.12) need to be assessed [23]. The pathologist needs to be informed that the specimen is an endoscopic mucosal resection and the margin needs to be assessed (if a single intact specimen is procured). Typically the pathologist will use india ink to assess the margin microscopically (Fig. 9.13). However, if the specimen is removed in a piecemeal fashion, the margins of the resection will be difficult, if not impossible to assess. If these types of specimens are not submitted regularly to the pathologist, a discussion about how the specimen is procured needs to occur with the pathologist prior to the first case.

Core biopsy

Core biopsies are typically handled by surgical pathologists, although they are starting to be used as an adjunct to fine-needle aspiration [24,25]. The indications are typically the same as for fine-needle aspiration. Where they appear to have the greatest utility is in mesenchymal tumors (GI stromal tumors, leiomyomas, etc.), which are typically poorly sampled with traditional fine-needle aspiration. They are handled by the pathology laboratory similar to endoscopic biopsies and should be fixed in the usual fixative for endoscopic biopsies.

Regular stains

Most biopsy specimens, with the exception of cytology and fine-needle aspiration specimens, will be stained routinely with a hematoxylin and eosin (H&E)

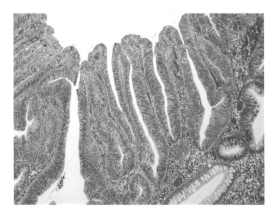

Fig. 9.14 Medium-power view of a villous adenoma of the colon. The routine stain used in pathology is the hematoxylin and eosin (H&E) stain. The nuclei stain blue with the hematoxylin and the cytoplasm has a pink (eosinophilic) appearance with the eosin.

stain (Fig. 9.14). The hematoxylin stains the nuclei of the cell blue while the eosin is a counter-stain that stains the cytoplasm of the cell pink. This is the standard stain used by the pathologist for all tissues. Additional (special) histochemical and immunohistochemical stains can also be performed and will be discussed later.

Exfoliative and fine-needle cytology

Cytology plays an important role in the evaluation of many gastrointestinal processes. Its most important use currently is in the evaluation of the pancreatobiliary tree and as an adjunct to endoscopic ultrasound in the evaluation of mass lesions.

There are a number of different sampling techniques that are used. Aspiration of fluid, brushing a lesion or duct, and fine-needle aspiration can all obtain cells for cytological analysis. Key to all these techniques is the use of imaging (visual, ultrasound, fluoroscopic) to guide the needle or brush to the area of interest. If the needle is not in the mass, or the brush not on the tumor, the entire procedure is completely worthless and may even cause harm. Sampling accuracy is one of the key components in cytology.

Once the specimen is obtained or reaches the laboratory there are a number of different preparation methods. A brush can be smeared onto a slide (Fig. 9.15), or during a fine-needle aspiration a drop of material can be placed on a slide and then a second slide used to smear the material onto the slide (Fig. 9.16). Alternatively, some newer techniques are available that put the material into a fixative (one example is ThinPrep) which is transported to the lab and a monolayer smear of the material is made (Fig. 9.17). This has the advantage of avoiding some of the common artefacts.

Fig. 9.15 Slide view of a smear using a brush from a pancreatic duct brushing. The brush was smeared onto the slide, depositing cells, the slide fixed in alcohol and stained with a Pap stain.

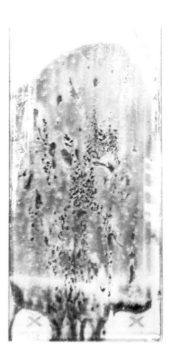

Fig. 9.16 Slide view of a smear made from a fine-needle aspiration. A drop of material was placed at the top of the slide and smeared with a second slide to spread the cells. The material was allowed to air dry and stained with Romanovsky stain.

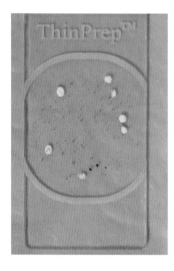

Fig. 9.17 Slide view of a ThinPrep. The material is placed into a fixative and transported to the lab. The ThinPrep machine creates a monolayer of cells on a slide that are then stained with Pap stain.

Specimen handling; staining and fixation

Two stains are primarily used in cytology, Papanicolaou (Pap) stain and the Romanovsky stain. Each has advantages and provides different information. Papanicolaou stain is the primary stain of cytology (used in evaluating pap smears of the cervix). The cells are first fixed with alcohol, which is a coagulative fixative. This causes the cells to contract and appear more rounded, almost spherical, like a boiled egg. The stain contains three cytoplasmic dyes: orange G, eosin Y (pink), light green, and hematoxylin (dark blue) nuclear stain (Fig. 9.18). With the Romanovsky stain (Fig. 9.19) the slides are allowed to air dry, which tends to spread out and flatten the cells, similar to a fried egg. The stain is a metachromatic stain (also used for blood smears) that is relatively quick and often used for rapid assessment. The Papanicolaou stain is a transparent type of

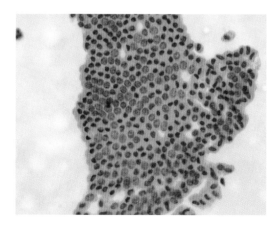

Fig. 9.18 Medium-power view of Pap-stained slide. Image of a cluster of normal glandular epithelial cells. Similar to a H&E-stained histology slide, the nuclei are stained blue (from hematoxylin). There are three cytoplasmic stains: light green (which stains the majority of the cytoplasm in this image), eosin (a pink stain), and orange G.

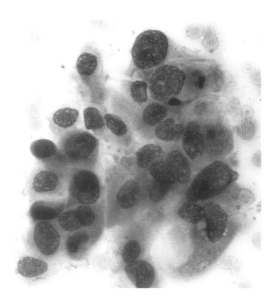

Fig. 9.19 High-power image of a Romanovsky (metachromatic stain). These slides are allowed to air dry with subsequent enlargement of the cells' cytoplasm and nuclei.

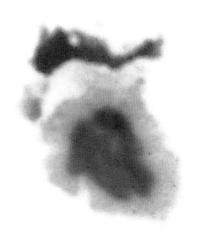

Fig. 9.20 High-power view of an air-drying artifact in a Pap-stained slide. The nuclei breakdown and the nuclear contours become indistinct. There is irregularity to the cytoplasmic borders as well.

stain and allows wonderful assessment of the nuclear detail. The Romanovsky stain, on the other hand, provides nice staining of the cytoplasmic cellular features, background substances, mucin, and microbiological organisms. The adage in cytology is that the nuclear features allow one to determine if a cell is benign or malignant, while the cytoplasmic features tell one where the cell originated.

Artefacts

A number of artefacts (usually induced at the time of collection) canmake cytological diagnosis difficult or impossible. Air drying [26] (Fig. 9.20) of a

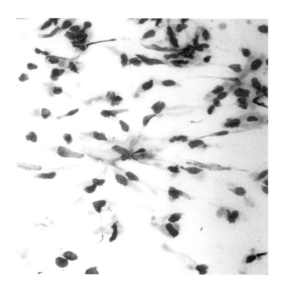

Fig. 9.21 Medium-power view of a cytological crush artifact. The cells can become spindled (as in this example) and may be mistaken as a sarcoma. The nuclei become elongate and, if crushed enough, can be uninterpretable.

Papanicolaou-stained smear occurs when the smear is not placed into fixative quickly enough. The cell nuclei may enlarge and take on the appearance of malignant cells. Cytoplasmic distortion also occurs. Crushing of the cells (Fig. 9.21) may occur when spreading the cells on the slides. Certain cell types (lymphocytes and small cell carcinoma) are especially vulnerable to crush artifact. Crushed cells lose their cytoplasm (naked nuclei) and the nuclei are elongated, precluding cytological evaluation. Obscured smears occur when the material is not smeared adequately or in very bloody specimens. Ideally a specimen should have tissue and very little blood. Excessive blood or cells on top of one another (Fig. 9.22) makes it very difficult to analyse the features of a single cell. Displaced epithelium [27] (Fig. 9.23) refers to cells being picked up from another site. Virtually every fine-needle aspiration will pick up cells as one goes through the gut wall, even with the stylet in place. It is for this reason that one does not biopsy lymph nodes through the tumor. A positive node might be the result of displaced epithelium and not a true positive lymph node. We looked at a number of test needles with a very tight gap, but were still unable to avoid displaced epithelium. Displaced epithelium can also contaminate brush specimens.

Cytological diagnosis

The final task for the pathologist/cytologist is stating a diagnosis. Remember that a diagnosis is just another name for an opinion. The diagnostic categories typically used are unsatisfactory, benign, reactive, atypical, suspicious, and malignant, regardless of site of origin. The diagnostic categories can be viewed

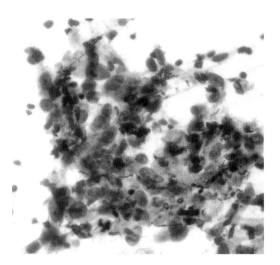

Fig. 9.22 High-power view of Pap-stained slide with cells on top of one another. The three dimensional nature of this preparation makes it very difficult to evaluate the cytological features of each individual cell. The features are obscured by other cells on top of one another.

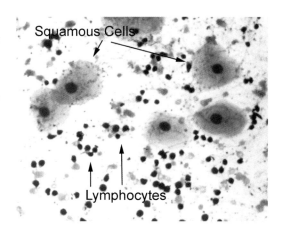

Fig. 9.23 Medium-power view of Romanovsky-stained cytology slide with displaced epithelium. Squamous cells (the large purple cells with centrally placed nuclei) are present in this aspirate from a lymph node. The squamous cells are picked up by the fine-needle aspiration through the esophagus lined by squamous epithelium. This is not a significant problem in this case; however, aspirating a lymph node through a malignancy is very problematic, as one may pick up malignant cells going through a tumor and get a false positive lymph node.

statistically, although it depends on the site biopsied and the likelihood of a positive test. Also remember that sampling errors will come into play as well.

Unsatisfactory (Fig. 9.24): Insufficient tissue to make a diagnosis or the artifacts obscures the cells.

Benign (Fig. 9.25): The cells on the slide are not malignant.

Reactive (Fig. 9.26): The cells on the slide have some changes not seen in normal cells, but are unlikely to be malignant.

Atypical (Fig. 9.27): The cells have more unusual features than seen in reactive cells but are not definitely malignant. About 60% of these cases will be malignant.

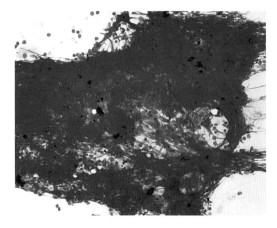

Fig. 9.24 A medium-power view of an unsatisfactory smear (Romanovsky stain). In this case the thickness of the preparation makes it impossible to render a cytological diagnosis.

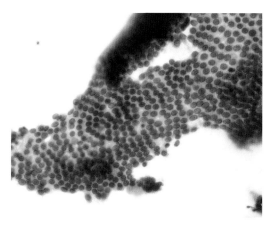

Fig. 9.25 A medium-power view (Pap stain) of a benign aspirate of a pancreas. There is a cohesive group of cells present in a 'honeycomb-like' arrangement of cells. The nuclei are relatively homogenous and small. The cells respect each others borders.

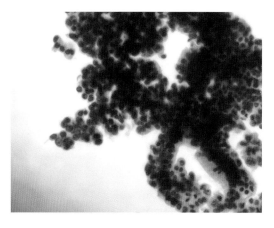

Fig. 9.26 A medium-power view (Pap stain) of a reactive aspirate of the pancreas. Pancreatic ductal epithelial cells are present. The nuclei are enlarged with single prominent nucleoli. These features are typically seen in inflammatory (reactive) conditions.

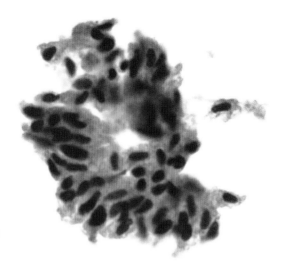

Fig. 9.27 A medium-power view (Pap stain) of an atypical smear of pancreatic ductal epithelial cells. The cells are clustered together; however, there is nuclear enlargement and elongation of the nuclei. This is not definitive for malignancy; however, these features are often seen in dysplasia and present in many malignant cases.

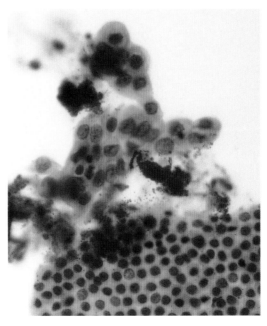

Fig. 9.28 A medium-power view (Pap stain) of a smear suspicious for malignancy. Two cell populations are present in this smear: the inferior aspect of the picture has normal epithelial cells with a nice homogenous appearance. In the superior cluster, the cells are larger. The nuclei are irregular and there is loss of the normal architecture. If this were all that were seen in a smear, the diagnosis of suspicious would be used. The majority of these lesions are malignant; however, there are typically too few diagnostic cells to feel comfortable with the diagnosis.

Suspicious (Fig. 9.28): The cells are worrisome for malignancy. Often this diagnosis is used when there are too few cells to feel comfortable with a malignant diagnosis. About 90% of these cases will be malignant.

Malignant (Fig. 9.29): The cells have all the characteristics of malignancy; 99% of these cases will be malignant.

Table 9.1 lists the typical features of malignancy by cytology.

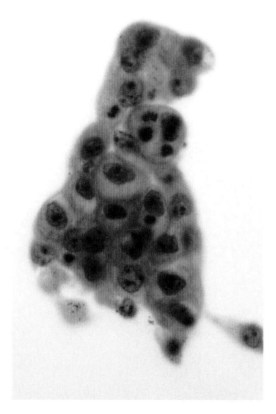

Fig. 9.29 A high-power view (Pap stain) of a malignant smear. The cells are enlarged. The nuclei are irregular with focal prominent nucleoli. There are nuclear contour irregularities and loss of the typical architecture. Necrotic individual cells are present as well.

Fine-needle aspiration

This involves the use of a fine needle (22 gauge or smaller) to remove a sample of cells. There must be a target, 'mass', that is identified initially by endoscopic vision, or through imaging methods, such as ultrasound, CT, or endoscopic ultrasound. The needle typically has a stylet to diminish the amount of displaced tissue. Once the needle is in the lesion, the stylet is removed, and suction is typically applied. A cutting motion is crucial with long 'piston-like' excursions and quick strokes (three strokes per second) [28]. Aspiration by suction alone, with the needle at rest, is not sufficient to draw tissue into the needle; some aspirations are performed with the cutting motion alone and no suction [29].

Major indications for FNA are mass lesions, hypertrophic folds, and lymph nodes. In general the diagnosis of metastatic tumor in lymph nodes and primary epithelial, endocrine, and lymphoid malignancies is very good (with an accuracy of 85–89% at our institution) [30]. Where FNA is limited is in diagnosis of mesenchymal lesions. The cells in these lesions are difficult to aspirate (sticky) and our diagnostic accuracy has been 38% [30]. We have begun to experiment

Table 9.1 Summary of diagnostic features of malignancy

Cells
    Increased number
    Increased nuclear/cytoplasmic ratio
    Overlapping nuclei
    Crowded groups
    Single atypical cells
Nuclei
    Nuclear contour irregularity
    Chromatin clearing and/or clumping
    Nuclear enlargement
    Multinucleation
    Pleomorphism (different sizes)
    Nuclear molding of nuclei to nuclei
    Macro-nucleoli
    Nucleoli irregularities
    Mitotic figures
Cytoplasm
    Loss of cell boundaries
    Pleomorphism
    Inclusions
Background
    Necrosis
    Blood

---

with EUS-guided core biopsy; however, it does not appear to be much better for these lesions [25].

Organ system overview

Esophagus

Histological evaluation of mucosal biopsies of the esophagus (as elsewhere in the gastrointestinal tract) allows one to distinguish between inflammatory, infectious, and malignant lesions. A few of the most common lesions are illustrated.

    The information that the pathologist needs from the endoscopist is the location of the biopsy (typically given in centimeters from the incisors); however, additional information is needed. The location of the gastroesophageal junction (or most proximal location of the gastric folds) and location of the z-line (squamocolumnar junction) must also be provided in order for the pathologist to accurately interpret the histopathological changes. Additionally, gross endoscopic findings should also be conveyed to the pathologist.

Where and when to biopsy

Number of biopsies and where to biopsy depends on the type of lesion encountered and will be discussed with each specific entity. A biopsy is typically performed to evaluate an endoscopic abnormality, patients with no endoscopic abnormality will typically not have histological abnormalities either. Special care must be taken in evaluating erosions and ulcers, especially in the setting of gastroesophageal reflux or Barrett's esophagus. Endoscopic biopsy can be useful to diagnose infectious lesions such as cytomegalovirus (CMV) and herpes simplex. However, in the setting of Barrett's esophagus and GERD, I typically suggest not to biopsy erosions or ulcers. Rather, treat the patient with proton pump inhibitors and bring the patient back for repeat endoscopy. The reason for this is that the inflammatory changes are often extreme and can occasionally be interpreted by pathologists as features of malignancy.

Gastroesophageal reflux disease

Endoscopic biopsy is probably not necessary for the diagnosis of GERD, with 24 h pH monitoring probably representing the gold standard. The histological changes seen with reflux are erosions, acute inflammatory cells (neutrophils and/or eosinophils) in the surface epithelium, basal cell hyperplasia, and elongation of the rete papilla [31] (Fig. 9.30). Additional features include capillary dilatation and numerous intraepithelial lymphocytes. Acute inflammatory cells are the most specific feature; unfortunately they are seen in less than 40% of patients [32]. Attention should be paid to the total number of eosinophils per high power field. Greater than 20 per high power field suggest a diagnosis of eosinophilic esophagitis (Fig. 9.31) and not reflux [33]. The basal cell hyperplasia and elongation of the rete papilla are sensitive for reflux (80% prevalence) (Fig. 9.32), however, not very specific (especially within 3 cm of the gastroesophageal junction) as they can be seen in asymptomatic patients [34].

Barrett's esophagus

The characteristic histological feature of Barrett's esophagus is the finding of goblet cells (intestinal metaplasia) within the tubular esophagus [35] (Fig. 9.33). These goblet cells are also found in association with cardia type mucosa and fundic type mucosa (typically seen in the stomach). One can find intestinal metaplasia of the gastric cardia in association with *Helicobacter pylori* infection [36]. Again, the site of the biopsy in relation to the gastroesophageal junction is crucial in the diagnosis. The goal of the biopsy should be to establish a

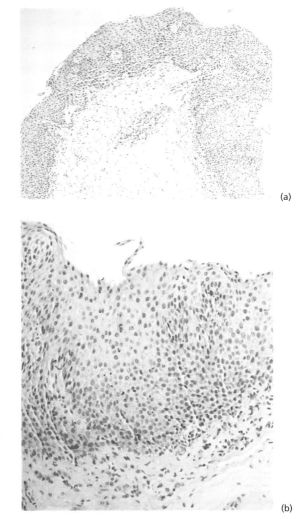

(a)

(b)

Fig. 9.30 H&E images of reflux esophagitis. These are (a) low- and (b) medium-power images of the squamous mucosa in reflux esophagitis. There is basal cell hyperplasia (expansion of the basal proliferative zone) and elongation of the rete papilla of the squamous epithelium. In image B, a central eosinophil can be seen in the squamous mucosa.

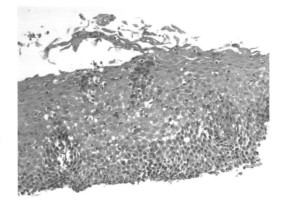

Fig. 9.31 H&E image of eosinophilic esophagitis. There is some basal cell hyperplasia and elongation of the rete papilla (as seen in reflux esophagitis); however, in contrast there are numerous eosinophils (typically greater than 20 per high-power field) in the squamous mucosa.

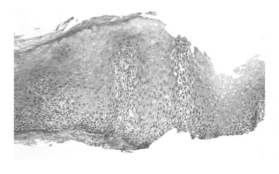

Fig. 9.32 H&E image of marked elongation of the rete papilla (greater than 90% of the mucosal thickness) and basal cell hyperplasia.

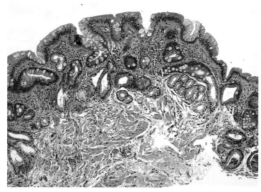

(a)

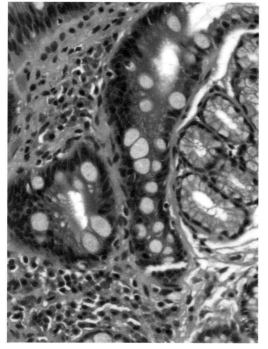

(b)

Fig. 9.33 Low- and high-power H&E images of Barrett's esophagus. (a) There is replacement of the normal squamous epithelial lining of the esophagus by a glandular mucosa (typically gastric type with the presence of goblet cells). (b) is a high-power view of intestinal metaplasia with numerous goblet cells.

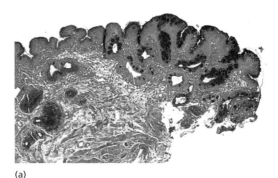

(a)

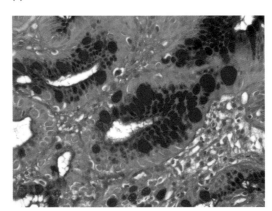

Fig. 9.34 Combination Alcian blue at pH 2.5 and PAS stain on the same biopsy seen in Fig. 9.33. The goblet cells stain deep blue with the Alcian blue stain, while the gastric-type epithelium with neutral mucins stains pink with the PAS stain. (a) is a low-power view, while (b) is a high-power image.

(b)

diagnosis of Barrett's esophagus, verify its length, and identify any dysplasia. Biopsies should be taken from the following sites:

1   2 cm below the gastroesophageal junction.
2   Gastroesophageal junction.
3   2 cm intervals above the GE junction (four quadrant biopsies).
4   Proximal margin (z-line).
5   Target lesion, nodules, plaques.

Histologically the goblet cells have an acid mucin (as opposed to the neutral mucins of the stomach) that can be identified using an Alcian blue stain at pH 2.5 [37] (Fig. 9.34).

Infective esophagitis

The primary infections identified histologically are candida, herpes simplex virus (HSV) and CMV. Each organism infects a different cell or region within the mucosal biopsy and may require a biopsy from a different area within the esophagus.

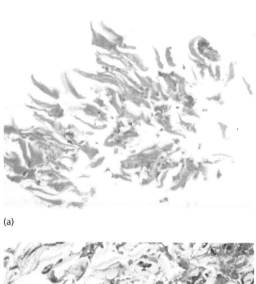

(a)

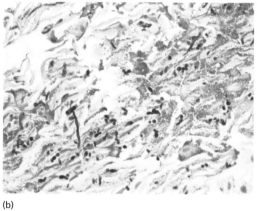

(b)

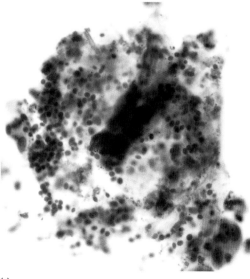

(c)

Fig. 9.35 High-power images of candida in the esophagus. (a) An H&E stain. (b) A PAS stain. (c) A cytology specimen stained with Pap. All show, with varying degrees of clarity, squamous epithelial cells and candidal spores and hyphae (pink on H&E, purple on PAS, and red on Pap).

Candida. Candida (Fig. 9.35) typically appears as raised white plaques. The organism is identified in the superficial squamous epithelium, often associated with a neutrophilic inflammatory response. These areas may be lost if one attempts to orientate or mount these biopsies, so these biopsies should just be placed into fixative without attempt at orientation. Histochemical stains (periodic acid–Schiff or Gomori's methenamine silver stains) may be used to better identify the organisms.

Herpes simplex virus. Herpes simplex virus [38] (Fig. 9.36) infects the squamous epithelial cells and will be best identified at the edge of an ulcerative lesion. The histological features are multiple intranuclear inclusions with nuclear molding and margination of the chromatin. An immunohistochemical stain can be used to highlight the virus.

Cytomegalovirus. CMV (Fig. 9.37) typically infects endothelial cells and thus can be best found in the center of ulcers [39]. The diagnostic cell is an enlarged cell with a single 'owl's eye' eosinophilic intranuclear inclusion. Additionally, numerous small, basophilic, cytoplasmic inclusions may also be seen. Again, an immunohistochemical stain can confirm the presence of CMV.

Adenocarcinoma and squamous cell carcinoma

Diagnosis of esophageal carcinoma using endoscopic biopsy is highly accurate. As few as two biopsies from the lesion will give a diagnosis in 96% of the cases [40]. The two major carcinoma types are squamous cell carcinoma (Fig. 9.38) and adenocarcinoma (Fig. 9.39). Squamous cell carcinoma will typically have intercellular bridges, ample eosinophilic cytoplasm, and evidence of keratinization, while adenocarcinomas will form glands and have mucin production. Typically, in the well and moderately differentiated tumors there is no difficulty differentiating the two entities. However, the poorly differentiated tumors (Fig. 9.40) can pose a diagnostic dilemma and there may be no way to differentiate the two types on the basis of the biopsy.

Stomach

Where and when to biopsy

The important landmarks are the region of the stomach from which the biopsy came: antrum, body/fundus, cardia, greater curvature, lesser curvature, and angularis. This is especially important for the pathologist to determine the degree of glandular atrophy as the thickness of the glands is different in the

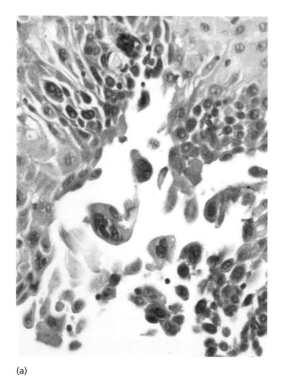

(a)

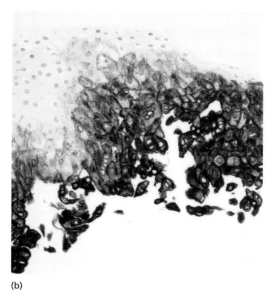

(b)

Fig. 9.36 Herpes esophagitis. (a) An H&E high-power view of the base of the epithelium adjacent to an ulcer. There are enlarged multinucleated cells (representing the intranuclear inclusions of the virus). (b) An immunohistochemical stain, with the herpes infected squamous cells staining brown.

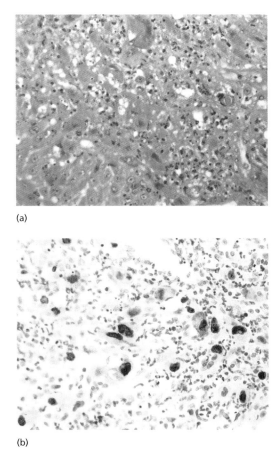

(a)

(b)

Fig. 9.37 Cytomegalovirus esophagitis. (a) An H&E high-power view of the base of the ulcer. There are enlarged cells with single eosinophilic intranuclear inclusions (representing the intranuclear inclusions of the virus). (b) An immunohistochemical stain, with the CMV-infected endothelial cells staining brown.

various areas of the stomach. It is at its thickest in the mid portion of the body along the greater curvature. Additional useful information for the pathologist is the patient's drug therapy. Specifically, the use of antibiotics for *H. pylori* eradication (which will make the hunt for organisms much more difficult and may suggest to the pathologist to do one of the many special stains for *H. pylori*), non-steroidal anti-inflammatory drugs (NSAIDs), and proton pump inhibitors. If a lesion is identified in the stomach and a biopsy taken of the lesion it is also worthwhile taking a second (separately labelled) biopsy of the adjacent 'normal' mucosa to see the 'soil' in which the lesion is arising.

Inflammatory conditions; gastritis

Inflammatory and reactive changes of the gastric mucosa compose the bulk of gastric biopsy findings encountered in the surgical pathology laboratory. The

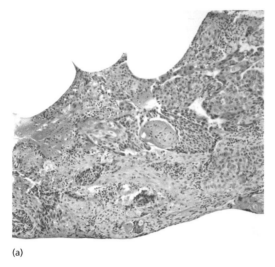

(a)

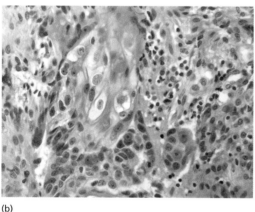

(b)

Fig. 9.38 Invasive squamous cell carcinoma. (a) is a medium- and (b) a high-power H&E-stained slide. The lesion consists of infiltrating nests of tumor cells. The cells have intercellular bridges and focal keratinization, characteristic of squamous differentiation.

most common causes of gastric injuries are *H. pylori* and NSAIDs. There are numerous different nomenclatures. The Houston gastritis workshop proposal [2], expanded on the previous Sydney classification and took into account the topographical distribution, histology, and etiological factors. In general, gastric lesions can be divided into three broad categories: acute, chronic, and special forms. Each of these categories is then subdivided by specific causes, distribution, and histological characterization. With this classification system, clinical information and interaction of the pathologist and endoscopist is crucial. Lesions are also characterized as either gastritis, where the inflammatory infiltrate predominates the histological features, or gastropathy, where the epithelial or vascular changes predominate.

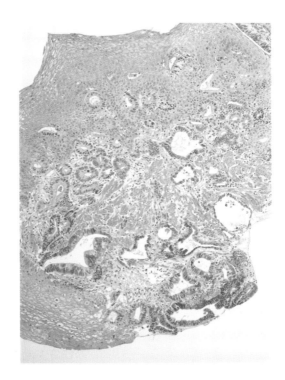

Fig. 9.39 Adenocarcinoma of the esophagus. Medium-power H&E section with overlying squamous mucosa and infiltration of the lamina propria and muscularis mucosa by a gland-forming tumor. The nests of tumor cells have enlarged hyperchromatic nuclei and irregular contours.

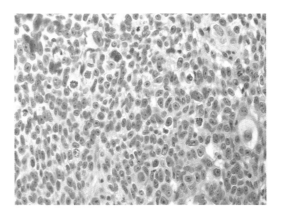

Fig. 9.40 Poorly differentiated tumor of the esophagus. Medium-power H&E section of a poorly differentiated malignancy of the esophagus. Immunohistochemical stains would be required to exclude sarcomas, lymphomas from carcinoma. No distinguishing elements (gland or mucin formation for an adenocarcinoma or keratinization for a squamous cell carcinoma) are present.

NSAIDS. The typical finding as a result of NSAID injury is reactive gastropathy [41] (Fig. 9.41). Histologically one sees foveolar hyperplasia, cytologically reactive epithelial cells, edema, and congestion of the lamina propria, and smooth muscle proliferation in the lamina propria. There may also be surface erosions. The inflammatory infiltrate is typically minimal, although neutrophils may be present adjacent to an erosion.

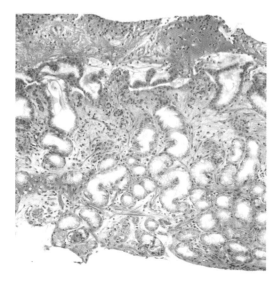

Fig. 9.41 Reactive gastropathy. Medium-power H&E section of gastric antral type mucosa. There is elongation of the foveolar (surface epithelium) with focal erosion and an inflammatory exudate. The inflammatory cells present are predominately neutrophils, with a relative paucity of lymphocytes (chronic inflammatory infiltrates).

H. pylori gastritis. *H. pylori* has a characteristic histological features [2] (Fig. 9.42). The *H. pylori* organisms can be identified on the surface epithelium (either on the basic H&E or using special stains [42] such as Giemsa, Genta, modified Warthin–Starry, and an immunohistochemical stain). There typically is a neutrophilic inflammatory infiltrate both in the lamina propria and glandular epithelium (active inflammation), an increased mononuclear (lymphocytes and plasma cells) infiltrate in the lamina propria, and lymphoid follicles with reactive germinal centers. Glandular atrophy and intestinal metaplasia may also be present. In areas with extensive intestinal metaplasia it may be more difficult to identify the *H. pylori* organisms, as they do not live in the acid mucins of the intestinal metaplastic cells.

Hypertrophic folds

In patients with enlarged (hypertrophic) folds the differential diagnosis [43] includes infiltrating malignancy (carcinoma [Fig. 9.43] and lymphoma [Fig. 9.44]), infections, granulomatous inflammation (Fig. 9.45), and primary epithelial hyperplasia. Endoscopic biopsy is usually adequate for the evaluation of this lesion, although occasionally endoscopic ultrasound fine-needle aspiration may help in the evaluation. If lymphoma is a concern, additional biopsies can be obtained to use for flow cytometry, which will better evaluate the lymphoid process. In general, this is probably best used in those patients who have a diagnosis of an atypical lymphoid infiltrate and a second endoscopy is scheduled to obtain tissue for flow cytometry.

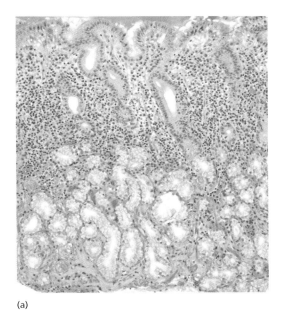

(a)

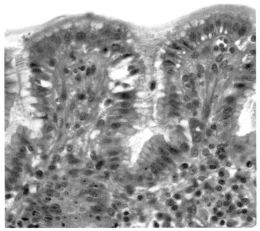

(b)

Fig. 9.42 *H. pylori*-associated chronic active gastritis. (a) Medium-power H&E section with a superficial infiltrate of lymphocytes and plasma cells in the lamina propria (what was once called a superficial gastritis). (b) High-power H&E of the superficial foveolar epithelium to illustrate some *Helicobacter* organisms. (*Contd. p. 224*)

Polyps

A number of neoplastic and non-neoplastic lesions can present as polyps in the stomach. These can additionally be classified as epithelial or non-epithelial. Biopsy is relatively accurate, except in the submucosal mass type lesions. A biopsy of the adjacent mucosa is often very helpful to identify whether the lesion is arising in a general pathological process or is focal. It also serves as a control when the architectural abnormality of the polyp is relatively subtle. The most common polyp encountered in the antrum is a hyperplastic polyp (Fig. 9.46), while the most common encountered in the gastric body is a fundic

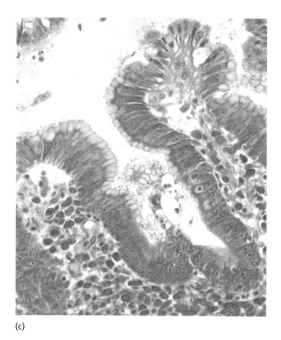

(c)

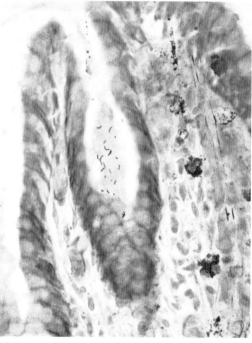

(d)

Fig. 9.42 (*cont'd*) (c) High-power Giemsa stain of *Helicobacter* organisms (staining blue). (d) High-power silver stain (Steiner stain) where the *Helicobacter* organisms are black.

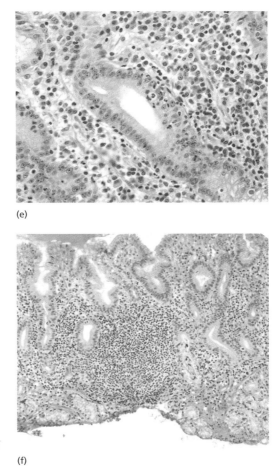

(e)

(f)

Fig. 9.42 (*cont'd*) (e) High-power H&E revealing the infiltration of the gastric epithelium by neutrophils (acute or active gastritis). (f) Medium-power H&E revealing a lymphoid aggregate at the base of the epithelium, typical of *Helicobacter* infection.

gland polyp [44] (Fig. 9.47). Both of these lesions are non-neoplastic. Neoplastic polyps (adenomas) are relatively uncommon; however, they should be removed in their entirety.

Mass lesions

Tumors of the stomach are among the most common neoplasms in the world, and the majority are epithelial (adenocarcinomas) (Fig. 9.48). Neoplasms of endocrine (Fig. 9.49), lymphoid (Fig. 9.50), and mesenchymal (Fig. 9.51) tissue occur in the stomach less commonly. In general, endoscopic biopsy will permit diagnosis of the majority of these lesions, the exception being mesenchymal tumors. These lesions often arise in the submucosa or muscularis propria and are not sampled by endoscopic biopsy. Fine-needle aspiration may be more helpful in these cases.

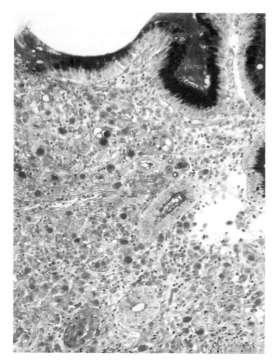

Fig. 9.43 Medium-power PAS-stained section of an infiltrative signet ring carcinoma of the stomach. There is loss of the normal glandular architecture. Residual normal surface epithelium (staining pink at the top) is present and there is an infiltration of single malignant cells in the lamina propria. These cells are filled with mucin that stains pink with the PAS stain.

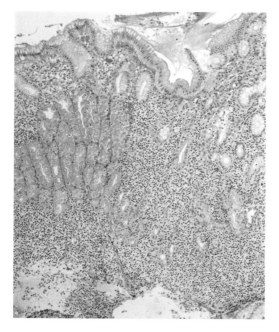

Fig. 9.44 Mucosal associate lymphoid tissue (MALT) lymphoma. H&E medium-power view with intense infiltration of the lamina propria by a lymphoid infiltrate (blue) with associated parietal gland (pink) loss on the right hand portion of the image.

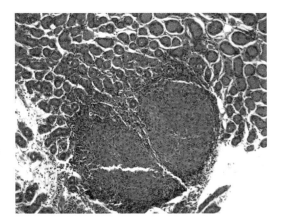

Fig. 9.45 Stomach with granuloma: H&E medium-power view with two large epithelioid granulomas at the base of the mucosa, surrounded by a lymphoid aggregate in a Crohn's patient.

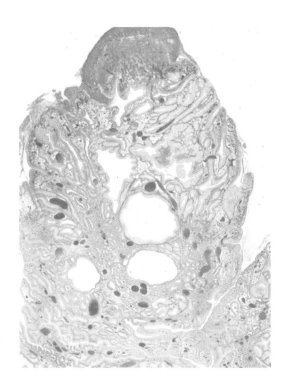

Fig. 9.46 Hyperplasic polyp: H&E low-power image of antral mucosa with surface erosion (*top of image*), foveolar hyperplasia, and glandular dilatation lined by mucinous cells.

Small bowel

Biopsies of the small bowel are typically obtained from the duodenum or terminal ileum, which is the reach of standard upper and lower endoscopy. In general these biopsies are done in the work-up of diarrhea and malabsorption. Orientation of the small bowel biopsies in this case is very important as evaluation of the villus-to-crypt ratio plays a prominent role in the pathological

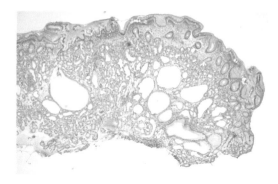

Fig. 9.47 Fundic gland polyp. H&E low-power image of fundic-type mucosa with glandular dilatation lined by a mixture of parietal, chief, and mucinous cells.

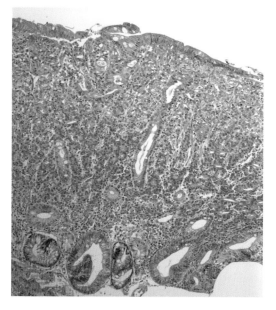

Fig. 9.48 Gastric adenocarcinoma. H&E medium-power image of an adenocarcinoma of the stomach. There is an increased number of glands with enlarge nuclei and relatively little cytoplasm. The normal gastric glands are not present.

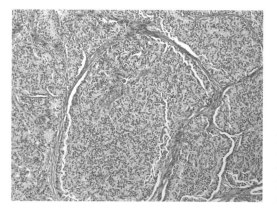

Fig. 9.49 Endocrine (carcinoid) tumor. H&E medium-power image with tumor comprised of nests and lobules of cells. Gland formation is not identified.

Fig. 9.50 Lymphoma. H&E medium-power image of a high-grade lymphoma. The cells are enlarged with prominent vesicular nuclei and prominent nucleoli. Numerous mitotic figures are present.

Fig. 9.51 Gastrointestinal stromal tumor. H&E medium-power image of a spindle cell neoplasm with numerous admixed lymphocytes. There is relatively little mitotic activity. Immunohistochemical stains are needed to subclassify this mesenchymal neoplasm. The primary prognostic factors are tumor size and mitotic activity.

classification of small bowel lesions (Fig. 9.52). Duodenal biopsies should be taken distal to the duodenal bulb. Biopsies from the bulb may be difficult to interpret secondary to artifactual blunting of the villi by the Brunner's glands. Most findings in the bulb are secondary to peptic-acid disease and there is often a 'mild chronic duodenitis' [45]. Usually 2–3 biopsies obtained with a regular-sized forcep from the second or third part of the duodenum should be sufficient for evaluation.

Small bowel mucosal lesions are categorized as specific (diagnostic) or non-specific and the severity of mucosal injury is subjectively expressed as the degree of abnormality (or loss) of the villous architecture. Normal small bowel should have a villus-to-crypt ratio of at least 3:1, fewer than 25 intraepithelial lympho-cytes [46], and one should have at least 3–4 villi in a row to feel confident of the findings.

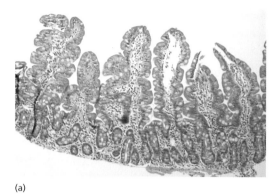

(a)

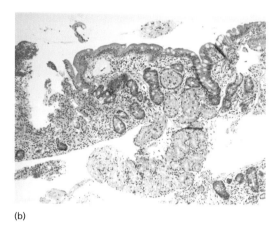

(b)

Fig. 9.52 Normal small bowel mucosal biopsies. H&E medium-power image. (a) has the normal gland-to-villus ratio of 3:1, while (b) is a biopsy from the duodenal bulb with Brunner's glands and relative villous blunting, but no increased inflammatory infiltrate.

Celiac sprue

Celiac sprue is one of the more common lesions encountered in biopsies of patients with diarrhea and malabsorption. The histological features are not specific; however, with the appropriate clinical information (improvement with gluten-free diet), they are diagnostic. The typical histological lesion is absence of villi (total or subtotal villous atrophy), an abnormal surface epithelium, increased numbers of intraepithelial lymphocytes, and an increased lymphoplasmacytic infiltrate in the lamina propria (Fig. 9.53). This typical flat mucosa represents one end of the spectrum of pathologic abnormalities in gluten-sensitive individuals. The 'infiltrative lesion' of latent sprue [47] (more than 40 lymphocytes per 100 epithelial cells) characterizes the earliest recognizable pathological change.

Infective enteropathies

Infectious lesions of the small bowel are typically categorized as specific (diagnostic) lesions with appropriate identification of the organism. Common lesions

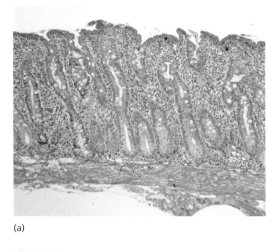

(a)

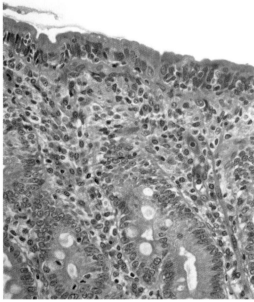

Fig. 9.53 Celiac sprue. This is a severe mucosal lesion with almost total villous atrophy ((a) medium-power H&E), an increased lymphoplasmacytic infiltrate in the lamina propria, and increased numbers of intraepithelial lymphocytes ((b) high-power H&E).

(b)

identified include Whipple's disease, *Mycobacterium avium–intracellulare*, and *Giardia*.

Whipple's disease. Whipple's disease is a rare bacterial infection with *Tropheryma whippelii* that affects the small intestine in a diffuse fashion but can involve many other organ systems. The typical histological feature [48] is massive infiltration of the lamina propria with foamy macrophages (Fig. 9.54). The macrophages contain the Whipple bacilli and will stain with a periodic

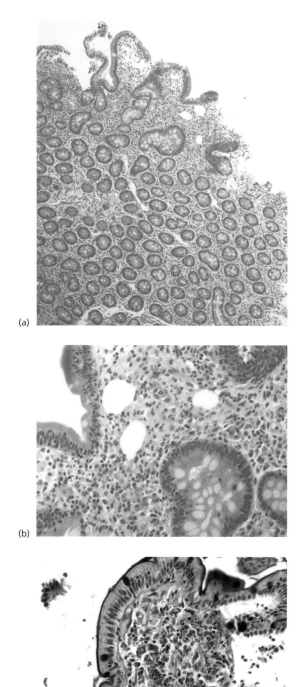

(a)

(b)

(c)

Fig. 9.54 Whipple's disease.
There is a lamina propria
infiltration by histiocytes. Focal fat
(clear spaces) are present as well.
(a) is a medium-power H&E,
(b) a high-power H&E, and
(c) a high-power PAS-stained section.
The histiocytes are positive (pink)
with the PAS stain.

acid–Schiff (PAS) stain. Additionally, small collections of fat may be present in the lamina propria (the original name coined by Whipple was lipodystrophy).

Mycobacterium avium–intracellulare. Have become more prominent in immuno-suppressed patients [49]. Histological evaluation reveals sheets of macrophages within the lamina propria. There is often thickening of the folds. The macro-phages are stuffed with organisms, which can be identified with acid fast stains (Fite) (Fig. 9.55).

Giardia lamblia. Is an extracellular parasite present on the surface epithelium, and easier to recognize in cytological smears. Histologically the organisms appear slightly basophilic or grayish in the mucus adherent to villus tips or between villi [50] (Fig. 9.56). They are approximately the size of an enter-ocyte nucleus and have a characteristic pear-shaped profile. The prominent paired 'owl's eye' central nuclei and indistinct flagella attached to the tapered end are usually visible only in smears. Trichrome or Giemsa stains make the organism more prominent.

Polyps

The majority of polypoid lesions in the duodenum consist of benign hetero-topic or hamartomatous lesions. Heterotopic gastric mucosa, including gastric surface metaplasia (Fig. 9.57) with or with out gastric gland, is the most common lesion [51]. Brunner's gland nodules and hamartomas are also com-mon in the first portion of the duodenum [52] (Fig. 9.58). Neoplastic lesions (adenomas) do occur, predominately in the second portion of the duodenum. Many of these lesions are found in patients with familial adenomatous coli [53]. The criteria for the diagnosis of small intestine adenomas is the same as that for adenomas elsewhere in the gastrointestinal tract, namely, the pres-ence of dysplastic epithelium (Fig. 9.59). These may be virtually indistinguish-able from adenomas elsewhere in the GI tract, but Paneth cells are often prominent.

Mass lesions

Tumors of the small bowel are relatively uncommon, however; similar to the rest of the gastrointestinal tract the majority are still epithelial (adenocarcinomas). Compared to the colon, the relative proportion of neoplasms of endocrine, lymphoid [54], and mesenchymal tissue occur more commonly.

In general, endoscopic biopsy can diagnose the majority of these lesions, the exception being mesenchymal tumors. These lesions often arise in the

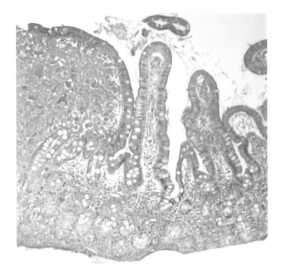

(a)

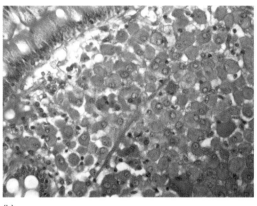

(b)

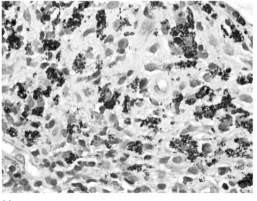

(c)

Fig. 9.55 *Mycobacterium avium–intracellulare* (MAI). Similar to Whipple's disease, there is a significant infiltration of histiocytes in the lamina propria. These are filled with the organisms and can be identified on a modified acid fast stain (Fite). (a) medium-power H&E, (b) high-power H&E, and (c) high-power fite stain.

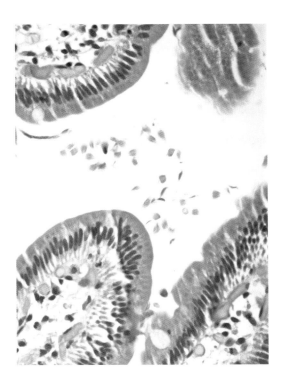

Fig. 9.56 *Giardia*. High-power H&E of small bowel mucosa. The organisms can be seen in the lumen adjacent to the surface epithelium. They are purple concave or pear shaped.

submucosa or muscularis propria and are not sampled by endoscopic biopsy. Fine-needle aspiration may be more helpful in these cases.

Colon

Colonoscopic endoscopic biopsy specimens are one of the most frequent specimens encountered in the pathology laboratory. Typically they are obtained in the work-up of a patient with diarrhea or colon cancer screening, or the work-up of bleeding. A few clinical/endoscopic findings are typically found with these biopsies: a normal endoscopy in a patient with diarrhea, abnormal endoscopy (redness, ulceration, friability), or polyp/mass lesion. Each will be addressed separately.

The diagnostic yield of lower endoscopy and biopsy is very good in the work-up of diarrhea. It is recommended that representative biopsies be taken in all cases (both endoscopically normal and abnormal). Patel *et al.* [55] looked at the diagnostic outcome in 205 consecutive study patients with lower endoscopy for diarrhea. Of these, 152 (74%) had a normal endoscopy and biopsy, 37 (18%) had a specific diagnosis based on endoscopy and biopsy (Table 9.2) reveals a list of the abnormal endoscopy and biopsy findings), and 16 (8%) had either an endoscopy or biopsy inconsistent with the final clinical diagnosis.

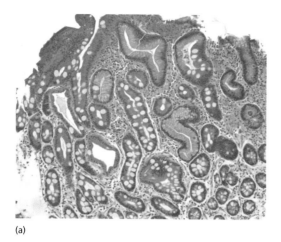

(a)

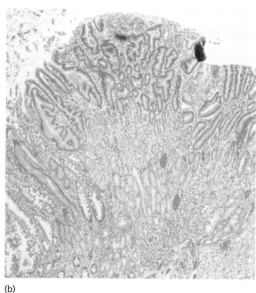

(b)

Fig. 9.57 Gastric metaplasia. (a) Medium-power H&E of duodenal mucosa with the typical goblet cells. In the center of the picture the surface epithelium has the foveolar epithelium typically seen in gastric mucosa (gastric surface metaplasia). (b) Low-power H&E of duodenal mucosa with gastric surface metaplasia and gastric fundic-type glands.

When the endoscopy diagnosis (typically colitis) was inconsistent with the final clinical diagnosis the biopsies were normal (7 cases). The biopsy diagnoses that were inconsistent with the final clinical diagnosis usually had a diagnosis of 'non-specific colitis' (7 of 9 cases).

Defining 'normal'

Pathologists should not use the diagnosis of 'non-specific colitis'. Usually this is an overcall of normal colonic mucosa. The diagnosis of normal colonic mucosa or an unremarkable colonic mucosal biopsy is an important one. It helps the

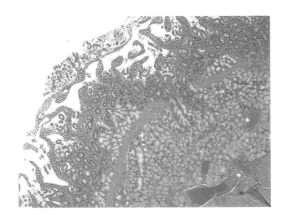

Fig. 9.58 Brunner's gland nodule.
Low-power H&E image of surface
duodenal mucosa and prominent
submucosal Brunner's glands
(endoscopically a nodular
appearance).

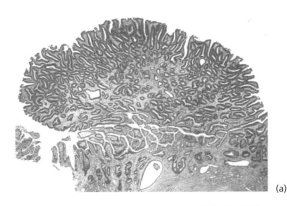

(a)

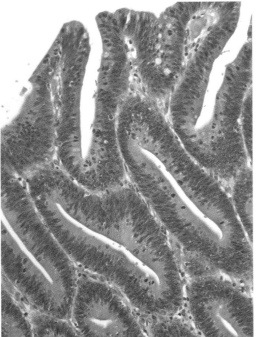

Fig. 9.59 Adenoma.
(a) Low-power H&E image of an
adenomatous polyp. The lesion is
blue from low power due to the
enlargement and hyperchromasia
of the epithelium (dysplasia).
(b) Higher-power H&E of the
dysplastic epithelium with
enlargement and stratification
of the nuclei typical of adenoma
(dysplasia, low grade in this
instance).

(b)

Table 9.2 Abnormal endoscopy and biopsy findings in 205 patients with diarrhea

Diagnosis	Number of patients
Pseudomembranous colitis	7
Ulcerative colitis	4
Crohn's disease	2
Indeterminate colitis	2
Villous adenoma >5 cm	3
Melanosis coli	1
Rectal prolapse	1
Collagenous colitis	1
Peridiverticulitis	1
Ischemic colitis	1

endoscopist to rule out an inflammatory colonic lesion as the cause of the diarrhea. There is often the feeling that the pathologist must make some sort of diagnosis, since the endoscopist took the biopsy for 'some reason'. Unfortunately this gives the clinicians two options: treat everyone and over-treat the patients, or ignore the diagnosis and miss those patients with true inflammatory disease.

Biopsies of the normal colonic mucosa typically are comprised of parallel crypts lined by colonocytes, similar to test tubes in a row if the biopsy is properly orientated. As in the small bowel there is a lymphoplasmacytic infiltrate in the lamina propria and lymphoid aggregates (follicles) present [8]. It is this normal baseline inflammatory infiltrate that is often over-interpreted as 'chronic non-specific colitis'. The inflammatory infiltrate is typically concentrated in the upper third of the mucosa (Fig. 9.60).

Inflammatory colitides

Normal colonoscopy. The majority of biopsy specimens taken in individuals with diarrhea with a normal endoscopy will be normal, however, approximately 1–10% will have a microscopic colitis [56]. The term microscopic colitis is an unfortunate one as it typically encompasses the diagnosis of collagenous colitis (Fig. 9.61) and lymphocyte colitis (Fig. 9.62), but is occasionally used as a diagnosis on its own. In general the specific diagnoses should be used and not the ambiguous term 'microscopic colitis'. Both lymphocytic and collagenous colitis can be seen in association with NSAIDs, celiac disease, and autoimmune diseases. Their causes are unknown, their histological appearances are similar [57], with the differentiating feature being basement membrane thickening (greater than 10 µg) in collagenous colitis. This basement membrane thickening can be highlighted with a trichrome stain. The common histological features are increased intraepithelial lymphocytes (IEL), increased numbers of eosinophils, flattening and detachment of the surface epithelium, and an increased number

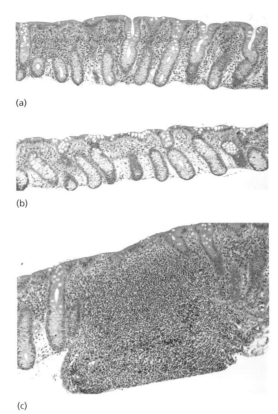

(a)

(b)

Fig. 9.60 Normal colonic mucosa, H&E stains. (a) Low-power image of the right side of the colon and left side of colon. (b) The architecture is similar with the crypts lined up as 'test tubes' in a rack. There is a difference in the inflammatory infiltrate, with more lymphocytes, plasma cells, and eosinophils typically present on the right side of the colon. (c) There is some mild architectural distortion adjacent to this normal lymphoid aggregate in the center of this biopsy.

(c)

of lymphocytes and plasma cells in the lamina propria. With collagenous colitis the collagen thickening is patchy and typically best identified from biopsies in the transverse colon [58].

Abnormal colonoscopy. In patients with diarrhea and an abnormal endoscopy, the differential diagnosis includes the idiopathic inflammatory bowel diseases (ulcerative colitis and Crohn's disease), ischemia, and infectious colitis. The endoscopic appearance of the bowel and clinical history are very important in this differential diagnosis and need to be communicated to the pathologist.

Inflammatory bowel disease

The idiopathic inflammatory bowel diseases (IBDs) are chronic lesions and are characterized by chronic histological mucosal findings. There is typically marked crypt architectural distortion (Fig. 9.63): irregularities of the crypts (loss of the typical parallel test tube architecture), crypt atrophy, lifting of the crypts from the muscularis mucosa, and a basal plasmacytosis (plasma cells below the base of the crypts). These features are very useful in differentiating

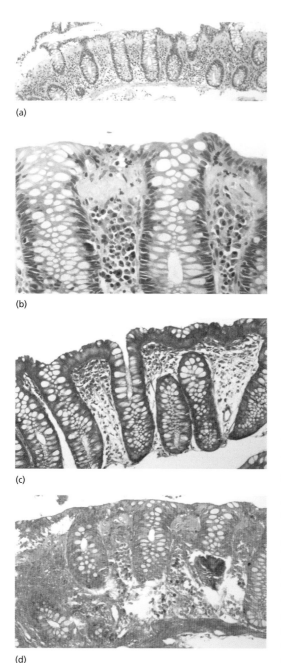

Fig. 9.61 Collagenous colitis. (a) Low-power H&E view of a colonic biopsy in collagenous colitis. The architecture is similar to the normal mucosa (Fig. 9.60a) with crypts arranged parallel to one another and extending to the base of the biopsy. There is a mild increase in the lymphocytes in the lamina propria. A prominent acellular band is present below the surface epithelium. This 'collagenous' expansion of the basement membrane is the characteristic finding in collagenous colitis. (b) High-power H&E view of the thickened basement membrane. This basement membrane should be thicker than 15 μm (a normal lymphocyte is 7 μm, so at least the thickness of two lymphocyte nuclei). There are often entrapped lymphocytes and blood vessels in the collagen band. Additionally there are increased numbers of lymphocytes, eosinophils, and plasma cells in the lamina propria. There is focal epithelial detachment from the basement membrane and some epithelial apoptosis. (c) Medium-power trichrome stain of normal colonic epithelium. The blue strip below the epithelium is the normal basement membrane thickness. This is to be contrasted with (d), a trichrome stain in collagenous colitis that highlights the marked basement membrane thickening (blue) below the surface epithelium.

IBD from acute self-limited colitis (ASLC) [59] (Fig. 9.64), especially in adults. In children these features may be less prominent. There is also goblet cell mucin depletion, infiltration of neutrophils and eosinophils in the lamina propria and glands, and reactive epithelial hyperplasia. However, these features overlap with those of ASLC.

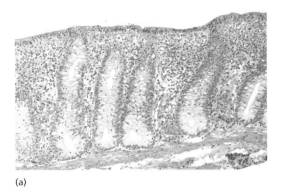

(a)

Fig. 9.62 Lymphocytic colitis.
(a) Medium-power H&E view of
lymphocytic colitis. Similar to
normal and collagenous colitis, the
architecture of the mucosa is intact,
with parallel crypts that extend to
the muscularis mucosa. There is an
increased lymphocytic infiltrate in
the lamina propria, no thickening of
the basement membrane, and a
characteristic increase in the
number of intraepithelial
lymphocytes (lymphocytes above
the basement membrane and
between the colonic epithelial cells).
This increase in the number of
intraepithelial lymphocytes is best
identified in (b), a high-power H&E
view of the mucosa. There should be
greater than one lymphocyte per five
epithelial cells.

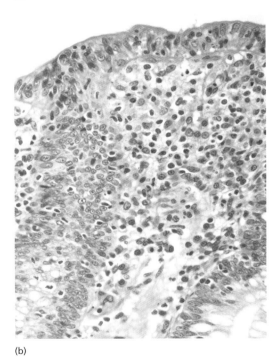

(b)

Differentiation of ulcerative colitis and Crohn's disease can be problematic
on endoscopic mucosal biopsy. The characteristic feature of Crohn's disease
is the presence of epithelioid granulomas (Fig. 9.65). Unfortunately these are
typically only seen in approximately 20% of biopsies from patients with Crohn's
disease. Additionally, microgranulomas and granulomas associated with a ruptured crypt can be seen in ulcerative colitis (and other lesions) (Fig. 9.66). The
other useful differentiating histological feature is a microscopic patchiness to
the inflammatory infiltrate (similar to the endoscopic skip lesions) (Fig. 9.67). The
best time to differentiate these two lesions is on initial endoscopy and biopsy
with communication of the endoscopic findings (diffuse vs. patchy, presence of

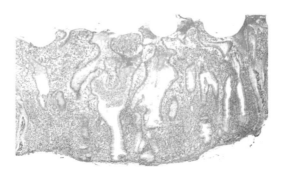

Fig. 9.63 Crypt architectural changes in idiopathic inflammatory bowel disease. Medium-power H&E view of a biopsy from a patient with ulcerative colitis. The normal crypt architecture is disrupted. There is crypt branching. Some of the crypts are markedly expanded with the presence of neutrophils in the lumen (crypt abscess). A number of the crypts are foreshortened with the base of the crypt not extending all the way to the muscularis mucosa at the base of the biopsy. The surface of the biopsy has an undulating, almost villiform appearance, not the typical flat surface.

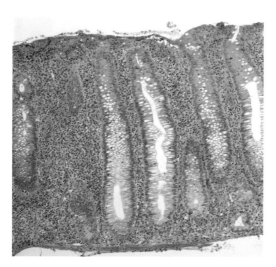

Fig. 9.64 Acute self-limited colitis (infectious colitis). A medium-power H&E view of colonic mucosa with an increase in the number of lamina propria inflammatory cells. The majority of inflammatory cells are in the upper half of the lamina propria (as opposed to the predominance of deep inflammatory cells in typical inflammatory bowel disease. There is no crypt architectural distortion.

rectal sparing) and representative biopsies of both normal (if present) and abnormal areas. Like biopsies should be labelled and separately submitted. If a patient has patchy disease (suspicious for Crohn's endoscopically), biopsies should be taken from the normal and abnormal areas and be put in separate containers. In biopsies from a diffuse colitis (suspicious for ulcerative colitis), biopsies should be taken from the involved colon (no more than four biopsies per container) and a separate container used with biopsies of the normal terminal ileum and proximal colon (if present). Differentiating the two lesions after the initial biopsy becomes more difficult, as treatment of ulcerative colitis

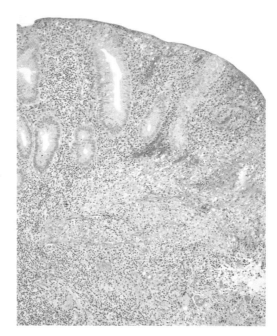

Fig. 9.65 Crohn's disease. Medium-power H&E view of mucosa and superficial submucosa with an epithelioid granuloma, typical of that seen in Crohn's disease. The granuloma is seen in the middle of the image, at the base of the crypts. There is an increase in the number of inflammatory cells in the lamina propria and some crypt architectural distortion.

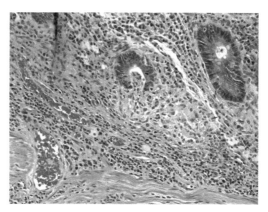

Fig. 9.66 Granuloma associated with a ruptured crypt. High-power H&E image of a ruptured crypt in the center of the image with an associated granuloma composed of epithelioid histiocytes. These lesions can be seen in both ulcerative colitis and Crohn's disease and are not the characteristic granuloma (Fig. 9.65) virtually diagnostic of Crohn's disease.

can give patchiness, rectal sparing, and even histologicalal and endoscopic reversion to normal [60–63].

Pseudomembranous colitis. Pseudomembranous colitis (Fig. 9.68) can be seen associated with antibiotics (*Clostridium difficile*-associated colitis) and ischemia (Fig. 9.69). Pseudomembranes can be present with ischemia; however, in the majority of cases they are not present [64]. Both lesions have a predominantly neutrophilic inflammatory infiltrate (as opposed to the prominent lymphoplasmacytic infiltrate in the inflammatory bowel lesion) and a collection of

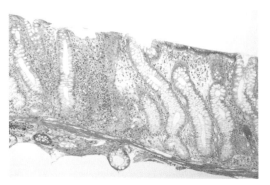

Fig. 9.67 Crohn's disease. Medium-power H&E view of colonic mucosa illustrating patchy microscopic inflammation typical of Crohn's disease. In addition to the gross patchiness present on endoscopic examination, microscopic patchiness is also present. There is a focus of inflammation on the left side of the image, while the right side of the image has a normal inflammatory component.

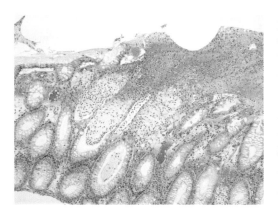

Fig. 9.68 Pseudomembranous colitis. Medium-power H&E view of colonic mucosa with pseudomembrane formation. There is a predominantly neutrophilic (acute) inflammatory infiltrate present in the biopsy. The pseudomembrane is present on the right upper portion of the image. There is a loss of the surface epithelium and the pseudomembrane is comprised of inflammatory cells and pink fibrin.

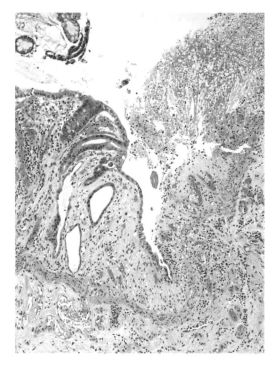

Fig. 9.69 Ischemic colitis. Medium-power H&E view of colonic mucosa in ischemia. There is surface erosion and a pseudomembrane present in the top right portion of the image. In contrast to Fig. 9.68, there is atrophy (loss) of the crypt glandular epithelium and the lamina propria has a pink hyalinized quality.

neutrophils, fibrin, and necrotic cells making up the pseudomembrane on the surface epithelium.

Ischemic colitis Ischemic colitis can be histologically very similar to pseu-domembranous colitis, due to the presence of a pseudomembrane. However, ischemia typically has a hyalinized lamina propria, is localized on endoscopy, and has atrophic crypts, often with full-thickness mucosal necrosis. The hyalin-ization of the lamina propria (Fig. 9.69) is the most characteristic feature and best differentiates this lesion from pseudomembranous colitis.

Polyps

Polyps are typically sampled to identify the patient's risk for subsequent carci-noma, and removed to prevent progression to malignancy [65]. There are many types of polyps; however, the focus here will be on those most commonly encountered, i.e. adenomas and hyperplastic polyps.

Adenomatous. Adenomatous polyps are by definition neoplastic and dysplastic. All have a malignant potential; however, only a very few will actually become malignant. A good demonstration of this is patients with familial adenomatous polyposis. These patients have thousands of polyps, which usually begin to become apparent in the teens, and typically, by the age of 30 one or two of the thousands of polyps will have become an invasive carcinoma. Thus with a given adenomatous polyp, the likelihood that it will become malignant is low and it will take many years. All adenomatous polyps have dysplastic epithelium (Fig. 9.70) (characterized by nuclear enlargement and hyperchromasia) and thus appear basophilic (or blue) on the microscopic slide. The lesion is confined by the basement membrane and there is no invasion into the adjacent tissue, so there is no possibility of metastatic disease to the lymph nodes. Histologically the lesions are divided into tubular (Fig. 9.71), villous (Fig. 9.72), and mixed

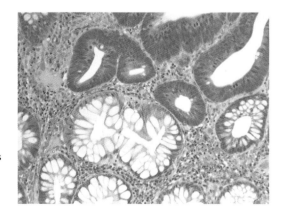

Fig. 9.70 Tubular adenoma. High-power H&E image of tubular adenoma. The top of the image has the adenomatous (dysplastic) epithelium and is to be compared with the normal colonic mucosa in the lower portion of the image. The dysplasia is characterized by a dark blue appearance to the tissue. This is secondary to the increased size of the nuclei, stratification of the nuclei, and a loss of pale mucin.

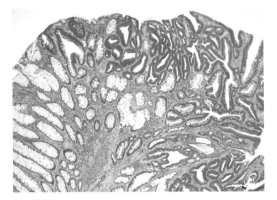

Fig. 9.71 Tubular adenoma. Low-power H&E image of tubular adenoma. The extreme left portion of the image contains normal colonic mucosa and the remainder of the darker glandular tissue is the (dysplastic) tubular adenoma. This image should be compared to Fig. 9.72, of a villous adenoma. The tubular adenoma is comprised of tubular forms of the dysplastic glands.

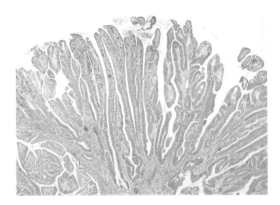

Fig. 9.72 Villous adenoma. Low-power H&E image of a dysplastic (adenomatous) epithelium with tall finger-like projections. The architecture is similar to the villi present in small bowel mucosa (Fig. 9.52), however, there are increased nuclear atypia and enlargement.

tubulovillous [66] based on the architecture of the polyp. Tubular lesions have crypt type architecture, while villous lesions mimic the finger-like projections (villi) found in the small bowel mucosa. Traditional teaching is that there is a higher risk of carcinoma in villous adenomas; however, this probably has more to do with the larger size of these lesions than the architecture seen. The degree of dysplasia (low and high-grade) can be designated; however, for an individual polyp it has no prognostic value and is not a feature upon which I typically comment [67]. These lesions can be polypoid (with a stalk) or sessile. Recently, flat (Fig. 9.73) and depressed adenomas [68] have been described. These had been thought to perhaps have a higher incidence of carcinoma in smaller lesions; however, this has not been confirmed by studies in the United States.

Serrated Lesions. Ten years ago serrated lesions were very simple. They we all hyperplastic polyps and were thought to be benign, no malignant potential. Histologically they have epithelial hyperplasia with a serrated (sawtooth) appearance. On cross-section the glands look like a starfish (Fig. 9.74). By definition these lesions should not have any dysplasia. Recently at least two subsets of these

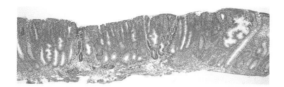

Fig. 9.73 Flat adenoma. Low-power H&E view of colonic mucosa with dysplastic epithelium. On the far right of the image there are a couple of normal crypts present. Unlike usual adenomatous polyps, there appears to be no protrusion of the dysplastic epithelium above the normal mucosa (the lesion appears flat, or even depressed).

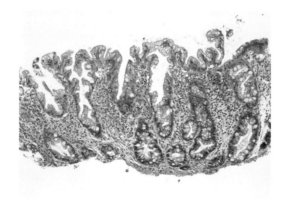

Fig. 9.74 Hyperplastic polyp. Medium-power H&E view of a typical hyperplastic polyp. There is an increased number of epithelial cells, giving a serrated (saw-like) appearance to the surface epithelium and into the crypts. There is no increase in the nuclear size (no dysplasia).

lesions have been described that appear to have a malignant potential [69]. These lesions are different from the typical adenomas from a histological and molecular standpoint. They appear to have a defect in the DNA mismatch repair genes, the same defect found in patients with hereditary non-polyposis colon cancer (HNPCC) and a minority of sporadic colon cancers [70]. This is in contrast with the typical dysplasia–carcinoma sequence that begins with defects in the APC gene for most adenomas and carcinomas (and familial adenomatous polyposis). The first lesion to be described was the serrated adenoma (Fig. 9.75). This lesion has the architecture of a hyperplastic polyp but with dysplastic nuclear changes. An additional distinct lesion called a sessile serrated adenoma (or sessile serrated polyp) (Fig. 9.76) has also been described without the nuclear dysplasia, but with more architectural changes than seen in the usual hyperplastic polyp (basal crypt dilatation and architectural distortion).

Mass lesions

The majority of mass lesions within the colon are adenocarcinomas (Fig. 9.77). One frustration for many endoscopists is that they will biopsy a mass lesion that they are certain is a carcinoma and the pathology report will just refer to an

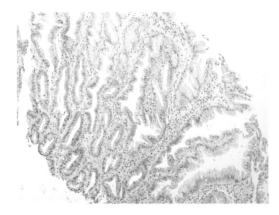

Fig. 9.75 Serrated adenoma. Medium-power H&E view of a lesion that has the architecture of the hyperplastic polyp (Fig. 9.74), but nuclear atypia and hyperplasia (dysplasia) typically seen in a tubular adenoma (Fig. 9.70).

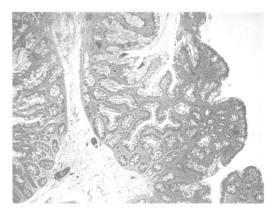

Fig. 9.76 Sessile serrated adenoma. Medium-power H&E view of a lesion with architecture of the hyperplastic polyp (Fig. 9.74), but more architectural distortion (dilatation of the basal glands and arrangement of the glands parallel to the muscularis propria). There should not be significant dysplasia (nuclear atypia) in contrast to a serrated adenoma (Fig. 9.75).

adenoma or use words such as 'invasion cannot be excluded'. Many biopsies of these lesions will just obtain tissue from the surface of the tumor or from the pre-existing adenoma often present at the edge of the lesion. The tissue obtained may not show the deeper invasive component of the cancer with its associated desmoplastic reaction. The endoscopist should realize that this is not an indication for a second endoscopy to obtain 'diagnostic material'. Regardless of the diagnosis (adenoma vs. invasive carcinoma), in a mass lesion the patient is most likely going to have the lesion resected. In truth the biopsy is really done to exclude a non-surgical etiology for the lesion, such as an infection or a lymphoma. Thus a diagnosis of adenoma in a mass lesion should be referred for excision (endoscopic or surgical).

Special stains

A number of special studies can be applied to tissue obtained for both histological and cytological evaluation. This includes histochemical stains, immunohistochemical stains, *in situ* hybridization, flow cytometry, molecular pathology, cytogenetics, and electron microscopy.

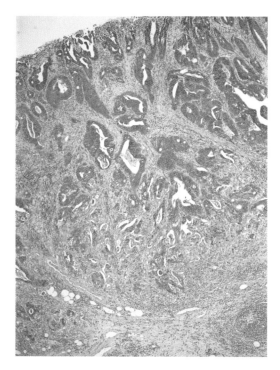

Fig. 9.77 Adenocarcinoma of the colon. Medium-power H&E view of a moderately differentiated invasive adenocarcinoma. The lesion is forming glands (best seen in the top of the image). At the base of the image, the glandular cells are infiltrating into the lamina propria. There is a characteristic desmoplastic response to the tumor, comprised of a fibroblastic response around the tumor cells.

Histochemical stains

These are the traditional stains used by pathologists for decades (H&E and Pap stains are examples). They essentially apply chemistry and chemical reactions to a slide to highlight types of tissue of interest.

Immunohistochemical stains

These are the application of antibodies to a specific protein with the use of some type of colorimetric (fluorescent or chromogen) reporter to a slide.

In situ hybridization

This is similar to immunohistochemical stains; however, instead of using antibodies, complementary DNA or RNA is used to identify a specific sequence on a slide.

Flow cytometry

In contrast to the techniques above, which are slide based, this involves measuring multiple characteristics of single cells in a moving fluid stream. Cell size, internal structures, antigens, DNA ploidy, and cell cycle can all be analyzed. It requires the specimen to be collected fresh or in a balanced media (RPMI) and run within 24 h of collection.

Electron microscopy

A technique that allows examination of intracellular architecture. It allows much higher magnification of individual cells and can be helpful in determining the type of tumor. It is rarely done due to the availability of immunohistochemical stains. These specimens should be fixed in glutaraldehyde fixative for optimum fixation.

Cytogenetics

In order to obtain a cytogenetic analysis one must grow the cells and get them to divide. Cytogenetics is essentially a gross evaluation of the chromosomes of the cells. It allows one to look for major molecular abnormalities such as deletions, translocations, and aneuploidy. Similar to flow cytometry, it requires fresh specimens. This technique is not currently in routine use.

Molecular pathology

This includes PCR and extraction of DNA for various analyses. It is typically best done on fresh tissue, but can be performed on formalin-fixed tissue. As the molecular bases of many diseases are becoming evident, this type of analysis is becoming more common.

Outstanding issues and future trends

Pathology continues to evolve. The integration of proteinomics and genomics will change the way we view pathology information, in terms of risk stratification and management for individual patients. Interestingly, the more we learn about the molecular changes present in both inflammatory and malignant diseases, the more they support the different phenotypic changes seen under the microscope by the pathologist.

An important parallel development is the increasing sophistication of enodoscopic imaging. Techniques such as zoom endoscopy, vital staining, narrow band imaging, confocal microscopy and endocytoscopy bring endoscopists ever closer to the dream of 'optical' biopsy, i.e. the ability to make a firm diagnosis without removing tissue [71]. A number of different techniques are resulting in images approaching the quality and resolution of unstained histological slides. The potential for added information from *in vivo* changes (as opposed to the static slide-based images a pathologist currently views) is very exciting. The traditional boundaries between radiologists, endoscopists, and pathologists are becoming blurred. Close collaboration will ensure that optimal diagnostic techniques will be developed and enter routine GI practice.

References

1 Lewin DN, Lewin KJ, Weinstein WM. Pathologist–gastroenterologist interaction: the changing role of the pathologist. *Am J Clin Pathol* 1995; 103 (4) (Suppl. 1): S9–12.

2 Dixon MF, Genta RM, Yardley JH *et al.* Classification and grading of gastritis: the updated Sydney System. International Workshop on the Histopathology of Gastritis, Houston 1994. *Am J Surg Pathol* 1996; 20 (10): 1161–81.

3 Lundell LR, Dent J, Bennett JR *et al.* Endoscopic assessment of oesophagitis: clinical and functional correlates and further validation of the Los Angeles classification. *Gut* 1999; 45 (2): 172–80.

4 Riddell RH, Goldman H, Ransahoff DF *et al.* Dysplasia in inflammatory bowel disease: standardized classification with provisional clinical applications. *Hum Pathol* 1983; 14 (11): 931–68.

5 Lauwers GY, Shimizu M, Correa P *et al.* Evaluation of gastric biopsies for neoplasia: differences between Japanese and Western pathologists. *Am J Surg Pathol* 1999; 23 (5): 511–18.

6 Theodossi A, Spiegelhalter DJ, Jass J *et al.* Observer variation and discriminatory value of biopsy features in inflammatory bowel disease. *Gut* 1994; 35 (7): 961–8.

7 Stamm B, Heer M, Buhler H *et al.* Mucosal biopsy of vascular ectasia (angiodysplasia) of the large bowel detected during routine colonoscopic examination. *Histopathology* 1985; 9 (6): 639–46.

8 Levine DS, Haggitt RC. Normal histology of the colon. *Am J Surg Pathol* 1989; 13 (11): 966–84.

9 Lazenby AJ, Yardley JH, Giardiello FM *et al.* Pitfalls in the diagnosis of collagenous colitis: experience with 75 cases from a registry of collagenous colitis at the Johns Hopkins Hospital. *Hum Pathol* 1990; 21 (9): 905–10.

10 Lewin KJ, Riddell RH, Weinstein WM (1992). Dialogue, handling of biopsies and resected specimens. *Gastrointestinal pathology and its clinical implications*, pp. 15–18. Igaku-Shoin, New York.

11 Driman DK, Preiksaitis HG. Colorectal inflammation and increased cell proliferation associated with oral sodium phosphate bowel preparation solution. *Hum Pathol* 1998; 29: 972–8.

12 Zwas FR, Cirillo NW, El-Serag HM *et al.* Colonic mucosal abnormalities associated with oral sodium phosphate solution. *Gastrointest Endosc* 1996; 43: 463–6.

13 Oh JK, Meiselman M, Lataif LE. Ischemic colitis caused by oral hyperosmotic saline laxatives. *Gastrointest Endosc* 1997: 319–22.

14 Pockros PJ, Foroozan P. Golytely lavage versus a standard colonoscopy preparation: effect on normal colonic mucosal histology. *Gastroenterology* 1985; 88 (2): 545–8.

15 Kliebeuker JH, Cats A, Zwart N *et al.* Excessively high cell proliferation in sigmoid colon after an oral purge with anthraquinone glycosides. *J Natl Cancer Inst* 1995; 87: 452–3.

16 Meisel JL, Bergman D, Graney D *et al.* Human rectal mucosa: proctoscopic and morphological changes caused by laxatives. *Gastroenterology* 1977: 1274–9.

17 Ji X, Shen M, Jeng Y *et al.* Diagnosis of mucosa-associated lymphoid tissue (MALT) lymphoma in gastroendoscopic biopsy specimens. *J Environ Pathol Toxicol Oncol* 1999; 18 (1): 61–3.

18 Woods KL, Anand BS, Cole RA *et al.* Influence of endoscopic biopsy forceps characteristics on tissue specimens: results of a prospective randomized study. *Gastrointest Endosc* 1999; 49 (2): 177–83.

19 Bernstein DE, Barkin JS, Reiner DK *et al.* Standard biopsy forceps versus large-capacity forceps with and without needle. *Gastrointest Endosc* 1995; 41 (6): 573–6.

20 Cooper HS, Deppisch LM, Gourley WK *et al.* Endoscopically removed malignant colorectal polyps: clinicopathologic correlations. *Gastroenterology* 1995; 108 (6): 1657–65.

21 Coverlizza S, Risio M, Ferrari A. *et al.* Colorectal adenomas containing invasive carcinoma: pathologic assessment of lymph node metastatic potential. *Cancer* 1989; 64 (9): 1937–47.
22 Masaki T, Muto T. Predictive value of histology at the invasive margin in the prognosis of early invasive colorectal carcinoma. *J Gastroenterol* 2000; 35 (3): 195–200.
23 Kondo H, Gotoda T, Ono H *et al.* Early gastric cancer: endoscopic mucosal resection. *Ann Ital Chir* 2001; 72 (1): 27–31.
24 Farmer KD, Harries SR, Fox BM *et al.* Core biopsy of the bowel wall: efficacy and safety in the clinical setting. *AJR Am J Roentgenol* 2000; 175 (6): 1627–30.
25 Varadarajulu S, Fraig M, Schmulewitz N *et al.* Comparison of EUS-guided 19-gauge Trucut needle biopsy with EUS-guided fine-needle aspiration. *Endoscopy* 2004; 36 (5): 397–401.
26 Smith MJ, Kini SR, Watson E. Fine needle aspiration and endoscopic brush cytology: comparison of direct smears and rinsings. *Acta Cytol* 1980; 24 (5): 456–9.
27 Young NA, Mody DR, Davey DD. Misinterpretation of normal cellular elements in fine-needle aspiration biopsy specimens: observations from the College of American Pathologists Interlaboratory Comparison Program in Non-Gynecologic Cytopathology. *Arch Pathol Lab Med* 2002; 126 (6): 670–5.
28 DeMay RM 1996 Fine needle aspiration biopsy. *The Art and Science of Cytopathology*, pp. 464–87. American Society for Clinical Pathology Press, Chicago.
29 Wallace MB, Kennedy T, Durkalski T *et al.* Randomized controlled trial of EUS-guided fine needle aspiration techniques for the detection of malignant lymphadenopathy. *Gastrointest Endosc* 2001; 54 (4): 441–7.
30 Williams DB, Sahai AV, Aabakken L *et al.* Endoscopic ultrasound guided fine needle aspiration biopsy: a large single centre experience. *Gut* 1999; 44 (5): 720–6.
31 Ismail-Beigi F, Horton PF, Pope CE. Histological consequences of gastroesophageal reflux in man. *Gastroenterology* 1970; 58 (2): 163–74.
32 Winter HS, Madara JL, Stafford RJ *et al.* Intraepithelial eosinophils: a new diagnostic criterion for reflux esophagitis. *Gastroenterology* 1982; 83 (4): 818–23.
33 Ahmad M, Soetikno RM, Ahmed A. The differential diagnosis of eosinophilic esophagitis. *J Clin Gastroenterol* 2000; 30 (3): 242–4.
34 Weinstein WM, Bogoch ER, Bowes KL. The normal human esophageal mucosa: a histological reappraisal. *Gastroenterology* 1975; 68 (1): 40–4.
35 Goldblum JR, Richter JE, Vaezi M *et al.* Helicobacter pylori infection, not gastroesophageal reflux, is the major cause of inflammation and intestinal metaplasia of gastric cardiac mucosa. *Am J Gastroenterol* 2002; 97 (2): 302–11.
36 Goldblum JR. The significance and etiology of intestinal metaplasia of the esophagogastric junction. *Ann Diagn Pathol* 2002; 6 (1): 67–73.
37 Gottfried MR, McClave SA, Boyce HW. Incomplete intestinal metaplasia in the diagnosis of columnar lined esophagus (Barrett's esophagus). *Am J Clin Pathol* 1989; 92 (6): 741–6.
38 Bonacini M, Young T, Laine L. Histopathology of human immunodeficiency virus-associated esophageal disease. *Am J Gastroenterol* 1993; 88 (4): 549–51.
39 Goodgame RW, Genta RM, Estrada R *et al.* Frequency of positive tests for cytomegalovirus in AIDS patients: endoscopic lesions compared with normal mucosa. *Am J Gastroenterol* 1993; 88 (3): 338–43.
40 Lal N, Bhasin DK, Malik AK *et al.* Optimal number of biopsy specimens in the diagnosis of carcinoma of the oesophagus. *Gut* 1992; 33 (6): 724–6.
41 El Zimaity HM, Genta RM, Graham DY. Histological features do not define NSAID-induced gastritis. *Hum Pathol* 1996; 27 (12): 1348–54.
42 Laine L, Lewin DN, Naritoku W *et al.* Prospective comparison of H & E, Giemsa, and Genta stains for the diagnosis of Helicobacter pylori. *Gastrointest Endosc* 1997; 45 (6): 463–7.
43 Chusid EL, Hirsch RL, Colcher H. Hypertrophic gastropathy: a clinical review. *Am J Gastroenterol* 1965; 43: 303–10.
44 Deppisch LM, Rona VT. Gastric epithelial polyps: a 10-year study. *J Clin Gastroenterol* 1989; 11 (1) (1989): 110–15.
45 Kreuning J, vd Wal AM, Kuiper G *et al.* Chronic nonspecific duodenitis: a multiple biopsy study of the duodenal bulb in health and disease. *Scand J Gastroenterol Suppl* 1989; 167: 16–20.

46 Hayat M, Cairns A, Dixon MF *et al*. Quantitation of intraepithelial lymphocytes in human duodenum: what is normal? *J Clin Pathol* 2002; 55 (5): 393–4.

47 Weinstein WM. Latent celiac sprue. *Gastroenterology* 1974; 66 (4): 489–93.

48 Dobbins WO, III. The diagnosis of Whipple's disease. *N Engl J Med* 1995; 332 (6): 390–2.

49 Roth RI, Owen RL, Keren DF *et al*. Intestinal infection with Mycobacterium avium in acquired immune deficiency syndrome (AIDS): histological and clinical comparison with Whipple's disease. *Dig Dis Sci* 1985; 30 (5): 497–504.

50 Brandborg LL, Tankersley CB, Gottieb S *et al*. Histological demonstration of mucosal invasion by Giardia lamblia in man. *Gastroenterology* 1967; 52 (2): 143–50.

51 Kreuning J, Bosman FT, Kuiper G *et al*. Gastric and duodenal mucosa in 'healthy' individuals: an endoscopic and histopathological study of 50 volunteers. *J Clin Pathol* 1978; 31 (1): 69–77.

52 Walk L. Nodular hyperplasia of duodenal Brunner's glands: does it exist? *Endoscopy* 1982; 14 (5): 162–5.

53 Jagelman DG, DeCosse JJ, Bussey HJ. Upper gastrointestinal cancer in familial adenomatous polyposis. *Lancet* 1988; 1 (8595): 1149–51.

54 Taggart DP, Imrie CW. A new pattern of histologic predominance and distribution of malignant diseases of the small intestine. *Surg Gynecol Obstet* 1987; 165 (6): 515–18.

55 Patel Y, Pettigrew NM, Grahame GR *et al*. The diagnostic yield of lower endoscopy plus biopsy in nonbloody diarrhea. *Gastrointest Endosc* 1997; 46 (4): 338–43.

56 Goff JS, Barnett JL, Pelke T *et al*. Collagenous colitis: histopathology and clinical course. *Am J Gastroenterol* 1997; 92 (1): 57–60.

57 Lazenby AJ, Yardley JH, Giardiello FM *et al*. Lymphocytic ('microscopic') colitis: a comparative histopathologic study with particular reference to collagenous colitis. *Hum Pathol* 1989; 20 (1): 18–28.

58 Offner FA, Jao FV, Lewin KJ *et al*. Collagenous colitis: a study of the distribution of morphological abnormalities and their histological detection. *Hum Pathol* 1999; 30 (4): 451–7.

59 Nostrant TT, Kumar NB, Appelman HD. Histopathology differentiates acute self-limited colitis from ulcerative colitis. *Gastroenterology* 1987; 92 (2): 318–28.

60 Bernstein CN, Shanahan F, Weinstein WM. Histological patchiness and sparing of the rectum in ulcerative colitis: refuting the dogma. *J Clin Pathol* 1997; 50 (4): 354–5.

61 Kleer CG, Appelman HD. Ulcerative colitis: patterns of involvement in colorectal biopsies and changes with time. *Am J Surg Pathol* 1998; 22 (8): 983–9.

62 Levine TS, Tzardi M, Mitchell S *et al*. Diagnostic difficulty arising from rectal recovery in ulcerative colitis. *J Clin Pathol* 1996; 49 (4): 319–23.

63 Odze R, Antonioli D, Peppercorn M *et al*. Effect of topical 5-aminosalicylic acid (5-ASA) therapy on rectal mucosal biopsy morphology in chronic ulcerative colitis. *Am J Surg Pathol* 1993; 17 (9): 869–75.

64 Dignan CR, Greenson JK. Can ischemic colitis be differentiated from C difficile colitis in biopsy specimens? *Am J Surg Pathol* 1997; 21 (6): 706–10.

65 Winawer SJ, Zauber AG, Ho MN *et al*. Prevention of colorectal cancer by colonoscopic polypectomy. The National Polyp Study Workgroup. *N Engl J Med* 1993; 329 (27): 1977–81.

66 Rubio CA. Colorectal adenomas: time for reappraisal. *Pathol Res Pract* 2002; 198 (9): 615–20.

67 Terry MB, Neugut AI, Bostick RM *et al*. Reliability in the classification of advanced colorectal adenomas. *Cancer Epidemiol Biomarkers Prev* 2002; 11 (7): 660–3.

68 Yao T, Tada S, Tsuneyoshi M. Colorectal counterpart of gastric depressed adenoma: a comparison with flat and polypoid adenomas with special reference to the development of pericryptal fibroblasts. *Am J Surg Pathol* 1994; 18 (6): 559–68.

69 Longacre TA, Fenoglio-Preiser CM. Mixed hyperplastic adenomatous polyps/serrated adenomas: a distinct form of colorectal neoplasia. *Am J Surg Pathol* 1990; 14 (6): 524–37.

70 Li SC, Burgart, L. Histopathology of serrated adenoma, its variants and differentiation from conventional adenomatous and hyperplastic polyps Arch Pathol Lab Med 2007; 131 (3): 440–5.

71 Nishioka NS. Optical biopsy using tissue spectroscopy and optical coherence tomography. *Can J Gastroenterol* 2003; 17 (6): 376–80.

CHAPTER 10

Pediatric gastrointestinal endoscopy

JONATHAN S. EVANS AND LORI MAHAJAN

Synopsis

The pediatric patient is different from the adult one not only in terms of his or her constitutional make-up but also in terms of the pathologies encountered. Although many of the basic principles and techniques are similar, the differences and needs are such that pediatric endoscopy has evolved into a specialized discipline unto itself. This relatively new discipline requires pediatric-specific training, instrumentation, and knowledge in order to accomplish procedures that are safe, comfortable, and ultimately of benefit to the child's well-being.

Introduction

Thirteen years after the introduction of the fiberoptic gastroscope by Basil Hirshowitz in 1957 [1] the first reports of flexible gastrointestinal endoscopy in children were published [2–6]. The earliest pediatric endoscopes were either ill-adapted to children or to the gastrointestinal tract itself (e.g. small caliber bronchoscopes). Since that period, an extraordinary evolution has occurred with the advent of progressively thinner and more flexible pediatric-dedicated instruments. Current technology permits safe visualization, tissue sampling, and therapeutic interventions of the upper and lower gastrointestinal tracts in even preterm newborns. It has transformed the practice of pediatric gastroenterology.

The old adage 'children are not small adults' applies especially to the field of pediatric gastroenterology. The pediatric patient must be viewed as an evolving, dynamic patient in terms of anatomy, physiology, and psychological make-up. In addition, pediatric gastroenterologists must be familiar with the multitude of congenital and acquired anomalies not seen in adult practice. This chapter will highlight the differences between the worlds of adult and pediatric endoscopy. It is organized under four major topics:
- the endoscopy facility and personnel;
- the pediatric patient and procedural preparation;

- endoscopic procedures currently performed in pediatric patients;
- selected gastrointestinal pathologies in pediatric patients.

The endoscopy facility and personnel

Endoscopy facility

Proper care of pediatric patients requires a child-friendly environment and medical personnel specifically trained in the care of children and adolescents. Pediatric endoscopic procedures, like those performed in adult patients, are routinely performed in a variety of locations. In dedicated pediatric procedural suites and in procedural units shared with adult colleagues, the safe and efficient flow of patients should be assured through the careful organization of the structure and function of these areas. This information, specific to each facility, should be detailed in a policy and procedures manual.

The pediatric endoscopist may also be called to patient areas that are not primarily designed for endoscopy, such as the neonatal or pediatric intensive care units. In these instances, a mobile cart with the necessary equipment, including an endoscope of the appropriate size, a light source and monitor, and a complete panoply of diagnostic and therapeutic instruments together with their generating units (e.g. electrocautery unit), is necessary. The procedure and patient monitoring should be conducted no differently than in a dedicated endoscopy unit.

Equipment

Endoscopes

The design of gastrointestinal endoscopes continues to evolve, with video-endoscopes now largely supplanting their older fiberoptic counterparts. Video technology has brought about impressive advances in the field of optics, and innovations such as zoom technology and image processing. The three major manufacturers (Olympus, Fujinon, and Pentax) have pediatric product lines with similar characteristics. Each provides brilliant, high-resolution color views of the gastrointestinal mucosa through a wide angle. The depth of view ranges from 5 to 100 mm, with nearly a 30-fold magnification of the mucosa. Depending on the manufacturer, smaller-sized duodenoscopes, enteroscopes, and variable-stiffness colonoscopes can be found. Olympus recently introduced the EVIS EXERA II™ 180 platform of gastroscopes and colonoscopes which deliver both high-definition and narrow band imaging technologies. This provides the gastroenterologist with enhanced observation capabilities of the mucosal morphology and capillary pattern. The colonoscopes offer a panoramic 170-degree field of view, which not only enhances observation, but also possibly reduces hand and wrist fatigue related to manipulation of the scope. In addition, adult therapeutic (two-channel) gastroscopes and 'zoom' gastroscopes allowing magnification (up to 150×) of the mucosal image have occasional applications in children.

For most pediatric gastroenterologists, the instrument chosen to perform an endoscopic procedure is based upon personal preference, clinical experience, and level of comfort for both the patient and endoscopist alike. Outer tip diameter and working channel diameter are the two specifications that are of greatest importance in the selection of an endoscope for the smaller child. Outer tip diameters currently range from 5.0 to 12.8 mm in gastroscopes and 11.3 to 13.3 mm in colonoscopes and sigmoidoscopes. Working channel diameters range from 2.0 mm in the slimmest instruments (generally less than 5.9 mm outer diameter) up to 4.2 mm for the largest adult therapeutic endoscopes. Published guidelines for the choice of the appropriate-sized endoscope for a child based on size are few [7,8], perhaps because issues other than size need to be considered. These may include the weight and height of the child, indications for the procedure, and the type of sedation used. For example, a 5 mm gastroscope, passed through a pacifier, has been used in minimally sedated nursing infants by the authors, while we have also used adult-sized endoscopes in ventilated infants (over 6 kg) for therapeutic procedures such as foreign body removal.

Some authors feel that an adult colonoscope may be safely used in patients as small as 15 kg [9]. Because the external diameter of most adult colonoscopes ranges between 13 and 14 mm and they are significantly stiffer than pediatric instruments, they must be used with extreme caution in young patients to minimize the risk of colonic laceration or perforation. Several years ago, Olympus introduced a colonoscope with variable stiffness of the insertion tube, the PCF 160 AI/L. The stiffness of the colonoscope may be adjusted during the procedure by turning a dial on the upper portion of the shaft. This has been shown to decrease looping in the sigmoid and transverse colon upon insertion; however, stiffening of the colonoscope should be performed with caution [10]. Pediatric or adult gastroscopes with outer diameters ranging from 6 to 9 mm may also be substituted for standard colonoscopes for colonoscopy in smaller patients.

Endoscopy accessories

Adult endoscopic instruments are appropriate for children if an adult-sized endoscope is being used. Many of these instruments have been redesigned to pass through the smaller diameter (2.0 mm) working channels of the infant-sized endoscopes. These 5F-sized instruments include: biopsy forceps, grasping forceps (e.g. rat-toothed, 'penny pinchers', alligator, etc.), polypectomy snares, injection catheters, baskets, cautery probes (for argon plasma coagulation), and dilation guidewires. Currently lacking are band ligation devices, electrocautery probes, balloon dilators, and foreign body hoods.

Ancillary equipment

In addition to the necessary light sources, monitors, mobile carts, and monitoring equipment, many endoscopy units have access to software allowing image processing and electronic reporting of the endoscopic procedure. Photo-documentation of the procedure can be helpful from both a clinical and liability standpoint, and whenever possible should be appended to the endoscopic record. Software allowing reporting of an electronic endoscopic record is now available from both commercial and non-commercial sources. In particular, PEDS-CORI (www.peds-cori.org) is a non-commercial venture that supplies an electronic pediatric endoscopy-report software program in exchange for collecting outcomes data on endoscopic procedures in children. This banking of information is allowing important outcome studies to be performed. Regardless of the source, these programs should allow accurate and complete recording of the procedure as well as generate data for billing and quality improvement purposes. It is imperative that they be adapted to the pediatric practice.

Personnel

The endoscopist

'Endoscopy in children requires appropriate cognitive and technical skills necessary to diagnose and treat disorders of the gastrointestinal tract, liver and pancreas' [11]. Professional societies in both Europe and North America have set forth processes that will allow trainees in pediatric gastroenterology to acquire these skills [11,12]. These processes assume competence in general pediatrics and completion of a fellowship in which two levels of endoscopic competency can be achieved: basic and advanced. Minimum numbers of supervised procedures have been described and procedural proficiency tools are currently under development to help the trainee achieve competency. Guidelines for the maintenance of acquired skills and development of new skills beyond training are also being discussed.

Pediatric practice guidelines have also been issued for adult endoscopists [13]. Adult endoscopists may be called upon by pediatric primary care providers to render basic services when a pediatric gastroenterologist is not available, or to provide advanced services not routinely performed by a pediatric gastroenterologist (e.g. ERCP). Although the indications for endoscopy in children may be similar to those for adults, a team approach is recommended whenever possible to avoid potentially unnecessary or even deleterious procedures.

Any gastroenterologist performing pediatric procedures should have thorough knowledge of the pediatric airway and be certified in PALS (Pediatric Advanced Life Support, offered by the American Heart Association/American Academy of Pediatrics) unless assisted by a qualified anesthesiologist.

Nursing and ancillary personnel

Nurses and endoscopy technicians play an integral role in pediatric endoscopy. They must be specifically trained and comfortable in the field of endoscopy and in meeting the needs of children. In addition, they must be adept at communicating with families and patients, with specific attention to the developmental and cognitive levels of the latter. Safe and efficient endoscopy, when utilizing conscious sedation, is best performed with the help of two assistants. One assistant monitors the patient during the procedure while the other assists the endoscopist with tissue sampling and therapeutic interventions. The assistant assigned to monitoring the patient continually assesses the patient's vital signs and comfort level, can physically and emotionally provide support for the patient, monitors patient positioning, and can give the endoscopist periodic updates on the patient's degree of abdominal distension. When general anesthesia is employed, only one endoscopy assistant is usually necessary to assist with biopsies and therapeutic interventions.

Most institutions require that nursing personnel involved in sedated pediatric procedures maintain skills and certification in PALS (see above). These highly specialized procedural nurses now have their own professional organizations through which more information can be obtained (www.naspgn.org/sub/apgnn.asp and www.sgna.org).

The pediatric patient and procedural preparation

Patient preparation

Preparation of the pediatric patient for an endoscopic procedure requires two equally important components: psychological preparation and medical preparation.

Psychological preparation

It has been well demonstrated that appropriate preparation prior to an endoscopic procedure will reduce patient distress and anxiety, thereby reducing overall use of sedative medications and enhancing patient safety [14,15]. Information regarding the need for the procedure, how and where it will be performed, and the process of recovery is given to both the patient and parents. Information given should be honest and accurate, and that communicated to the child should be done in a sensitive manner appropriate to his or her developmental level. Ideally, this is done by the endoscopist well in advance of the procedure and away from the procedural unit.

Often, innovative techniques are used to help prepare the child. For example, placement of an IV catheter for sedation is especially anxiogenic for children [14]. It may be reduced by using a preprocedural nursing unit where the catheter is placed by skilled pediatric phlebotomists after application of a topical anesthetic such as EMLA™. Furthermore, a 'cooling off' period after the IV has been placed has been found to be helpful. Additional techniques used to reduce preprocedural anxiety include the use of illustrative pictures and dolls, preparatory videos, diagrams, visits to the endoscopy suite, and distribution of written materials. Explanatory pamphlets can be downloaded from www.NASPGHAN.org and many pediatric units have produced their own personalized guides. These approaches require additional time, effort, and personnel but are ultimately found to be helpful.

Medical preparation

This begins with a careful history, physical examination, and assessment of patient ASA classification [16] (Table 10.1). These will determine the type of procedure needed, its appropriateness, procedure location (e.g. operating or endoscopy suite), personnel and equipment support needed, and level of sedation required. In addition, laboratory assays, imaging tests, and assessment of parental or patient expectations may be helpful in making these decisions.

Recommendations for fasting. The need for preprocedural fasting continues to be an evolving issue. Traditionally, and based upon little data, children

Table 10.1 ASA physical classification status system

ASA class	Status
1	Normal healthy patient
2	Patient with mild systemic disease
3	Patient with severe systemic disease
4	Patient with severe systemic disease that is a constant threat to life
5	Moribund patient not expected to survive without operation

ASA, American Society of Anesthesiologists.

Table 10.2 Preprocedure fasting guidelines

Ingested material	Minimum fasting period (h)
Clear liquids	2
Breast milk	4
Infant formula	6
Non-human milk	6
Light meal	6

Adapted from American Society of Anesthesiologists task force on sedation and analgesia by non-anesthesiologists. Practice guidelines for sedation and analgesia by non-anesthesiologists. *Anesthesiology* 2002; 96: 1004–17.[Ref 20]

undergoing a sedated endoscopic procedure have been required to fast for a minimum of 8 h. This practice is uncomfortable for infants, young children, and parents alike. It can also lead to dehydration in very young infants and hypoglycemic events in children with underlying metabolic disorders. A body of evidence now supports more lenient fasting guidelines [17–19] and is supported by the American Society of Anesthesiologists [20] (Table 10.2). These guidelines should be followed for any child who is to receive sedation and/or undergo an esophagogastroduodenoscopy (EGD).

Bowel preparation. Bowel preparation for lower intestinal endoscopy has been well standardized for adults [21]. It is usually based upon a large volume lavage with oral polyethylene glycol (PEG) in an electrolyte-balanced solution. Pediatric gastroenterologists have long recognized that these protocols fail miserably in most children due to the poor taste and large volumes of solution required. Some children may be hospitalized and a nasogastric tube placed for instillation, but this adds an extra degree of cost and discomfort that is most often unacceptable. Consequently, most institutions use a variety of agents combined into 'home-grown recipes' (Tables 10.3, 10.4). Few of these have been studied and compared. Consensus on the best colonic lavage preparations in pediatric patients has yet to be reached [22–25].

Antibiotic prophylaxis. The American Heart Association and the American Society for Gastrointestinal Endoscopy have published guidelines for antibiotic prophylaxis prior to endoscopic procedures [26]. The overall risk of bacterial endocarditis as a direct result of an endoscopic procedure is small. Transient bacteremia may occur during or immediately following endoscopy, however, the organisms typically identified are unlikely to cause endocarditis. The rate of

Table 10.3 Common cathartic agents, used alone or in combination, for preparation of children for lower bowel endoscopy

Agent	Brand name	Dose*
Clear liquids		
PEG balanced electrolyte solution	Golytely, Nulytely	20 ml/kg/h (max 1 l/h) till clear
PEG unbalanced solution	Miralax	0–17.5 gm PO BID × 1–2 days
Magnesium citrate		2–4 ml/kg PO BID; max 300 ml
Milk of magnesia		5–30 ml PO BID × 1–2 days
Bisacodyl	Dulcolax	5–15 mg PO/PR × 1–2 days
Oral sodium phosphate	Fleets Phospho Soda	15–45 cc PO × 1–2 doses
Rectal sodium phosphate	Fleets Enema (adult)	1 PR × 1–2 doses q 12–24 h

* Suggested doses, which should be adjusted based upon age, size, comorbidities, etc.

Table 10.4 Example of a colonoscopy prep for a child aged 6 years*

2–3 days before the procedure	Milk of magnesia 1 TBS PO BID
36 h before the procedure	Clear liquid diet
Evening before the procedure	Magnesium Citrate followed by 2–3 glasses of clear fluids
4–6 h before the procedure	NPO

* Other regimen examples can be found in Refs 23 and 24.

bacteremia associated with routine upper endoscopy, colonoscopy, or sigmoidoscopy is between 2 and 5%, and does not increase with mucosal biopsy or polypectomy. Thus, endocarditis prophylaxis is not routinely recommended for 'negligible risk' patients undergoing these endoscopic procedures with or without mucosal biopsy and/or polypectomy. In addition, antibiotics are not recommended for immunocompromised patients or those with pacemakers or prosthetic joints. Other endoscopic procedures such as varix sclerosis, stricture dilation, and ERCP can be associated with bacteremia in up to 45% [27]. High-risk patients include those with prosthetic heart valves, a prior history of endocarditis, a surgically constructed or congenital systemic–pulmonary shunt, or a synthetic vascular graft that is less than 1 year old. These patients should receive antibiotic prophylaxis prior to all endoscopic procedures associated with increased risk of bacteremia, as mentioned. In these patients, however, there are not sufficient data to make recommendations regarding antibiotic prophylaxis prior to routine endoscopy with mucosal biopsy or polypectomy, and the decision is left with the patient's endoscopist and cardiologist, to decide on a case-by-case basis.

Recommended antibiotics and dosages for bacterial endocarditis prophylaxis are as follows: ampicillin 50 mg/kg IM/IV (not to exceed 2.0 g) and gentamicin 1.5 mg/kg IV/IM (not to exceed 120 mg), given 30 min prior to the procedure; 6 h later, ampicillin 25 mg/kg IM/IV or amoxicillin 25 mg/kg po is given. If the patient is penicillin-allergic, vancomycin is administered in place of the ampicillin and is used in combination with the aforementioned dose of gentamicin. Vancomycin 20 mg/kg IV (not to exceed 1 g) is administered over 1–2 h and completed within 30 min of starting the endoscopic procedure [26].

It should also be noted that all children undergoing percutaneous endoscopic gastrostomy tube placement should be given prophylactic antibiotics to decrease the risk of soft tissue infection from skin pathogens.

Informed consent

As with other invasive procedures, it is mandatory to obtain informed consent prior to endoscopic procedures in pediatric patients according to institutional guidelines. If the patient is under the age of 18 years, the custodial parent or legal guardian must render the informed consent. Although they are unable to provide informed consent, the procedure should also be explained to the patient in an age-appropriate manner.

Endoscopic procedures currently performed in pediatric patients

Indications and limitations

Indications for gastrointestinal endoscopy and colonoscopy in pediatric patients are summarized in Tables 10.5 and 10.6. They are adapted from a 1996 medical position statement issued by NASPGHAN (North American Society for Pediatric Gastroenterology, Hepatology and Nutrition) [28]. The primary indications for upper endoscopy in pediatric patients include evaluation of gastrointestinal bleeding, recurrent epigastric pain, nausea or vomiting, feeding or growth abnormalities, and caustic or foreign body ingestion. Additional indications are listed in Table 10.5.

The primary indications for colonoscopy in pediatric patients include gastrointestinal blood loss, unexplained chronic diarrhea, abdominal pain with systemic symptoms suspicious for inflammatory bowel disease (IBD), and dysplasia screening in patients with IBD or polyposis syndromes. Additional indications are listed in Table 10.6.

In contrast to adult patients, colonoscopy is typically not indicated in the pediatric patient with constipation or chronic abdominal pain without other

Table 10.5 Indications for pediatric upper gastrointestinal endoscopy

Diagnostic
- Caustic ingestion
- Chest pain
- Dysphagia or odynophagia
- Early satiety or anorexia with weight loss
- Food refusal
- Gastrointestinal blood loss
- Iron deficiency anemia
- Nausea or persistent vomiting
- Persistent or recurrent dyspepsia or heartburn
- Tissue/fluid sampling
- Epigastric pain
- Evaluation of imaging abnormality

Periodic/Surveillance
- Barrett's esophagus
- Familial adenomatous polyposis syndrome
- Gardener's syndrome
- Grading of varices
- Hereditary flat adenoma syndrome
- Intestinal transplantation
- Polyposis syndromes
- Selected mucosal disease
- Selected ulcers

Therapeutic
- Enteral or feeding tube placement or change
- Foreign body removal
- Injection therapy: Botulinum toxin, corticosteroid, sclerosants
- Variceal ligation
- Pneumatic dilation
- Polypectomy
- Stricture dilation
- Control of bleeding: injection, cautery, 'clip' placement

clinical 'red flags' in the history, examination, or laboratory findings, or a 'change in bowel habits', as the incidence of colorectal cancer is exceedingly low in children without underlying predisposing conditions. In addition, a follow-up colonoscopy is not indicated for an asymptomatic pediatric patient found to have fewer than five juvenile polyps.

Absolute and relative contraindications for both upper and lower endoscopies are listed in Tables 10.7 and 10.8, respectively. It should be noted that

Table 10.6 Indications for pediatric lower gastrointestinal endoscopy

Diagnostic
- Chronic diarrhea
- Evaluation of imaging abnormality
- Gastrointestinal blood loss
- Intraoperative lesion localization
- Iron deficiency anemia
- Marking a lesion for surgical localization
- Placement of motility catheter
- Suspected inflammatory bowel disease (diagnosis/determination of extent of disease)
- Tissue/fluid sampling

Periodic/Surveillance
- Determination of response to IBD therapy
- Dysplasia/malignancy
- Intestinal transplantation

Therapeutic
- Control of bleeding (persistent): injection, cautery, 'clip' placement
- Foreign body removal
- Placement of percutaneous cecostomy
- Polypectomy
- Sigmoid volvulus/intussusception reduction
- Stricture dilation

Table 10.7 Contraindications to EGD in pediatric patients

- Partial or complete intestinal obstruction
- Peritonitis
- Recent bowel surgery
- Severe injury to hypopharynx
- Severe shock or respiratory distress
- Suspected perforation
- Uncooperative patient
- Uncorrected bleeding diathesis

children with connective tissue disorders such as Ehler–Danlos syndrome are at increased risk of perforation [29]. Endoscopy should always be avoided when similar results can be obtained in a less invasive manner. Although not contraindicated, endoscopy is generally not helpful in patients with hypertrophic pyloric stenosis or uncomplicated gastroesophageal reflux disease, or for pre-emptive control of varices prior to the first episode of bleeding. Similarly,

Table 10.8 Contraindications to colonoscopy in pediatric patients

Absolute
- Peritonitis
- Suspected bowel perforation

Relative
- Cardiovascular instability
- Massive colonic bleeding
- Neutropenia/suspected typhlitis
- Partial or complete intestinal obstruction
- Poor bowel preparation
- Recent bowel surgery
- Toxic megacolon
- Uncorrected bleeding diathesis

colonoscopy is not indicated in the setting of acute self-limited diarrhea and may only serve to confuse the clinical picture.

The main limitation in pediatric endoscopy continues to be size, both as it relates to the patient and to instrumentation. As manufacturers continue to develop smaller and smaller endoscopes and their associated instruments, neonatal endoscopic pathology is being described with increasing frequency [30–33]. Gastroscopes with an outer diameter of 5.0 mm have been used for diagnostic endoscopy in children weighing 900 g [32], and for percutaneous endoscopic gastrostomy (PEG) placement in children approaching 2100 g (personal experience, JSE).

Patient sedation

In pediatric patients, the need for an endoscopic procedure is often synonymous with the need for sedation. The patient-specific goals of sedation include anxiolysis, analgesia, and amnesia for the procedure. Endoscopist-specific goals for sedation include patient safety, adequate endoscopic examination and therapeutic intervention, equipment safety, time efficiency, and patient cost [34]. As the types and complexity of pediatric endoscopic procedures have increased, the type of sedation (general anesthesia, deep, moderate, and mild sedation) has become a more complex issue for the pediatric gastroenterologist [35].

The best method for achieving procedural sedation remains the subject of ongoing debates and is under constant evolution. This is perhaps due to the variety of sedation modalities available, and the complexity and number of

Table 10.9 Factors other than medications needing consideration in choosing an appropriate sedation protocol

Patient-related
- Age
- Level of maturity
- Past experiences
- Underlying condition
- Comorbidities

Endoscopist-related
- Level and type of sedation training
- Past experience
- Efficiency

Procedure-related
- Type (e.g. EGD vs. ERCP)
- Complexity (e.g. diagnostic vs. therapeutic)
- Duration

Institution-related
- Site (e.g. OR vs. outpatient GI suite)
- Availability of nursing and ancillary personnel
- Policy (e.g. JCAHO-mandated protocols)

issues that need to be taken into consideration when choosing the most appropriate sedation protocol (Table 10.9).

Occasionally, no sedation is administered to pediatric patients undergoing endoscopic procedures. Sedation has traditionally been withheld in very young infants undergoing upper endoscopy, perhaps due to our poor knowledge base of the pharmacokinetics of sedative agents in these patients. This position is becoming increasingly hard to defend [36,37]. Sedation practices in the very young are changing, but require further study [38].

Recently, unsedated upper endoscopies were studied in 21 motivated and consenting children over 8 years of age with good outcomes in terms of tolerance and safety [39]. These patients, however, constituted a very small proportion of the total patients undergoing EGD in that institution. Most pediatric gastroenterologists recognize other instances when sedation may not be required (e.g. small infants or mature children undergoing flexible sigmoidoscopy).

The use of sedation and analgesia, however, remains the norm for most pediatric endoscopic procedures. The choice of an appropriate sedation protocol is complex and takes into account the patient's age, maturity level, disease state, the type and expected duration of the procedure, the risks and benefits of each sedation protocol, and the wishes of the patient and patient's family.

Other important issues that enter the decision-making process are outlined in Table 10.9. Consequently, pediatric endoscopists must remain knowledgeable and flexible in their abilities to design different sedation protocols that will meet the many needs of their patients.

A variety of agents can be used by physicians trained in their administration. These physicians should be competent in dose titration to achieve the expected level of sedation, the monitoring of pediatric patients, and the ability to recognize and treat complications as they arise. The choice of appropriate agents should take into account their ability to provide sedation, analgesia, and amnesia. Detailed descriptions of these agents and guidelines for their use go beyond the scope of this chapter and have been well described elsewhere [16,35].

Most endoscopists will use the combination of a narcotic (e.g. fentanyl or meperidine) and a benzodiazepine (e.g. midazolam) to achieve a state of moderate sedation. Over the past several years, 'non-traditional' agents for pediatric endoscopy have been increasingly used, including propofol [40,41], ketamine [42,43], and sevoflurane [44]. Although effective, they often achieve deep sedative states or can be responsible for specific airway issues requiring monitored anesthesia care for safe usage.

Endoscopic technique

The overall technique of pediatric endoscopy is similar to that used in adults, but significant differences exist and must be kept in mind. The following is not intended to be an in-depth description of pediatric endoscopic technique, as excellent descriptions can be found elsewhere [9,45]. Rather, it will highlight the differences between pediatric and adult practice. The reader is reminded that any written description of endoscopic technique can only complement and should not replace a hands-on, well-mentored training program.

Esophagogastroduodenoscopy

Esophagogastroduodenoscopy (EGD) is the most common endoscopic procedure performed by pediatric gastroenterologists. In experienced hands, pediatric upper endoscopy is a safe and minimally invasive procedure. As in adults, EGD in children is often an outpatient procedure and typically takes 15–20 min to complete, depending on procedural findings. The advent of ultra-thin endoscopes, such as the Olympus N30 endoscope with an external diameter of 5.3 mm, allows examination of premature infants as small as 1.5 kg [46].

Preparation for upper endoscopy may differ somewhat in infants. Bite blocks are usually not required in edentulous infants. Nursing infants may use the endoscope itself as a pacifier or the instrument may be passed through a formula bottle nipple in which the tip has been cut away. Also, it has been our practice to avoid the use of topical anesthetic sprays in the pharynx of young infants. We have found its application distressing and usually not worth the small benefit.

Intubation of the esophagus under direct visualization is preferred over blind intubation. It is more comfortable in children receiving moderate levels of sedation but importantly, allows examination of the hypopharyngeal structures to look for signs of gastroesophageal reflux disease, foreign bodies, and laryngeal malformations.

Applying a short puff of air to the hypopharynx may facilitate intubation. This will often produce a cough followed by a swallow which opens the esophageal introitus. The esophagus, from the cricopharyngeus to the thoracic inlet, is narrow and difficult to examine, especially in infants. It is the most frequent site of foreign body entrapment. The distance in centimeters from the gum line to the gastroesophageal junction should be noted in addition to the location of the gastric Z-line in relation to the gastroesophageal junction.

After aspiration of gastric secretions and insufflation until there is near complete effacement of the gastric rugae, the endoscope is advanced through the body of the stomach and into the antrum, carefully observing the mucosa. It should be noted that the junction between the body and antrum, forming the incisura, often makes a more acute angulation than in adults and requires filling the greater curvature of the stomach with the endoscope to allow passage. This places some degree of pressure on the greater curvature that the patient may experience as discomfort.

Retroflexion views of the cardioesophageal junction are a necessary component of the procedure but often difficult in small children, especially when a larger endoscope is used. This maneuver, which can also be performed after examination of the duodenum, requires withdrawal of the tip to the incisura. The up-dial is then turned maximally, often combined with either action of the right/left dial and/or torquing of the instrument. The tip is then withdrawn proximally with frequent twisting of the instrument to provide 360° views of the cardioesophageal junction.

Passage through the pylorus should not be forceful as it will cause the tip of the endoscope to abruptly abut against the distal wall of the duodenal bulb, placing the pediatric patient at increased risk of duodenal hematoma or perforation. This is due to the relatively short pediatric bulb and release of tension on the endoscope that was caused by loading of the greater curvature. After examination of the bulb, the endoscope is passed into the second portion of the duodenum using the same maneuvers as for an adult. Greater care should be taken, however, due to the exiguity of this area. The distal duodenum can then be examined using a straightening maneuver (i.e. a short withdrawal of the endoscope resulting in a paradoxical advancement of the tip).

Biopsies are usually taken upon withdrawal of the instrument. The quality of tissue for histologic evaluation is determined by the size of the biopsy specimen and the choice of location for collection [47,48]. In general the largest possible biopsy forceps for the working channel is chosen. The choice of location for biopsy collection is more problematic. Biopsies should be taken in areas that are visually abnormal or in areas where a suspected diagnosis is most likely to be found (e.g. proximal esophagus in suspected eosinophilic esophagitis).

Even when the procedure is visually normal, it is still advisable to obtain biopsies to confirm normality at a histologic level. In these instances it has been recommended that samples be obtained from the distal duodenum, antrum, or prepyloric area, the body of the stomach along the greater curvature, and in the distal esophagus 2–5 cm above the Z-line [47].

Pediatric gastroenterologists tend to be generally more liberal with mucosal biopsies due to poor correlation between endoscopic and histological abnormalities [49,50]. For example, it is routine to biopsy the distal duodenum in pediatric patients to rule out celiac disease, as creases or notches in the valvulae conniventes are oftentimes not apparent until adolescence.

Upon withdrawal from the stomach, remaining gastric air should be aspirated to facilitate breathing and prevent gaseous discomfort. At the conclusion of the procedure, the abdomen should be manually examined for excessive distension, crepitus, or tenderness.

Colonoscopy

Understanding the anatomy of the colon and its potential variations is essential for repeated performance of safe and efficient colonoscopic examinations. The degree of difficulty encountered during the examination is in large part determined during fetal development. In 15% of individuals, the ascending and descending colon do not become fixed retroperitoneally in the paravertebral gutters. Instead, they remain free on mesocolons identical to those that are normal for the transverse and sigmoid colon [51]. This results in a potentially mobile colon that may move unpredictably within the abdomen during the procedure. Such anatomy may promote loop formation.

The thickness of the colonic wall and the length of the colon are also key considerations during colonoscopy. The colonic wall is extremely thin, varying in thickness from only 1.7 to 2.2 mm. At birth, the colonic length measures approximately 50 cm, reaching a typical adult length of 90–120 cm in late adolescence.

During colonoscopy to the cecum, this translates into an instrument insertion length of 40–50 cm in young children and 60–80 cm in adolescents and adults once all loops have been successfully removed. Careful monitoring of insertion depth throughout the procedure is even more important in pediatric gastroenterology, especially since the introduction of longer instruments. An insertion length that is significantly beyond the expected colonic length typically signals the presence of a large loop, which may increase the risk of colonic perforation.

Prior to starting the procedure, the height of the examination table should be positioned at the waist level of the endoscopist to optimize control of the colonoscope. In addition, some pediatric patients may require the ambient room temperature to be increased to maintain the patient's core body temperature. This is especially true of young anesthetized infants undergoing a prolonged colonoscopy.

Patient positioning often begins in the left lateral decubitus position, unless general anesthesia is used, in which case a supine, frog-legged position may facilitate the anesthesiologist's care. The procedure should always begin with a careful perianal and digital rectal exam. The presence of perianal disease such as skin tags or fissures, in the absence of constipation, should be considered a sign of inflammatory bowel disease until proven otherwise.

The digital rectal exam, in addition to providing valuable clinical information (e.g. the presence of a stricture, polyp, etc.) will also give an indication as to the adequacy of sedation and bowel preparation. A brief examination of the patient's abdomen prior to the beginning of the procedure is also essential to assess for baseline abdominal distension and tone.

The colonoscope should be advanced through the entire colon, keeping the following general recommendations in mind [45,52]:

• The colonic lumen should be visualized at all times, recognizing that this may not be always possible, at least for short times and distances (e.g. passage of the rectosigmoid junction or splenic flexure).

• Minimizing air insufflation will facilitate passage while lessening loop formation.

• Loop formation should be avoided whenever possible; loops should be reduced as soon as they are formed.

• Frequent short advancements and withdrawals of the colonoscope will allow the colon to 'accordion' onto the instrument, again facilitating passage and the avoidance of loop formation.

Correct colonoscopic technique can often be judged by a child who remains comfortable throughout the procedure, a cecum that is reached in most children and adolescents according to the distances described above, and lack of mucosal trauma seen upon withdrawal.

Examination of the rectal mucosa in infants and small children may reveal many small submucosal nodules. They tend to efface with insufflation but may not disappear completely. These nodules represent lymphonodular hyperplasia and are not pathologic.

Endoscopic landmarks, such as the blue silhouettes of the liver and spleen or the triangular contour of the transverse colon, may not always be apparent in very young children. Radiologic confirmation of position, however, is rarely indicated. Verifying successful cecal intubation can be achieved by identifying appropriate structures (e.g. the appendiceal orifice, the ileocecal valve, or the characteristic triradiate haustral folds of the cecal bas-fond), visualization of the instrument's light over the right lower abdominal quadrant, and observing a sharp cecal indentation upon palpation with the index finger in this same area [9].

Intubation of the ileocecal valve and examination of the terminal ileum are important maneuvers. It is especially useful in the evaluation of IBD and unexplained hematochezia. Intubation of the ileocecal valve is perhaps one of the most difficult colonoscopic skills to acquire but is always facilitated by straightening of the instrument. Both indirect [45] and direct visualization [9] intubation techniques have been described. To the adult endoscopist, the terminal ileum of the child often appears abnormal, carpeted by a multitude of submucosal nodules (Fig. 10.1). This again is a normal finding represented by an exuberance of Peyer's patches. This lymphonodular hyperplasia tends to decrease with age, but may be present even in older adolescents. Occasionally, it may mimic Crohn's disease on small bowel radiologic images. Endoscopically with Crohn's disease, overlying exudates and/or ulceration will also be seen (Fig. 10.2).

Distension of the colonic lumen with air allows examination of the entire mucosal surface upon withdrawal of the instrument. It is also upon withdrawal that tissue sampling should be obtained following the same principles as

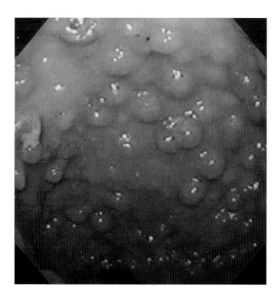

Fig. 10.1 Lymphonodular hyperplasia of the terminal ileum in a pediatric patient.

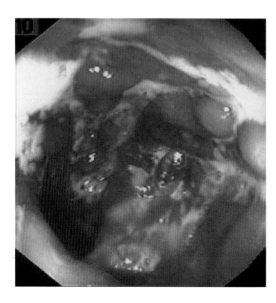

Fig. 10.2 Crohn's disease of the terminal ileum in an adolescent patient. (Courtesy of Marsha Kay, MD.)

described above [47,48]. Even when the mucosa is visually normal it is still advisable to collect biopsies. It is not unusual, even in experienced hands, to have discrepancies between the visual and histologic findings. Random biopsies are usually taken from the cecum, the transverse, descending, and sigmoid colons, and the rectum, and should be placed in separate containers. Retroflexion views of the distal rectum should be performed when possible prior to final withdrawal of the instrument.

Sigmoidoscopy

The techniques used for successful sigmoidoscopy are the same as for colonoscopy, recognizing that only the distal large intestine requires examination. Consequently, the required degree of bowel preparation and sedation may be less. In nursing infants, for example, clear liquids for 6–8 h and a formula bottle during the procedure may be all that is needed. If there is a probability that the sigmoidoscopy findings are likely to result in a second procedure (e.g. finding a juvenile polyp in a toddler with hematochezia) then a full colonoscopy should be performed first. This will avoid a second bowel preparation and sedation.

Therapeutic endoscopy

Therapeutic endoscopy has become a required component of the pediatric gastroenterologist's skills. It has the ability to supplant traditional surgical techniques requiring more invasive and time-needy approaches. Almost all therapeutic techniques, with the exception of percutaneous endoscopic gastrostomy (PEG) placement [53], originated from the adult experience and have been adapted to children. Consequently, general techniques, indications, and contraindications for pediatric therapeutic endoscopy are the same as for adults with, however, several limitations. These limitations include the size of the child, but especially the availability of the specialized instruments that fit through the smaller working channels of the pediatric endoscopes (see above). A list of therapeutic modalities that have been adapted to children are given in Tables 10.5 and 10.6.

Other endoscopic modalities

A number of additional, specialized endoscopic modalities need to be presented. Although they are indicated less frequently than the basic procedures described above or fit into the realm of emerging technologies, they nonetheless have increasingly become part of the pediatric gastroenterologist's armamentarium. An example is wireless capsule endoscopy which is now routinely used in many pediatric gastroenterology practices. Because the numbers for some of these procedures are small, the issue of who is best able to perform them continues to be discussed. It is clear that several pediatric referral centres see enough volume to ensure ongoing competency, but in many institutions the procedures require the assistance of trained adult colleagues.

Small bowel enteroscopy. There has always been a need and interest in being able to examine endoscopically the entire small bowel mucosa. This is especially valuable when tissue for diagnosis or therapeutic modalities are needed such as in cases of obscure intestinal bleeding, Crohn's disease, or polyposis syndromes. Three modalities have been traditionally used to examine endoscopically the small bowel: sonde enteroscopy, push enteroscopy, and intraoperative assisted push enteroscopy. Sonde enteroscopy, a passive, per nasal technique, is being largely abandoned for newer, quicker techniques with limited therapeutic capabilities. Push enteroscopy involves peroral passage of a long flexible endoscope beyond the ligament of Treitz. In experienced hands 120–180 cm of small bowel can be examined [9,54]. Pediatric colonoscopes or specialized small bowel enteroscopes may be used. Limitations include increased procedural duration and discomfort, often requiring the use of general anesthetics, and the angulation of the duodenum. This acute angulation dissipates the propelling forces put on the endoscope, resulting in a large and uncomfortable gastric loop [45]. This can be overcome by use of a straightening overtube or newer, variable-stiffness enteroscopes. In addition to visual examination of the mucosa, biopsies may be taken. Therapeutic options are otherwise limited. Intraoperative assisted enteroscopy involves both a surgeon and an endoscopist. It allows for broader therapeutic options, including multiple polypectomies in children with familial polyposis syndromes and ablation of multiple intestinal vascular ectasias. In this procedure the peritoneal cavity is approached either laparoscopically or through an open incisional technique. The small bowel is intubated perorally using an enteroscope, and passage to the terminal ileum is facilitated by the surgeon who 'accordions' the small bowel onto the endoscope as it is advanced.

The procedure is further facilitated by placing a non-crushing clamp at the ileocecal valve and using minimal air insufflation. The mucosa is examined upon withdrawal of the instrument. Air insufflation can be used at this point, while always keeping the intestinal clamp 20–40 cm distal to the tip of the endoscope. It is at this time also that biopsies may be taken, lesions ablated, polyps snared and removed, or the mucosa tattooed for later localization at surgical enterotomy.

Recently a fourth modality, double balloon enteroscopy, has allowed visualization of the entire small bowel mucosa through either per oral or per rectum insertion of a specially designed endoscope currently marketed by Fujinon. This endoscope has inflatable latex balloons placed near the tips of both a long enteroscope and its overtube. Through serial advances and withdrawals of the apparatus, using the balloons to 'grasp' the small bowel and accordion it back over the enteroscope, a full diagnostic and therapeutic endoscopy of the small bowel may be performed. It is expected that double balloon entersoscopy will replace the three preceding techniques.

Wireless capsule endoscopy. Since its first description in 2000 [55] this modality has rapidly become a valuable means to diagnose small bowel mucosal disease. This technology is based upon complementary metal oxide image sensors, application-specific integrated circuit devices, and white light emitting diode illumination. Its use is now well described in adults [56] and its value to pediatrics is beginning to be studied [57,58]. The video-endoscopic capsule is of a size (11×26 mm) such that it may be swallowed by cooperative children.

In excess of 200 000 of these disposable devices have been used worldwide, with an exceptional safety record. Indeed, the device has been FDA approved for use in children as young as 10 years of age. Although lower-size limits in children have not been published, we have had children weighing 25 kg swallow the capsule without difficulty. In smaller children or those unable to swallow the device, a front-loaded capsule deployment device (patented and marketed by US Endoscopy, Mentor OH) is used routinely to endoscopically deploy the capsule into the distal duodenum.

The short focal length lens (1 mm) obviates the need for air insufflation and provides excellent images. Video images are radio-transmitted continuously over a 6-hour period to a recording device. The stored images are then downloaded to a desktop computer for analysis.

This technology was initially indicated to detect the origin of obscure gastrointestinal bleeding. More recently, several other indications have been justified or are in the process of evaluation, including celiac disease, small bowel polyposis syndromes and surveillance of intestinal rejection or graft-versus-host disease following transplantation.

Wireless capsule endoscopy is contraindicated in patients with known or suspected small bowel obstruction or strictures. Its limitations include an inability to obtain tissue or fluid samples, a lack of therapeutic capabilities, and an inability to 'steer' the capsule. Additionally, it requires approximately 1 hour of an experienced physician's time to adequately review and analyze the stored data. Ongoing software releases continue to enhance the reader's ability to accurately and rapidly interpret the data. The development of legged-capsules whose movement can be controlled is in progress.

Endoscopic ultrasonography. Although well implemented in adult practice, perhaps due to the greater needs for cancer diagnosis, endoscopic ultrasound has yet to be routinely employed in the study of pediatric gastrointestinal disease. Published studies are few [59–61], but demonstrate its usefulness in the study of digestive tumors, angiomatosis, and biliary, pancreatic, and proctologic disease.

Endoscopic retrograde cholangiopancreatography (ERCP). ERCP continues to be a highly specialized procedure for the evaluation and treatment of both adult and pediatric pancreatico-biliary disease.

Selected gastrointestinal pathologies in pediatric patients

Eosinophilic esophagitis

Eosinophilic esophagitis (EE) is becoming increasingly recognized in pediatric patients. Reflux esophagitis and EE may have similar endoscopic appearances such as circumferential rings and vertical grooves. The presence of white specks adherent to the esophageal mucosa has recently been found to be highly specific for EE [62] (Fig. 10.3).

The specks have been found to microscopically contain eosinophils. It has been recommended that, in order to distinguish EE from reflux esophagitis, two biopsies should be obtained from the distal esophagus approximately 3 cm

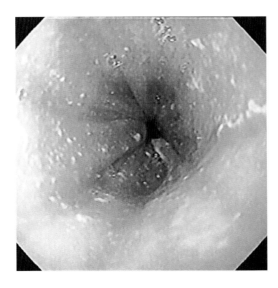

Fig. 10.3 Eosinophilic esophagitis. Note the white specks adherent to the mucosa. (Courtesy of Sandeep Gupta, MD.)

proximal to the squamocolumnar junction, and an additional two biopsies from the mid-esophagus.

The recommendation is based on the premise that reflux esophagitis is worse in the distal esophagus, while EE is a more diffuse process [63]. The distinction is critical clinically, as many patients with EE benefit from food allergy testing with subsequent elimination diets and topical corticosteroid therapy, as opposed to acid suppressants therapy alone.

Food allergic enteropathy and colitis

Gastrointestinal food allergy has gained recognition as a significant pediatric problem over the past several decades. Prospective studies looking at cow's milk protein allergy have reported a prevalence of 2.0% in cow's milk formula-fed infants while breastfed infants demonstrated an incidence of only 0.5% [64].

This is the most frequent form of food allergy during infancy. Typical symptoms include emesis, diarrhea, hematochezia, failure to thrive, malabsorption, and anaemia. Symptom onset may be at birth or delayed for months. There is a cross reactivity with soy protein in 40–60% of infants, thus necessitating use of a cow's milk protein hydrolysate formula or synthetic amino acid-based formula as therapy. The diagnosis is primarily based on clinical history.

Flexible sigmoidoscopy shows mucosal erythema, nodularity, and aphthous ulcers of the rectosigmoid region (Fig. 10.4). Typical biopsies show eosinophilic infiltrates. Patients typically respond well to dietary elimination programs.

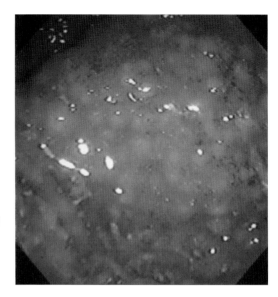

Fig. 10.4 Endoscopic appearance of rectal mucosa in an infant with cow's milk protein allergy. Note the nodular appearance and erosions.

Foreign body ingestion

This is a common problem faced by pediatric gastroenterologists. Over 80% of all ingestions occur in pediatric patients, with the majority being under the age of 3 years [65]. Symptoms associated with ingestion vary depending upon location of the foreign body and the age of the patient. They include dysphagia, odynophagia, chest pain, choking, drooling, feeding difficulty, respiratory difficulty, abdominal pain, and hematochezia. It is not uncommon that a foreign body is found incidentally on X-rays taken for other reasons such as cough or wheezing.

As many as 90% of ingested foreign bodies in pediatric patients are radiopaque; therefore, an X-ray is recommended in all suspected cases [66]. Of the foreign bodies that are brought to medical attention, up to 90% pass spontaneously, 10–20% require endoscopic removal, and less than 1% require surgical intervention [67].

Coins are by far the most common foreign body ingested by pediatric patients, with pennies ranking number one in the United States [68]. The most problematic coins are those trapped in the esophagus. It is important to note that coins in the esophagus will assume an *en face* appearance on the AP chest X-ray view while the edge of the coin is seen on a lateral film (Fig. 10.5).

If the opposite configuration is present, the coin is most likely in the trachea. Patients with a coin in the esophagus who are unable to swallow their secretions or those who are in respiratory distress require emergent endoscopic removal.

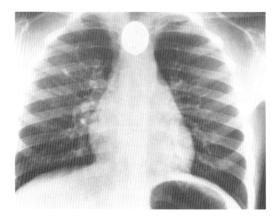

Fig. 10.5 AP chest X-ray demonstrating a coin in the esophagus.

Coins caught in the distal esophagus have a higher likelihood of spontaneous passage. In these instances a trial of glucagon or conservative management allowing the child to drink, with a repeat X-ray 12–24 h later, may be tried.

Coins trapped at the level of the thoracic inlet will not in most instances pass spontaneously and endoscopic removal should be scheduled within 24 h to minimize the risk of such complications as stricture, tracheal compression, pseudodiverticulosis, tracheo-/bronchoesophageal fistula, aortoesophageal fistula, or esophageal perforation. The endoscopic appearance of a coin in the esophagus is shown in Fig. 10.6.

We do not routinely recommend removal of coins distal to the gastroesophageal junction unless the patient is symptomatic or the coin has been retained for more than 4–6 weeks, in which case it is unlikely to pass spontaneously.

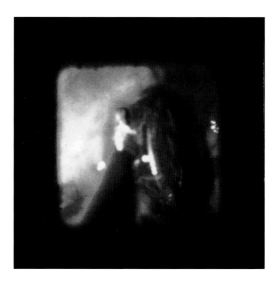

Fig. 10.6 Endoscopic appearance of esophageal foreign body—coin.

Although unlikely in adults, battery ingestions are common in pediatric patients. Button batteries are more commonly ingested than their cylindrical counterparts. Significant morbidity can occur if the battery lodges in the esophagus, making this clinical scenario an endoscopic emergency. Reported complications include delayed stricture development, esophageal perforation, fistula development, and even death [69].

Esophageal perforation may occur if the battery remains in the esophagus for as little as 6 h. Thus, rapid and precise distinction between button battery and coin ingestions must be made on X-ray. Button batteries have a 'double-density' appearance, as there is a step-off between the anode and cathode (Fig. 10.7). If the patient is asymptomatic and the battery is located in the stomach, observation is recommended.

If the battery remains in the stomach for over 48 h or if the patient becomes symptomatic at anytime, we recommend endoscopic retrieval. Such retrieval may be achieved with use of a basket, polypectomy snare, or forceps (tripod or pentapod) device. Cathartics are sometimes beneficial in hastening intestinal transit of the ingested battery. Meticulous screening of the patient's stool or repeat imaging is necessary to confirm passage.

Meat impactions and ingestions of sharp objects are treated the same in pediatric patients as they are in adults. A technique recently developed for

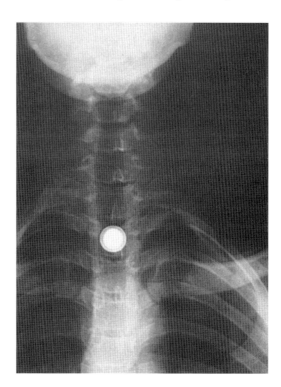

Fig. 10.7 Button battery in esophagus of an infant. Note the 'double-density' appearance. (Courtesy of Robert Wyllie, MD.)

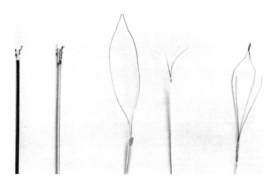

Fig. 10.8 Foreign-body retrieval equipment. From left to right: rat-tooth and alligator forceps, snare, tripod forceps, pentipod forceps.

management of objects not amenable to removal with standard forceps and baskets (Fig. 10.8) uses a string or suture placed endoscopically [70] (Fig. 10.9).

This technique has worked well in the removal of hair barrettes and washers, and should work well for other objects with a hole, such as a toothbrush if the bristles are not embedded in mucosa.

Helicobacter pylori gastritis

H. pylori infection is the most common cause of gastritis in pediatric patients, and recently appears to be associated with most primary ulcers in children over the age of 10 years [71,72]. Ulcers in children under the age of 10 years tend to be associated with stress events or medications such as corticosteroids or nonsteroidal anti-inflammatory medications. Infection during childhood with this organism has also been identified as a risk factor for mucosa-associated lymphoid tissue (MALT) lymphoma and gastric adenocarcinoma in adults. Transmission of the organism is by the fecal–oral and possibly oral–oral routes. Horizontal transmission within families has also been reported [73,74].

The prevalence of *H. pylori* appears to increase with age. Identified risk factors for infection include poor sanitation, crowding, lower socioeconomic status, poor nutrition, and a family history of peptic ulcer disease [75].

Presenting symptoms of *H. pylori* infection in pediatric patients includes upper abdominal pain and hematemesis. The upper endoscopy with biopsy remains the preferred diagnostic test for *H. pylori* in children. The sensitivity of breath urease testing in this population ranges from 75% to 100% in some reports, but is much less sensitive and specific in children under the age of 2 years [76,77].

The endoscopic appearance of the gastric and duodenal mucosa often correlates poorly with the presence or absence of histologic abnormalities in children. We therefore recommend that biopsies be obtained from the gastric

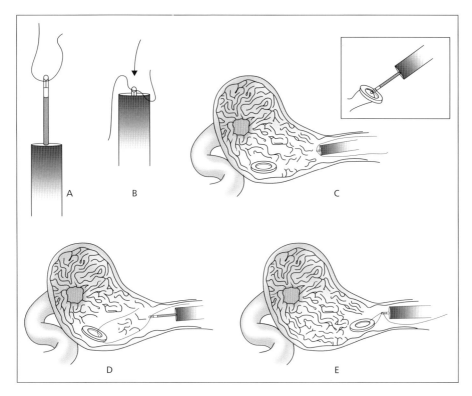

Fig. 10.9 Suture technique for removal of foreign bodies with a hole. (A) A long string or piece of suture material is loaded on the biopsy forceps and retracted into the endoscope channel (B). (C, D) The suture is firmly maintained in place on the outside of the endoscope until the region of the foreign body is reached. The suture is then threaded through the hole in the foreign body. (E) The suture is again grasped and secured upon withdrawal of the endoscope and foreign body. (Adapted from Kay M, Wyllie R. *Techniques in Gastrointest Endosc* 2002; 4 (4): 194 [70].)

antrum, gastric body, and duodenum in pediatric patients undergoing upper endoscopy.

Recently, diffuse antral nodularity has been found to be highly specific for *H. pylori* gastritis [78]. The characteristic histologic appearance shows chronic gastritis with the presence of mucosal lymphoid aggregates. *H. pylori* organisms are typically identified on the luminal surface or adherent to the apical surface of mucus cells in modified Giemsa stains, well-prepared hematoxylin-eosin stains, cresyl violet stains, or silver stains.

Triple therapy regimens, similar to those used in adults but modified according to patient weight, have been shown to eradicate the organisms in 70–95% of cases and have documented similar resolution of histologic and clinical abnormalities [79].

There remains, however, significant controversy surrounding the diagnosis and treatment of *H. pylori* in pediatric patients with non-ulcer dyspepsia. Repeat endoscopy to confirm eradication is generally not indicated unless the patient continues to be symptomatic and indirect diagnostic testing (e.g. stool antigen assay or C_{13} urea breath test) is negative.

Polyps in the pediatric patient

Polypectomy is the most common therapeutic application in both adult and pediatric patients undergoing colonoscopy. In contrast to adults, however, the vast majority of polyps in pediatric patients are juvenile polyps with negligible malignant potential unless they are part of a polyposis syndrome. Juvenile polyps account for more than 90% of polyps in children. They occur in approximately 1% of preschool and school age children [80]. This contrasts to adults where the incidence of adenomas is significantly greater. Juvenile polyps may be solitary or multiple, and typically present with painless rectal bleeding, recurrent abdominal pain, or intussusception. Because up to 60% of juvenile polyps are located proximal to the sigmoid colon, pediatric patients undergo a complete colonoscopy rather than flexible sigmoidoscopy when a polyp is clinically suspected [81]. Juvenile polyps may be sessile, but are often pedunculated and can measure up to several centimeters in length and diameter (Fig. 10.10).

Although the risk of developing malignancy in a solitary juvenile polyp is very small, discovery warrants removal. A single colonoscopy with polypectomy is

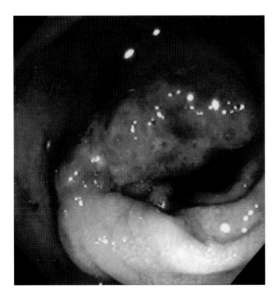

Fig. 10.10 Pedunculated juvenile polyp. (Courtesy of Robert Wyllie, MD.)

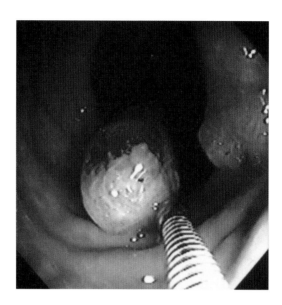

Fig. 10.11 Juvenile polyp status—postsnare polypectomy.

considered adequate treatment if the lesion is solitary and there is no family history of juvenile polyposis syndrome (Fig. 10.11).

If new symptoms arise, however, the patient needs reinvestigation. When indicated by the family history or when multiple polyps have been identified, updated routine screening guidelines must be followed.

Adenomas, too, may be found in pediatric patients, but are fortunately rare. They are most often encountered in families with a history of familial adenomatous polyposis (FAP) or hereditary non-polyposis colorectal cancer syndrome (HNPCC). The presence of a colonic adenoma in a patient under the age of 30 years should raise the suspicion for an inherited polyposis syndrome.

Appropriate genetic testing and counseling should be performed in such patients. An *APC* gene mutation may be detected in 60–80% of index cases.

For at-risk relatives with a negative gene test, FAP is excluded and the individual is considered to have an average population risk for the development of adenomas and colorectal cancer. A positive test in at-risk relatives confirms the diagnosis of FAP and patients should then undergo endoscopic assessment [82].

Annual flexible sigmoidoscopy is recommended from the age of 10–14 years until adenomas are found. Sigmoidoscopy is felt to be adequate because there is early rectal involvement in almost all patients. A complete colonoscopy is recommended by age 16 years to determine polyp load and location as well as the degree of dysplasia [83]. This information is used in combination with the psychosocial and educational needs of the patient to help make an informed decision regarding the timing and type of surgery.

In families in which the genotype is not known, protocols vary. We recommend annual sigmoidoscopy starting at age 10–14 years until rectal adenomas are identified, followed by routine colonoscopic surveillance as above. Some centres recommend that if no polyps are identified by age 20 years, the patient should then start undergoing colonoscopy with dye spray every 5 years [83].

Currently, the most common cause of cancer deaths in patients with FAP is duodenal and ampullary malignancies. Upper endoscopic surveillance of the stomach, duodenum, and periampullary region with a side-viewing scope is not routinely recommended for pediatric patients and should begin after age 20 years. If a pediatric patient with FAP develops unexplained upper abdominal pain, however, earlier investigation by an endoscopist trained in the use of side-viewing scopes is warranted [11].

Lymphonodular hyperplasia

Lymphonodular hyperplasia is a relatively common lymphoproliferative condition found in pediatric patients at the time of colonoscopy. It is typically most pronounced in the terminal ileum of pediatric patients, but is also commonly seen in the rectosigmoid or scattered throughout the colon. It does not appear to be related to any specific disease process. The submucosal lymphoid follicles typically range in size from 2 to 4 mm.

The condition may be responsible for intermittent hematochezia if located in the rectum or sigmoid. These nodules, either dense or sparsely distributed, usually tend towards effacement with air insufflation of the bowel. Gradual resolution with age is the rule. Stool softeners may help to decrease the amount of blood seen in the stool.

Outstanding issues and future directions

Pediatric gastrointestinal endoscopy continues to evolve favorably. Issues approached in this chapter requiring further investigation include:
* improved protocols for pediatric procedural preparation and sedation;
* evidence-based protocols for large bowel preparation in children;
* expanding the panoply of pediatric-dedicated endoscopy equipment;
* ongoing standardization of protocols for training and maintenance of proficiency to avoid the lack of a directed approach to the application of emerging technologies in pediatric gastrointestinal disease.

Future directions and initiatives should strive to create unified research and educational agendas that will address these issues and others as they arise. They can be established through the existing infrastructure of professional societies and institutions dedicated to these interests.

References

1 Hirshowitz BI, Peters CW, Curtiss LE. Preliminary reports on a long fiberscope for examination of the stomach and duodenum. *University Mich Med Bull* 1957; 23: 178–80.

2 Kawai K, Murakami K, Misak F. Endoscopical observations on gastric ulcers in teenagers. *Endoscopy* 1970; 2: 206–8.

3 Ottenjann R. Gastroscopic extraction of a foreign body. *Endoscopy* 1970; 3: 193–4.

4 Freeman NV. Clinical evaluation of the fiberoptic bronchoscope for pediatric endoscopy. *J Ped Surg* 1973; 8: 213–20.

5 Gleason PD, Tedesco FJ, Keating WA. Fiberoptic gastrointestinal endoscopy in infants and children. *J Pediatr* 1974; 85: 810–13.

6 Cremer M, Peeters JP, Emonts J *et al.* Fiberendoscopy of the gastrointestinal tract in children: experience with newly designed fiberscopes. *Endoscopy* 1974; 6: 186–9.

7 Fox VL. Pediatric endoscopy. *Gastrointest Endosc Clin N Am* 2000; 10: 175–94.

8 Seidman EG. Role of endoscopy in inflammatory bowel disease. *Gastrointest Endosc Clin N Am* 2001; 11: 641–57.

9 Thomson M. Colonoscopy and enteroscopy. *Gastrointest Endosc Clin N Am* 2001; 11: 603–39.

10 Brooker J, Saunders B, Shah S *et al.* A new variable stiffness colonoscope makes colonoscopy easier: a randomized controlled trial. *Gut* 2000; 46: 801.

11 Spolidoro JV, Kay M, Ament M *et al.* New endoscopic and diagnostic techniques: Working Group report of the first world congress of pediatric gastroenterology, hepatology and nutrition: management of GI bleeding, dysplasia screening, and endoscopic training—issues for the new millennium. *J Pediatr Gastroenterol Nutr* 2002; 35: S196–S204.

12 Hassal E. NASPGN Position Paper: requirements for training to ensure competence of endoscopists performing invasive procedures in children. *J Pediatr Gastroenterol Nutr* 1997; 24: 345–7.

13 Eisen GM, Chutkan R, Goldstein JL *et al.* Modification in endoscopic practice for pediatric practice. *Gastrointest Endosc* 2000; 52: 838–42.

14 Lewis Claar R, Walker LS, Barnard JA. Children's knowledge, anticipatory anxiety, procedural distress, and recall of esophagogastroduodenoscopy. *J Pediatr Gastroenterol Nutr* 2002; 34: 68–72.

15 Mahajan L, Wyllie R, Steffen R *et al.* The effects of a psychological preparation program on anxiety in children and adolescents undergoing gastrointestinal endoscopy. *J Pediatr Gastroenterol Nutr* 1998; 27 (2): 161–5.

16 Vasundhara T, Peters J, Gilger M. Sedation for pediatric endoscopic procedures. *J Pediatr Gastroenterol Nutr* 2000; 30: 477–85.

17 Ingebo KR, Rayhorn NJ, Hecht RM *et al.* Sedation in children: adequacy of two-hour fasting. *J Pediatr* 1997; 131: 155–8.

18 Schreiner MS, Triebwasser A, Keon TP. Ingestion of liquids compared with preoperative fasting in pediatric outpatients. *Anesthesiology* 1990; 72: 593–7.

19 Gleghorn EE. Preoperative fasting: you don't have to be cruel to be kind. *J Pediatr* 1997; 131: 12–13.

20 American Society of Anesthesiologists task force on sedation and analgesia by non-anesthesiologists. Practice guidelines for sedation and analgesia by non-anesthesiologists. *Anesthesiology* 2002; 96: 1004–17.

21 Faigel DO, Eisen GM, Baron TH *et al.* Guidelines: preparation of patients for GI endoscopy. *Gastrointest Endosc* 2003; 57: 446–50.

22 Gremse DA, Sacks AI, Raines S. Comparison of oral sodium phosphate to polyethylene glycol-based solution for bowel preparation for colonoscopy in children. *J Pediatr Gastroenterol Nutr* 1996; 23: 586–90.

23 Abubakar K, Goggin N, Gormally S *et al.* Preparing the bowel for colonoscopy. *Arch Dis Child* 1995; 73: 459–61.

24 Dashan A, Lin C-H, Peters J *et al.* A randomized, prospective, study to evaluate the efficacy and acceptance of three bowel preparations for colonoscopy in children. *Am J Gastroenterol* 1999; 94: 3497–501.

25 da Silva MM, Briars GL, Patrick MK *et al.* Colonoscopy preparation in children: safety, efficacy and tolerance of high- versus low-volume cleansing methods. *J Pediatr Gastroenterol Nutr* 1997; 24: 33–7.

26 Dajuni AS, Taubert KA, Wilson W *et al.* Prevention of bacterial condocarditis: recommendations by the American Heart Association. *JAMA* 1997; 277: 1794–801.

27 Neu HC, Fleischer D. Controversies, dilemmas, and dialogues: recommendations for antibiotic prophylaxis before endoscopy. *Am J Gastroenterol* 1989; 84: 1488.

28 Squires RH, Colletti RB. Indications for pediatric gastrointestinal endoscopy: a medical position statement of the North American Society for Pediatric Gastroenterology and Nutrition. *J Pediatr Gastroenterol Nutr* 1996; 23: 107–10.

29 Stillman AE, Painter R, Hollister DW. Ehler–Danlos syndrome type IV: diagnosis and therapy of associated bowel perforation. *Am J Gastroenterol* 1991; 86: 360–2.

30 Lazzaroni M, Petrillo M, Tomaghi R *et al.* Upper GI bleeding in healthy full-term infants: a case-control study. *Am J Gastroenterol* 2002; 97: 89–94.

31 Ojala R, Ruuska T, Karikoski R *et al.* Gastroesophageal endoscopic findings and gastrointestinal symptoms in preterm neonates with and without perinatal indomethacin exposure. *J Pediatr Gastroenterol Nutr* 2001; 32: 182–8.

32 Ruuska T, Fell JM, Bisset WM *et al.* Neonatal and infantile upper gastrointestinal endoscopy using a new small diameter fibreoptic gastroscope. *J Pediatr Gastroenterol Nutr* 1996; 23: 604–8.

33 deBoissieu D, Dupont C, Barbet JP. Distinct features of upper gastrointestinal endoscopy in the newborn. *J Pediatr Gastroenterol Nutr* 1994; 18: 334–8.

34 Nowicki MJ, Vaughn CA. Sedation and anesthesia in children for endoscopy. *Techniques in Gastrointestinal Endosc* 4 (4), 2002: 225–30.

35 Kaplan RF, Yang CI. Sedation and analgesia in pediatric patients for procedures outside the operating room. *Anesthiol Clin N Am* 2002; 20: 181–94.

36 Walco GA, Cassidy RC, Schecter NL. Pain, hurt and harm: the ethics of pain control in infants and children. *N Engl J Med* 1994; 331: 541–4.

37 Deboer SL, Peterson LV. Sedation for nonemergent neonatal intubation. *Neonatal Netw* 2001; 20: 19–23.

38 Ng E, Taddio A, Ohlsson A. Intravenous midazolam infusion for sedation of infants in the neonatal intensive care unit. *Cochrane Database Syst Rev* 2003: (1): CD002052.

39 Bishop PR, Nowicki MJ, May WL *et al.* Unsedated upper endoscopy in children. *Gastrointest Endosc* 2002; 55: 624–30.

40 Elitsur Y. Propofol sedation for endoscopic procedures in children. *Endoscopy* 2000; 32: 788–91.

41 Kaddu R, Bhattacharya D, Metriyakool K *et al.* Propofol compared with general anesthesia for pediatric GI endoscopy: is propofol better? *Gastrointest Endosc* 2002; 55: 27–32.

42 Law AK, Ng DK, Chan KK. Use of intra muscular ketamine for endoscopy sedation in children. *Pediatr Int* 2003; 45: 180–5.

43 Hostetler MA, Barnard JA. Removal of foreign bodies in the pediatric ED: is ketamine an option. *Am J Emerg Med* 2002; 20: 96–8.

44 Montes RG. Deep sedation with inhaled sevoflurane for pediatric outpatient gastrointestinal endoscopy. *J Pediatr Gastroenterol Nutr* 2000; 31: 41–6.

45 Wyllie and Kay chapter on technique. ?.

46 Fox VL, Walker WA *et al.* (2000) Upper gastrointestinal endoscopy in pediatric gastrointestinal disease. *Pathophysiology/Diagnosis/Management* (3/e) pp 1401–14 BC Decker Inc. Hamilton Ontario.

47 Gillett P, Hassall E. Pediatric gastrointestinal mucosal biopsy. *Gastrointest Endosc Clin N Am* 2000; 10: 669–711.

48 Gillett P. Pediatric gastrointestinal mucosal biopsy: special considerations in children. *Gastrointest Endosc Clin N Am* 2000; 10: 669–712.

49 Boyle JT. Gastroesophageal reflux in the pediatric patient. *Gastrointest Endosc Clin N Am* 1989; 18: 317–37.

50 Dahms BB, Rothstein FC. Mucosal biopsy of the esophagus in children. *Perspect Pediatr Pathol* 1987: 97–123.

51 Saunders BP, Phillips RKS, Williams CB. Intraoperative measurement of colonic anatomy and attachment with relevance to colonoscopy. *Br J Surg* 1995; 82: 1491–3.

52 Cotton PB, Williams CB. (1980) *Practical Gastrointestinal Endoscopy*. pp 99–141. Oxford, Blackwell.

53 Gauderer MWL, Ponsky JL, Izant RJ. Gastrostomy without laparatomy: a percutaneous endoscopic technique. *J Ped Surg* 1980; 15: 872–5.

54 Perez-Cuadrado E, Macenlle R, Iglesias J *et al*. Usefulness of oral push video enteroscopy in Crohn's disease. *Endoscopy* 1997; 29: 745–7.

55 Iddan G, Meron G, Glukhovsky A, Swain P. Wireless capsule endoscopy. *Nature* 2000; 405: 417.

56 Ginsberg GG, Barkun AN, Bosco JJ *et al*. Wireless capsule endoscopy: August 2002. *Gastrointest Endosc* 2002; 56: 621–4.

57 Seidman EG. Wireless capsule video-endoscopy: an odyssey beyond the end of the scope. *J Pediatr Gastroenter Nutr* 2002; 34: 333–4.

58 Mallet E, Cron J, Stoller J. Wireless capsule video-endoscopy: preliminary results in children. *Arch Pediatr* 2003; 10: 244–5.

59 Kato S, Fujita N, Shibuya H *et al*. Endoscopic ultrasonography in a child with chronic pancreatitis. *Acta Paediatr Jpn* 1993; 35: 151–3.

60 Roseau G, Palazzo L, Dumontier I *et al*. Endoscopic ultrasonography in the evaluation of pediatric digestive diseases: preliminary results. *Endoscopy* 1998; 30: 477–81.

61 Nadler EP, Novikov A, Landzberg BR *et al*. The use of endoscopic ultrasound in the diagnosis of solid pseudopapillary tumors of the pancreas in children. *J Pediatr Surg* 2002; 37: 1370–3.

62 Lim JR, Gupta SK, Fitzgerald JF *et al*. White specks in esophageal mucosa (WSEM): a true endoscopic manifestation of severe eosinophilic esophagitis (EE) in children? *J Pediatr Gastroenterol Nutr* 2001; 33: 411 (Abstract 164).

63 Liacouras CA, Wenner WJ. The quantity of esophageal eosinophils, not the location, is diagnostic of eosinophilic esophagitis in children. *Gastrointest Endosc* 2000: 51: AB133 (Abstract 3709).

64 Host A, Halken S. A prospective study of cow milk allergy in Danish infants during first three years of life. *Allergy* 1990; 45: 587–96.

65 Webb WA. Management of foreign bodies of the upper gastrointestinal tract. *Gastroenterology* 1988; 94: 204–16.

66 Macpherson RI, Hill JG, Othersen HB *et al*. Esophageal foreign bodies in children: diagnosis, treatment and complications. *Am J Roentgenol* 1996; 166: 919–24.

67 Arana A, Hauser B, Hachimi-Idrissi S *et al*. Management of ingested foreign bodies in childhood and review of the literature. *Eur J Pediatr* 2001; 160: 468–72.

68 Jefferson S. A thought for your pennies. *JAMA* 1999; 28: 122.

69 Litovitz T, Schmitz BF. Ingestion of cylindrical and button batteries: an analysis of 2,382 cases. *Pediatrics* 1992; 89: 747–57.

70 Kay M, Wyllie R. Techniques of foreign body removal in infants and children. *Techniques in Gastrointest Endosc* 2002: 4 (4): 188–95.

71 Drumm B, Sherman P, Cutz E *et al*. Association of Campylobacter pylori on the gastric mucosa with antral gastritis in children. *N Engl J Med* 1987; 316: 1557–61.

72 Gormally SM, Kierce BM, Daly LE *et al*. Gastric metaplasia and duodenal ulcer disease in children infected by Helicobacter pylori. *Gut* 1996; 38: 513–17.

73 Elitsur Y, Adkins L, Saeed D *et al*. Helicobacter pylori antibody profile in household members of children with H. pylori infection. *J Clin Gastroenterol* 1999; 29: 178–82.

74 Mitchell JD, Mitchell HM, Tobias V. Acute Helicobacter pylori infection in an infant associated with gastric ulceration and serologic evidence of intra-familial transmission. *Am J Gastroenterol* 1992; 87: 382–6.

75 Hassall E, Dimmick JE. Unique features of Helicobacter pylori disease in children. *Dig Dis Sci* 1991; 36: 417–23.

76 Rowland M *et al*. Carbon 13-labeled urea breath test for the diagnosis of Helicobacter pylori infection in children. *J Pediatr* 1997; 131: 815–20.

77 Madani S, Rabah R, Tolia V. Diagnosis of Helicobacter pylori infection from antral biopsies in the pediatric patient: is urease test that reliable? *Dig Dis Sci* 2000; 45: 1233–7.
78 Elitsur Y, Raghuverra A, Sadat T *et al.* Is gastric nodularity a sign for gastric inflammation associated with Helicobacter pylori infection in children? *J Clin Gastroenterol* 2000; 30: 286–8.
79 Dohil R, Israel DM, Hassall E. Effective 2 week therapy for Helicobacter pylori disease in children. *Am J Gastroenterol* 1998; 92: 244–7S.
80 Session R *et al.* Carcinoma of the colon in the first two decades of life. *Ann Surg* 1965; 162: 279.
81 Mestre JR. The changing pattern of juvenile polyps. *Am J Gastroenterol* 1996; 81: 312–14.
82 Peterson GM, Francomano C, Kinzler K *et al.* Presymptomatic direct detection of adenomatous polyposis coli (APC) gene mutations in familial adenomatous polyposis. *Hum Genet* 1993; 91: 307–11.
83 Hyer W. Polyposis syndromes: pediatric implications. *Gastrointest Endosc Clin N Am* 2001; 11 (4): 659–82.

CHAPTER 11

Training and credentialing in gastrointestinal endoscopy

JONATHAN COHEN

Introduction

Training in gastrointestinal endoscopy represents an ever increasingly important endeavor as procedures have become more complex and more therapeutic
in nature. In the USA, the bulk of this instruction now occurs during formalized
training programs of at least 3 years duration. Additional periods of dedicated
intensive training in certain specialized procedures such as ERCP and EUS are
available, although many practitioners routinely perform such procedures
without added formal training. In addition to the supervised instruction of
novices during fellowship, training also encompasses the activities of experienced practicing gastroenterologists trying to learn new techniques or refresh
certain skills that have become rusty from disuse.

The goal of all training is to become proficient in the techniques being
taught. A lot of effort is being made to define when someone is truly competent
to perform a procedure independently and to determine how much training is
required to reach this level of skill. In the past, the number of cases performed
under supervision has sufficed as a surrogate for actual demonstration of competency. A wide range of minimum case numbers have been recommended for
different procedures often based on expert opinion. More recently, investigators have attempted to correlate the number of cases performed with objective
criteria for success. At the same time, organizations such as the American
Society for Gastrointestinal Endoscopy (ASGE) have emphasized the importance of using such objective criteria in lieu of procedure numbers to determine
competency. The current focus on optimizing quality in the performance of
endoscopic procedures will no doubt influence thinking about how best to
train individuals to perform high quality endoscopy, and how to measure the
success of trainees to determine that they are, in fact, competent to perform procedures independently and well. Ultimately, the forces pushing this quality
agenda may drive changes in the way program directors credential their trainees
and the way in which hospitals grant individuals privileges to perform endoscopic procedures.

Novel methods of instruction have been introduced to accelerate the learning curve of certain techniques at various stages in the training process. Endoscopy simulators, including ex-vivo animal tissue, artificial tissue, and virtual reality computer-based models, have exciting potential to enhance the existing practice of teaching endoscopy. In addition, these simulators may provide a way to assess competency in a controlled environment that does not affect patient care and could one day be used to facilitate the process of credentialing and recredentialing for endoscopy privileges. However, the precise role and the optimal use of the various models have not yet been clearly defined, and only in certain applications to date has the presumed benefit been confirmed by controlled studies.

This chapter will first review general principles of endoscopy training and the specific skill sets required to gain proficiency. It will then address each of the major endoscopic procedures, the type and amount of training currently recommended to master each procedure, and the evidence which supports current recommendations. Criteria used to assess competency for each procedure will be discussed. This chapter will then address the role of a wide variety of alternative methods for teaching endoscopy, which are available to supplement standard training. Finally, current recommendations for hospital credentialing and privileging will be discussed. Where possible, areas in need of investigation will be highlighted.

General principles of endoscopy training

Traditional standard means of instruction

Hands-on supervised one on one instruction is the mainstay of endoscopy training. Successful teaching with this method depends on many factors. Perhaps the most important ingredient to effective teaching is the teaching skill of the endoscopy instructor and the quality of the communication that takes place between trainer and trainee [1]. Rather than just watch a trainee attempt a procedure and take over when they experience difficulty or when they have used up a pre-determined period of time, the instructor is supposed to engage in a dynamic process of mostly verbal description, feedback and inquiry with the trainee during each procedure. This is often difficult to do, even for expert endoscopists who must convey verbal instructions about maneuvers that they routinely perform without much thought. It requires the ability to breakdown the technical components into discrete steps for the novice. Just as it is difficult to tell someone how to tie a shoelace using only words, the instructor combines verbal instruction with brief demonstrations to illustrate a particular technique. Other important skills required of the endoscopy teacher include the patience to allow the trainee time to develop skills without endangering patient safety and the ability to give constructive feedback [2,3].

Apart from the quality of the instructor, optimal training conditions also depend upon a relaxed learning environment in the endoscopy unit with logistics that allow for the added time necessary for fellows to perform procedures. The training setting must also provide trainees with sufficient case volume for adequate repetition of skills, and a wide enough variety of pathology to allow them to develop cognitive assessment skills in parallel with technical expertise.

This supervised 'hands-on' training method has generally been an effective means of developing proficiency in a wide variety of procedures. It has largely supplanted the 'self-taught' method by which many of endoscopy pioneers learned and mastered endoscopic techniques before expert instruction became widely available. While some practitioners do attempt to perform new techniques with only perfunctory supervised hands-on instruction, this practice opens up a wide array of ethical and practical concerns.

What to teach and how to teach it

What skill sets must a trainee acquire in order to learn to perform endoscopic procedures? The novice endoscopist must develop both technical and cognitive proficiencies in the following areas:

1   Understanding of the indications and contraindications for endoscopic procedures, and risk factors for complications.
2   Knowledge of the endoscopic equipment and accessories and how to set this up equipment for use.
3   Familiarity with the endoscope control dials and buttons.
4   Dexterity in controlling the scope range of motion using the dials and torque applied to the endoscope shaft.
5   Hands–eye coordination to produce deliberate, precise manipulation of the scope within the lumen and the use of accessories.
6   Communication with nursing and technical staff regarding required assistance during the procedure.
7   Knowledge of normal anatomic landmarks and possible abnormal pathologies which might be encountered.
8   Interpretive skills to correctly identify abnormalities which are detected.
9   Judgment of how to manage appropriately those lesions encountered.
10   Familiarity with patient monitoring and the administration of conscious sedation.
11   Awareness of how to recognize and manage adverse events.
12   Understanding of risks and benefits of intended procedures and the ability to provide and document informed consent.

13 Documentation of findings.

14 Communication of results to patients and other physicians.

While many of these activities seem obvious, they are all critical skills which the endoscopic trainee must master before performing procedures independently. Some of this material may be included in a formal curriculum designed for the novice as an introduction to endoscopy. However, much is introduced to the new fellow more haphazardly as he or she begins to perform cases under supervision by one or more preceptors. While there has been increased focus within training programs on objective competency assessment, evaluation of fellows' progress is seldom broken down into such a detailed list of skill sets.

Defining competency and how to access it

Before determining how best to train fellows, it is necessary first to establish what constitutes the end product of successful instruction. Competency requires the consistent ability to meet safely the technical goals of the intended procedure and to correctly perform the cognitive aspects of the procedure.

The American Society for Gastrointestinal Endoscopy (ASGE) has published guidelines for training (http://www.asge.org) which emphasize several principles about the process of achieving competency in endoscopy [6]. First, all major procedures require formal preceptorship programs lasting more than several weeks which are best accomplished in a certified fellowship training program or residency. A minimum number of procedures must be performed before competency can even be assessed, and recent statements emphasize that the number alone does not guarantee competency. A body of data to be discussed later suggests that the published minimum numbers are too low to achieve acceptable success rates in most instances [7–9]. The endoscopist must be able to achieve a standard rate of technical success, but must also notice any abnormal pathology, identify it correctly, and decide upon the appropriate course of action. Specific training in the administration of conscious sedation and the management of patients receiving such medication is also required.

Increasingly, standard definitions of competency for diagnostic procedures demand proficiency in any related therapeutic maneuver that might be required during a diagnostic examination. For example, one cannot be considered competent to perform colonoscopy unless one can consistently reach the cecum, recognize and properly identify a polyp, and successfully remove the polyp during the examination. Next, competency in one procedure does not imply competency in another. Nor does competency in elective procedures constitute competency to perform an emergency therapeutic procedure.

How successful must a trainee be before qualifying as competent to perform a procedure independently? Data on procedure success rates by experts provides useful perspective in setting the bar. It is seldom possible for a trainee to be as good as a practitioner with several years of experience at the completion of formal training. The ASGE has suggested that trainees be able to demonstrate a minimum procedure success rate of 80–90% by the time they end their fellowship program [10]. The growing body of information detailed below on how many cases are required to reach this level of expertise for each procedure type serves not to obviate the measurement of actual success rates and personal outcomes, but to help ensure that training programs are designed with sufficient experience to achieve these goals. Given objective data available on the learning curve for endoscopic procedures and given the number of cases performed during the typical 3 year fellowship, an 80–90% success rate appears to be a feasible standard for most procedure types.

Fellows may learn at different rates and this may depend on case volume, quality of instruction, and on the intrinsic mechanical ability of the particular trainees. There is data to support this principle with regards to acquisition of competency in colonoscopy [Cass O, personal communication from ACES study data, manuscript in preparation]. The fact that some individuals take more or less time to learn skills than others strongly supports the trend within training programs to emphasize objective criteria for assessing competency rather than relying upon completion of a pre-set number of total procedures.

Data is limited proving that individuals who reach objective parameters of competency in training go on to have better patient outcomes than do individuals who begin to practice before such success rates are achieved. Optimal future validation of good training may need to assess not only success rates for intended procedures and complication rates but also patient satisfaction measures.

As more objective competency criteria are adopted for trainees in formal training programs, some attention needs to be given to address the issue of practicing endoscopists learning new techniques. They also need objective criteria of competency akin to standards set for fellows in formal training programs for the purpose of credentialing.

The recent effort on the part of gastroenterology societies to define evidence-based quality measures for different endoscopic procedures should serve to better set the bar for trainees and practitioners alike as to what constitutes competency. The two principle questions for each procedure type that gastroenterologists perform should be what factors matter when aiming to provide high quality service and how good does one need to be at each of these components in order to provide excellent care? [11–17] Future guidelines for training and assessing competency will likely call for the routine measurement of quality endpoints during training with increasing demand that appropriate benchmarks are met before individuals are credentialed to perform procedures independently.

Training and competency in specific endoscopic procedures

Esophagogastroduodenoscopy (EGD)

When new GI fellows begin their training, EGD is often the first procedure performed under supervision. During this time they must learn many things besides passing the instrument from the mouth to the duodenum. This is the time they learn about the care and handling of the instrument, the workings of the dials and channels, the preparation, monitoring, and sedation of the patient, as well as the technical and cognitive aspects of the EGD procedure itself. During the course of a 3 year training program, GI fellows invariably perform far more than the number of EGDs required to become proficient. However, a number of non-gastroenterologists also perform EGD in the USA. By some estimates, as much as 50% of all endoscopic procedures in this country are performed by non-gastroenterologist health care providers [18]. For this reason, the criteria for proper training in this procedure and evidence to define how much specific training is required to gain sufficient proficiency carry added importance.

Published guidelines for training in EGD

Most published guidelines for training in EGD are derived from expert opinion in the absence of objective data. Current ASGE recommendations reflecting some recent studies on the learning curve for endoscopic procedures state that at least 130 upper examinations are required before competency can be assessed for EGD [10]. There is a wide variation of in the minimum number suggested by various other professional societies and expert opinions ranging from 25 to 300 cases [19-30]. This degree of variation may result from differences in definition of what constitutes a competent examination and from lack of outcome data to support the recommendations. A summary of recommendations on minimum numbers of EGD, colonoscopy, and ERCP is shown in Table 11.1

Defining competence for EGD

Technical competence in EGD requires the consistent ability to intubate the esophagus with the endoscope and to traverse the pylorus into the duodenum. The entire stomach must be visualized, including turnaround view of the fundus and cardia. Any abnormal findings must be identified and correctly characterized. Patients must be adequately sedated and appropriately monitored. A trainee must be able to perform targeted mucosal biopsies when indicated [13].

Table 11.1 Variable recommendations of minimal training requirements

Source	Year	Ref	Minimum EGD	Minimum colonoscopy	Minimum ERCP
Expert opinion					
Internists	1989	13	25	25	
IM residency directors		14	25	25	
Gastroenterologists	1990	15	75	88	
ABIM survey GI program directors	1990	16	85	75	35
Professional societies					
Fed of Dig Dis Societies	1981	17	50	100	
SAGES	1991	18	25	50	
American Academy Family Practice	1993	19	<10	<10	
European Diploma Gastroenterology	1995	20	300	100	150
British Society Gastroenterology	1996	21	300	100	150
Conjoint Committee (Australia)	1997	22	200	100	200
ASGE	1998		100	100	100
ASGE (revised)*	2002	10	130	140	200

Adapted with permission from Freeman, ML. Training and competence in gastrointestinal endoscopy. *Rev Gastroenterol Disord.* 2001; 1: 73–86.
*Recently revised ASGE figures added to table as appeared in [19].

What technical success rate in constitutes an acceptable level of competency? Cass *et al.* conducted a single institution study of GI fellows and surgical residents and found that both groups of trainees achieved over 95% pylorus intubation rates after a mean of 120 cases, whereas experienced proctors completed the examination in over 99% of cases [8]. A review of 2500 EGDs performed by family practitioners in the USA reported a 93% rate of reaching the small intestine, perhaps reflecting less extensive time devoted to training and considerably lower cases volume than gastroenterologists, with an average caseload of 0.6 to 10.8 cases per month [31]. With readily available access to endoscopists with over 95% success rates, it is difficult to set the bar for achieving competency at technical success rates much lower than this level.

Data on acquisition of competency in diagnostic EGD

Two studies have addressed the question of the rate of skills acquisition in EGD. In the only published article on this subject, Cass *et al.* performed a prospective evaluation of 7 GI fellows and 5 fourth year surgical residents during their training in EGD and colonoscopy. Trainees were graded on standardized forms which tallied objective criteria of procedure success, including both technical and cognitive components. During this study, trainees were graded on a median of 113 EGDs (54–162). Esophageal intubation rates were 95% after 50 cases but then dipped to 75% until completing over 100 cases, reflecting the tendency of proctors to allow trainees to attempt more difficult cases only after increased experience. This finding illustrates a particular feature of objective analyses of learning curves during training, in which patient mix and case difficulty needs to be taken into consideration. For this reason, the authors elected to identify those threshold case volumes after which trainees maintained the success rates designated as minimum standards for competency. Sustained ability to traverse the pylorus was 100% after 90 procedures [8].

In a much larger multicenter study using the same grading form, Cass *et al.* prospectively studied 135 first year GI fellows from 14 centers. Preliminary results from this project are published in abstract form, and the manuscript containing the final results is currently in preparation [7; O. Cass, personal communication]. Both objective measures of procedure success and subjective rating of case performance were recorded. For the objective evaluations, competency for a particular procedure was defined as meeting all four of the following criteria: intubating the esophagus, intubating the pylorus, recognizing abnormalities, and correctly identifying any abnormalities. Competency for each trainee in a procedure was arbitrarily defined as ability to achieve 90% success in 2 successive blocks of 10 procedures. Similar assessments and definitions were used to evaluate the trainees' progress in colonoscopy, as will be discussed below in greater detail.

Data was collected on 13 195 EGDs. Over 160 EGDs were required before the average fellow met the definition of competency in diagnostic EGD by the objective criteria outlined above. Comparison of data sheet with fellows logs revealed approximately 30% of cases were not scored, suggesting that 160 is an underestimate of the true number of cases required to gain full proficiency in this procedure. Further, those cases which fellows were not allowed to attempt were not included in the evaluations. For EGD evaluation, scoring using the four objective criteria correlated well with subjective ratings of competency on a 5 point scale. These data establish that when the components of procedure competency are carefully assessed, the minimum number of supervised training cases far exceeds published guidelines.

This data should not affect GI fellowship programs where fellows routinely perform 500 or more EGDs within the 3 year experience. In contrast, this data directly challenges current practice by non-gastroenterologist providers, for whom far fewer cases are routinely performed during training. One review of experience in surgical training described that surgical residents performed an average of 75 EGDs and 75 colonoscopies during their residency. Family practitioners who perform EGD may undergo very limited training during short weekend courses involving in some instances fewer than 10 supervised procedures [32].

Competency and EGD outcome

Does additional training make a difference in terms of procedure outcome, complication rates, or patient satisfaction? It is intuitive that individuals with more extensive training and those with higher case volume will have different outcomes than those with less cumulative and ongoing experience. Some data supports this notion of variations in outcome. Data from Rodney describing a 93% duodenal intubation rate falls short of 99% success rates by experienced endoscopists in the Cass study [8,26]. One comparative prospective survey of EGD complications showed that internists had an over 3-fold higher rate than their GI counterparts [33].

Training in therapeutic EGD techniques

Biopsy, PEG placement, stricture dilation, achalasia dilation, hemostasis techniques, endoscopic mucosal resection, stent deployment, pneumatic dilation, tumor ablation.

Standard upper GI endoscopy techniques

The ability to perform targeted endoscopic mucosal biopsy should be considered integral to the performance of diagnostic EGD. Therapeutic procedures such as percutaneous endoscopic gastrostomy (PEG) placement, hemostasis of upper gastrointestinal hemorrhage, and stricture dilation require additional training. A strong argument can be made that individuals ought not be privileged in EGD without being capable of performing some or all of these interventions, to avoid the need for repeat therapeutic procedures by a second operator following a diagnositic-only EGD. There is not much data available on the amount of training needed to gain proficiency in the therapeutic interventions possible during upper endoscopy. In the absence of data to address the question of how many supervised cases are required to master each of these skills, current recommendations rely on expert opinion. The ASGE has provided guidelines for minimum number for some of these procedures [6,10,34,35] (Table 11.2). Typically, gastroenterology fellows receive ample experience during their training in such procedures as PEG placement, foreign body removal, stricture dilation, and hemostasis of variceal and non-variceal GI bleeding.

Table 11.2 Minimum number of procedures before competency can be assessed

Standard procedure	No. of cases required
Flexible sigmoidoscopy	30
Diagnostic EGD	130
Total colonoscopy	140
Snare polypectomy	30*
Nonvariceal hemostasis (upper and lower; includes 10 active bleeders)	25*
Variceal hemostasis (Includes 5 active bleeders)	20
Esophageal dilation with guide wire	20
PEG	15
Advanced procedures	
ERCP	200 #
EUS: Submucosal abnormalities†	40
Pancreaticobiliary†	75
EUS-guided FNA: Non-pancreatic‡	25
Pancreatic‡‡	25
Tumor ablation	20
Pneumatic dilation for achalasia	5
Laparoscopy	25
Esophageal stent placement	10
Enteroscopy	**

* Included in total number
# Includes at least 40 sphincterotomies and 10 stent placements
†For competence in imaging both mucosal and submucosal abnormalities, a minimum of 100 supervised cases is recommended.
For comprehensive competence in all aspects of EUS, a minimum of 150 supervised cases, of which 75 should be pancreaticobiliary and 50 EUS guided FNA is recommended.
‡ Intramural lesions or lymph nodes. Must be competent to perform mucosal EUS.
‡‡ Must be competent to perform pancreaticobiliary EUS.
** Data is not yet available on the minimum number of enteroscopies performed
From: ASGE Guidelines 2002 [10].

Hemostasis techniques

This topic warrants separate attention for several reasons. First, these cases represent some of the most emergent situations facing the endoscopist and can be accompanied by high risk of patient morbidity and mortality. During acute GI bleeding episodes, the endoscopist must combine a number of cognitive and technical maneuvers to successfully diagnose and control the hemorrhage while supervising the management of a potentially unstable patient. Time is a factor and the staffing conditions may be sub-optimal, requiring the endoscopist to possess a thorough understanding of equipment set up and accessory use. Cases present at variable rates and times, and conditions are not always conducive for a trainee to spend much time struggling with the endoscope as the mentor patiently provides advice. These factors, which require operator proficiency, also make the training process more difficult.

There is no published data yet on the learning curve for technical competency in hemostasis on real patients. The ASGE has published some minimum numbers for various techniques which are listed in Table 11.2, but there is little evidence to support that this amount of experience is sufficient for trainees to independently perform hemostasis with an acceptable rate of success.

Recent work with the compact-EASIE endoscopy simulator (Figs 11.1–11.3) has demonstrated that intensive workshops on this model can lead to significant improvement in trainees' hemostasis skills. This pilot study, presented at the 2002 Digestive Disease Week, characterized the learning curves on the simulator of 3 specific hemostasis techniques—band ligation, injection and coagulation of bleeding vessels, and hemoclip application—during 3 weekend workshops over 7 months. In this study, the model was used both as a means of providing repetitive, controlled, realistic practice with expert teaching and as a method of objectively evaluating those skills that were taught. Twenty-eight fellows were randomized to undergo either standard fellowship training or three 7-hour workshops in a 7 month period. Baseline skills were compared to final evaluations on the simulator after 7 months. Significant improvements were achieved in all techniques in the simulator group, but only for band ligation in the control group [36]. For the intensive group, the learning curves for the 3 specific techniques during the project are shown in Figs 11.4–11.5. Evaluations on the simulator after each session revealed a steady improvement in complex tasks such as hemoclip application and injection/coagulation. In contrast, band ligation skills reached maximal skill levels after only one intensive session. This data provides evidence that certain techniques require more repetitive training than others to master [36].

In this study, outcome data on a small number of real hemostasis cases demonstrated significant improvement in the group of fellows undergoing simulator training. While preliminary, such demonstation of improved real outcome provides the most compelling support for the benefit of incorporating work on ex-vivo animal models in routine hemostasis training.

What about using the animal simulators to assess competency in hemostasis? While this is a promising possibility, there is yet no validated measurement of skills on a simulator that has been correlated with successful performance on real bleeding cases. More work is needed in this area.

At some institutions, the creation of specialized bleeding teams direct the hemostasis cases to individuals who have considerable experience in these techniques [37]. Stevens *et al.* compared the rebleeding rates, need for surgery, hospital length of stay, and hospital charges for patients presenting with acute ulcer

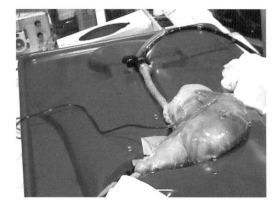

Fig. 11.1 Compact-EASIE porcine model hemostasis simulator.

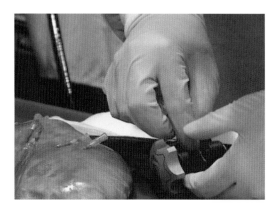

Fig. 11.2 Close-up view of porcine stomach with arteries sutured in attached to catheters for hook-up to tubing connecting vessels to pump. The trainee puts together band ligation devise for varices treatment simulation.

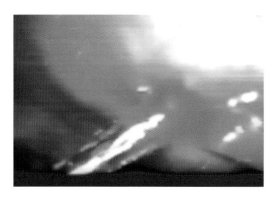

Fig. 11.3 Endoscopic image of spurting arterial bleeding realistic simulation using the EASIE model.

bleeding and found that those individuals treated by a specialized 'bleeding team' had significantly improved outcome for each variable as compared to those patients treated by other gastroenterologists at the institution [37].

Notwithstanding the potential benefits of sub-specialization, this development will certainly raise important question about competency in hemostasis

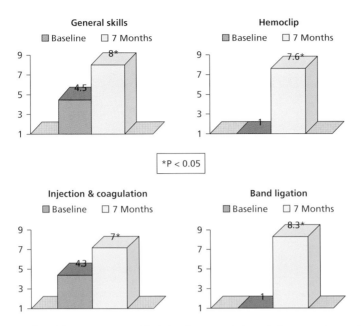

Fig. 11.4 Results of three intensive EASIE simulator workshops in hemostasis over 7 months on 10 point analogue scale to rate skill level. From Hochberger *et al.* [36].

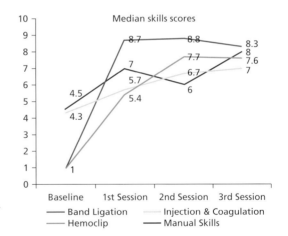

Fig. 11.5 Variable learning curves of different techniques on the EASIE simulator. From Hochberger *et al.* [36].

skills in the years to come. Who is competent to perform these procedures and how much ongoing experience is needed to *maintain* skills? [38] If data is just emerging about the training required to become competent in specific techniques, then data about experience and refresher courses needed to retain competency is even less available. The potential role of simulator based refresher courses on retraining and skills maintenance will be discussed below.

Other specialized therapeutic upper GI endoscopy techniques

Opportunities during fellowship to perform other procedures such as pneumatic dilation for achalasia, tumor ablation, endoscopic mucosal resection (EMR), and placement of esophageal stents may vary at different institutions depending on case volume and local expertise. Certain therapeutic techniques need not be mastered by every endoscopist. Nor is every fellow required to become proficient in every technique. For example, some practitioners may elect to refer cases of tumor palliation to individuals with a special interest in this field who are well versed in various endoscopic palliation modalities. Similarly, given the well recognized risk of esophageal perforation following pneumatic achalasia dilation, it is reasonable for a gastroenterologist with limited experience in this area to opt to send such procedures to a colleague who performs a higher case volume, in the interest of patient safety and improved outcomes. Future data on the learning curves for developing technical and cognitive expertise in these particular specialized procedures will be useful for individuals intending to pursue these interests.

Flexible sigmoidoscopy

Training in flexible sigmoidoscopy is a topic of particular importance given the applicability to many non-gastroenterologist practitioners, and even to certain non-physician providers. While a number of other endoscopic procedures are performed by non-gastroenterologists, flexible sigmoidoscopy by such groups is widespread. The future role of sigmoidoscopy in colorectal cancer screening, with the increasing practice of screening colonoscopy and the advent of virtual colonoscopy is somewhat uncertain. For the time being, given the logistic difficulties inherent with screening the population at risk with full colonoscopy, training in flexible sigmoidoscopy remains an important endeavor. It is unclear what percentage of medicine and family practice trainees currently get trained in this procedure during their residency.

Published guidelines for training in flexible sigmoidoscopy

The ASGE has recommended a minimum of 30 supervised examinations be performed in order to develop sufficient proficiency in flexible sigmoidoscopy to perform these procedures independently [6,10].

   The seminal paper on the subject of endoscopic training pertains to flexible sigmoidoscopy. In 1986, Hawes *et al.* conducted a study of 25 residents in internal medicine, surgery, and family practice in which the trainees were evaluated on consecutive supervised sigmoidoscopies [39]. In addition to grading trainees on a 6 point subjective scale, the authors scored the ability of each trainee to visualize each quadrant every 10 cm of the examination and the performance of the student to correctly make major and minor diagnoses. Eighty per cent of residents performing 26 examinations and 89% of those performing over 30 procedures were deemed sufficiently competent by the preceptors to perform independent screening sigmoidoscopies. Several analyses demonstrated that the individuals with more competent subjective grades performed significantly better on the various objective technical and cognitive parameters measured. For example, polyp detection was 93% once competence was reached. None of the trainees were followed much beyond 30 cases to determine whether any incompetent examinations occurred after a resident had already been determined to be competent by the instructor. There was no requirement in this study for a set number of consecutive competent grades to meet criteria for overall competency. Few of the procedures graded in the competent range achieved the top mark defined as comparable to a second year gastroenterology fellow, suggesting that the learning curve does not stop after 30 procedures [39]. The numbers reported in this study serve to define a minimum acceptable supervised case experience for trainees in flexible sigmoidoscopy. It is interesting that among teaching institutions in the US at which non-physicians perform flexible sigmoidoscopy, the individuals are required to perform far more than the 30 supervised examinations recommended by the ASGE, ranging from 25 to 150 procedures [40].

The Hawes study described the learning curve for flexible sigmoidoscopy. It also provided a template for subsequent investigation to study the acquisition of endoscopy skills during training using objective assessment of performance based on objective technical and cognitive parameters of procedure success.

Colonoscopy

Increased demand for screening colonoscopy warrants a greater focus on the training required to gain proficiency in this procedure. To the extent that better trained operators perform more complete examinations, cause less patient discomfort, miss fewer important lesions, and cause fewer complications than less well-trained individuals, colonoscopy training may have an important direct impact on patients. Further, these outcome variables influence patient behavior and may affect their compliance with screening recommendations. Inasmuch as debate about potential cancer screening strategies centers around these outcome parameters, training issues in colonoscopy take on added importance.

Published guidelines for training in colonoscopy

There has been considerable discrepancy in the number of supervised cases recommended by different societies. On the low end, internist and internal medicine training directors estimated that as few as 25 cases were required to gain proficiency [20,21]. Several gastroenterological societies, including the ASGE, the British Society of Gastroenterology, the European Diploma of Gastroenterology and the Conjoint Committee for Recognition of Training in Gastrointestinal Endoscopy of Australia have recommended that at least 100 supervised colonoscopies be performed during training [10,27–29]. The surgical society SAGES has suggested a minimum number of 50 procedures [25]. Most of these figures were derived from the opinion of practitioners and training directors prior to available data to support such guidelines. In fact, a body of evidence, which will be discussed below, now indicates that all of these minimum training numbers are gross underestimates of the amount of training required before trainees are able to perform colonoscopy at minimum acceptable success rates of 80–90 %. More recent ASGE statements reflect a growing consensus that competency in any endoscopic procedure requires the demonstration by trainees of actual proficiency in that procedure and that no preset number of supervised procedures guarantees that an individual is adequately trained to perform the procedure independently [6,35].

Defining competence for colonoscopy

Traditionally, endoscopy instructors have considered reaching the cecum without assistance to be the main indicator that a trainee has performed a competent examination. As noted above, the ASGE guidelines suggest a standard of 80–90% technical success rates for individuals completing formal training. Expert gastroenterologists reach the cecum in over 95% of examinations. In a prospective VA multicenter study, gastroenterologists were successful in reaching the cecum in 97.7% of 17 732 colonoscopies [41]. Similar results were reported in a prospective German study [33].

Technical components of standard colonoscopy include the following.
- Passing the splenic flexure.
- Intubating the cecum.
- Visualizing 360 degrees of the lumen on endoscope withdrawal.
- Providing safe conscious sedation and monitoring.
- Maintaining patient comfort during the examination.
- Performing targeted biopsies when indicated.
- Removing and retrieving polyps when present.

Cognitive objectives essential for competency in colonoscopy include the following:
- Recognizing an abnormality is present or that a normal examination is normal.
- Correctly identifying abnormal pathology.

- Correctly assessing proper management strategies for the abnormality.
- Recognizing and managing immediate complications, including perforation.

Probably the clearest indicator of competency is the ability to correctly identify polyps and cancer. Expert gastroenterologists should expect to detect colon cancer >97% of the time [42]. Besides the ability to correctly identify pathology, the proper recognition of cecal landmarks is essential to prevent the false impression of a complete examination. Much attention recently has been paid to the adenoma detection rate on screening colonoscopy as an indicator of a high quality examination. The rates vary, and in some reports depend on the average time spent in withdrawal from the cecum [14]. An average adenoma detection rate of 25% of screening examinations performed is a currently accepted benchmark.

Such benchmarking data is the basis for defining quality measures for colonoscopy, and to a large extent determine where the bar is set when aiming to provide training to the level of competency.

Minimum training requirements to achieve competency for colonoscopy

How much training is required to be able to consistently meet these specific objectives? The simple answer is far more actual supervised cases than have appeared in the listed minimum required numbers in the various guidelines discussed above. The published data is summarized in Table 11.3 [7,8,43–47]. The most comprehensive study addressing this question is the multi-center ACES study performed by Cass *et al.* [7]. In this study, 135 first year gastroenterology fellows from 14 training programs were evaluated prospectively on 8349 colonoscopies by 243 faculty preceptors. Subjective assessment of competency on a 5-point scale and objective measures of procedure success were

Table 11.3 Objective data on colonoscopy technical success learning curve

Author	Ref.	Year	Number of trainees	Cecal intubation rate	Objectively competency threshold
Cass *et al.*	8	1993	12	84% at 100 cases	n/a
Parry	43	1991	1	91% at 305 cases	
Marshall	44	1995	13	86% at 328 cases	
Chak	45	1996	12	64% at 123 cases	
Church	46	1995	10	72% at 125 cases	
Tassios	47	1999	8	77% at 180 cases	
Cass ACES study	7	1996	135	90% at 195 cases	195 cases 90% objective success

recorded for each colonoscopy on standardize data forms. The objective parameters assessed included not only ability to pass the colonoscope to the cecum
but ability to recognize and correctly identify abnormal pathology during the
examination. Learning curves were constructed. Technical success rates at
reaching the cecum of at least 90% did not occur until a median of 195
procedures. Comparison with fellow's log books indicated that up to 30% of
procedures were not recorded on data forms, implying that the numbers
obtained were underestimates of the true number of colonoscopies required to
achieve competency. In contrast to the objective measurements, subjective ratings
indicated competent ratings >90% after a median of only 70 cases. This is the
best evidence that objective measurement of procedure outcome in endoscopy
cannot be surmised by subjective assessment.

Cass performed a least-squares regression of logarithmic curve using the
published data in the literature of cecal intubation rates at increasing level of
experience and arrived at an estimate of 341 colonoscopies for the average trainee
to achieve a 90% technical success rate. [48]. As mentioned, competency in
colonoscopy also requires cognitive accuracy and ability to perform polypectomy. A recently published evaluation of colonosocopy simulator training of 45
fellows using the same evaluation form as used in the Cass study corroborated
these results as to the median number of cases required before competency was
achieved. [49] Therefore, strong evidence supports the conclusion that as long
as objective competency levels of 80–90% are the endpoint of training, then
previously published minimum supervised case numbers are far too low.

Competency and colonoscopy outcome

The best indication of successful colonoscopy training is good outcome data for
practitioners following their supervised period of instruction. The rate of technically complete examinations and complication rates of recent graduates can
be compared to published rates for expert endoscopists in the community.
Outcome databases generated from computerized procedure reports will make
rates of complete examinations easier to track. Other important outcome
parameters such as complication rates and rates of missed pathology will be
much harder to follow outside of a prospective study. Finally, patient satisfaction data is needed to look at the influence of greater operator experience on
this important influencing factor on future screening compliance.

With as many at 700 cases performed during gastroenterology fellowship,
the suggested 90% technical success guideline for practitioners at the end of
training should be feasible, and lower success rates by any practitioner, regardless of specialty, should no longer be considered acceptable. When practitioners
experience substandard colonoscopy outcomes, it suggests that either initial

training was insufficient or current case volume is too low to maintain adequate skills.

Data on non-gastroenterologist endoscopists indicates that adequate outcomes may be not be achieved until a very large cumulative experience is acquired. One family practitioner achieved only a 54% cecal intubation rate during his first 293 cases [50]. At this many cases most gastroenterology fellows reach the cecum over 90%. It is likely that the vastly different daily procedure volume and the benefit of much greater supervised training accounts for this difference. Other internists and family practitioners have reported complete examination rates ranging from 75–91% [33,51–53]. Hopper *et al.* achieved only a 75% cecal intubation rate during 1048 initial cases without formal training, but over 90% if sedation was used [52]. It is expected that recent trainees take time to go from 90% success rates on graduation to 97% success rates achieved by experienced endoscopists. However, while 90% is an acceptable competency level for a newly trained endoscopist, it is below community standards for an experienced practitioner. One large German study showed that internists had not only significantly lower cecal intubation rates (91% vs. 97%) but also higher complication rates (1 in 1539 vs. 1 in 5155 cases) than gastroenterologists [33]. One study by Rex *et al.* demonstrated significant differences in sensitivity in detecting colon cancer between gastroenterologists (97.3%) and other practitioners (87%) [42]. Haseman *et al.* observed a 5 fold increase in missed cases of colorectal carcinoma among non-gastroenterologist colonoscopists as compared to gastroenterologists; of the missed cases, approximately half were due to inability to reach the cecum [54].

Excellent outcomes are not limited to gastroenterologists, however. Wexner presented a procedure success rate of 96.5% for 4 expert surgeon colonoscopists [55]. In the initial single center study by Cass *et al.*, 7 GI fellows and 5 fourth year surgical residents had similar performance levels [8]. These data suggest that specialty does not influence objective measures of competency, as long as the quality of training and the case experience is comparable and sufficient to achieve acceptable success rates.

Rate of skills acquisition for colonoscopy

The issue arises that some trainees learn faster than others. As training program directors look for more efficient methods of training to meet increasing manpower needs for colonoscopy, factors which influence the *rate* of skills acquisition will be important to define. In the Cass, study, there were significant differences in the mean number of procedures performed before becoming competent between the fastest and slowest 5% of fellows. [O. Cass, personal communication, manuscript in preparation.]

The baseline hand-eye coordination of the trainee may influence the early part of the learning curve as the fellow learns to control the dials and torque the instrument. If this could be assessed at the start of training, those with less developed skills might benefit from additional exercises on simulators or static models to accelerate their learning rate, or at least to make their initial cases more tolerable for the patients.

The volume of cases performed per week may also influence the pace of skill development. The training environment is often shaped by the clinical activity of the endoscopy unit, but more information about the optimal case load per week from the trainee's perspective may reveal that some fellows are performing too few cases each week. Alternatively, given increased workloads in some endoscopy units, it is quite possible that some trainees actually spend too much of their time performing colonoscopy. At this authors' institution, data from fellows' logs indicate that the trainees perform close to 700 colonoscopies during their 3 year experience.

Much of the studies on training focus on the important question on how much procedure training is enough. This is most appropriate in a setting where non-gastroenterologists are interested in performing these procedures without completing a dedicated training program akin to that of the gastroenterology fellow. But an equally valid question which has not received much attention or investigation is how much is too much, when more time might be devoted to developing cognitive skills, knowledge base, or research interests.

Training in therapeutic colonoscopy techniques

Biopsy, polypectomy, hemostasis techniques, stricture dilation, stent deployment

There is scant literature on the specific amount of training required to gain proficiency in therapeutic techniques performed during colonoscopy. Published guidelines acknowledge that individuals require extra specific training to develop these skills. Past recommendations have specified a suggested minimum number of procedures for trainees to perform [10,34], but there is really no evidence to support that these numbers are sufficient (Table 11.2). Most of these therapeutic colonoscopy procedures are routinely taught to GI fellows, and training programs typically provide trainees with ample case volume to surpass these numbers during a 3 year fellowship.

Therapeutic techniques integral to performance of diagnostic colonoscopy

Given the widespread access to practitioners with the ability to perform targeted biopsy and polypectomy whenever the need arises during a diagnostic endoscopy, some have questioned the ethics of anyone performing diagnostic colonoscopy without sufficient training to take biopsies or remove polyps [56]. Non-gastroenterologists who provide colonoscopy services should be able to not only achieve cecal intubation rates that are comparable to community gastroenterologists but should also be able to perform these common therapeutic maneuvers to avoid unnecessary repeat procedures. It could also be argued that for very large polyps, if the endoscopist is not comfortable attempting to remove them endoscopically, then the individual must have the ability to mark the lesion with a tattoo to facilitate subsequent lesion localization by either an expert endoscopist or surgical consultant.

Advanced therapeutic colonoscopy techniques

Management of large polyps, saline assisted polypectomy, endoscopic dilation of colonic strictures, and placement of self-expanding metal stents for tumor palliation are procedures requiring specific training and expertise. Unlike the ability to remove polyps that are encountered routinely during the examination, it is not imperative than every practitioner performing colonoscopy be capable these advanced techniques. GI fellows typically receive some training in all of these procedures, although the extent of their experience during fellowship may vary. No data exists defining the amount of supervised training needed to become proficient in these specialized areas.

Diagnostic and therapeutic ERCP

Published guidelines for training in ERCP

The ASGE has recognized that certain endoscopic procedures such as diagnostic and therapeutic ERCP are more complex and entail greater risk than standard procedures. According this organization developed guidelines for advanced endoscopy training in 1994 and updated these in 2001 [57]. A revised ERCP curriculum guideline was published in 2006 [58]. Current minimum numbers of ERCPs which must be performed before competency can be assessed include 200 cases, including at least 40 sphincterotomies and 10 stent placements [10]. Notable among the general principles set forth in these recommendations are the following:

• Not all programs are suited to offer such training and not all fellows should receive this training.

• Those training programs which provide advanced endoscopic training must have sufficient case volume and local expertise.

• The former model of providing exposure to trainees with 100 or fewer procedures with subsequent additional supervised training during practice is no longer viewed as acceptable.

- Training should be focused upon trainees who will get to perform a large volume of cases with the expectation that they might develop sufficient skill to perform ERCP independently at the completion of the training period.
- Objective monitoring of performance should occur during training [57].

The published training guidelines emphasize the non-technical aspects of ERCP training and recommend that substantial time devoted to this pursuit. Time spent attending meetings and participating in endoscopic research is also advocated. While it is possible for someone with sufficient intrinsic ability and caseload to complete this training within a 3 year GI fellowship program, many trainees will require a dedicated 4th year of training to gain technical and cognitive proficiency in ERCP.

Defining competence for ERCP

ERCP involves a wide array of different diagnostic and therapeutic techniques. To be competent at ERCP, a trainee must be able to consistently perform the intended procedures without assistance. The ASGE guidelines suggest that trainees be able to perform all of the following tasks [6].

- Cannulation of desired duct.
- Opacification of desired duct.
- Stent placement.
- Sphincterotomy.
- Stone extraction.

ASGE recommendations are that trainees be able to perform these techniques with ≥80% success. Similar to other procedures, this must be accompanied by concomitant demonstration of appropriate interpretive and diagnostic proficiency. Unlike EGD and colonoscopy, the case volume per fellow at many programs does not always guarantee that a trainee will have sufficient training to reach the 80% benchmark by the completion of a 3 year program [9]. Some have also questioned the arbitrary level of 80% as too low an acceptable success rate at standard ERCP for credentialing individuals to perform ERCP independently. Given the higher risks associated with ERCP than other procedures and the usual availability within communities of practitioners performing at 90% success or better, does the limitation in available training case volume justify the standards for success to be set lower for ERCP than for EGD and colonoscopy? This topic on ongoing debate highlights the importance of accounting for procedure difficulty when tallying success rates.

As with colonoscopy, the appropriateness of outcome based definitions of competency in ERCP can be validated by examining the success rates of expert practitioners. Expert endoscopists have been shown to successfully cannulate the common bile date at a rate of >95%. [59–62]. One study from England described a range of biliary cannulation success rates among practitioners from 76% to 95% [63]. It is problematic to generalize results published from large academic centers, which are subject to referral bias in which more difficult cases are seen at expert centers. Such data may also be skewed in the opposite direction due to operator bias in which more experienced endoscopists at high volume centers are more willing to utilize aggressive techniques in order to achieve successful intervention than are less experienced colleagues in the community. All information on ERCP outcome looking at both procedure success and complication rates must consider these influential forces.

Limited information is available for standard benchmarks for specific technical aspects of ERCP apart from achieving biliary access. One can extrapolate from published series in the literature the specific procedure success rates at expert centers for sphincter of Oddi manometry, mechanical lithotripsy, deployment of metal biliary stents, pancreatic endotherapy, and minor papilla endotherapy. However, less information is available about success rates for these techniques by endoscopists in the community.

Measures of technical success, such as selective cannulation, can be recorded, but how does one rate a trainee when the expert proctor has difficulty with or fails to achieve the procedure objective? Schutz et al. have devised a rating scale to describe the degree of difficulty intrinsic to the procedure [64]. Both the nature of the intended procedure and the degree of difficulty actually experienced by the tutor when the trainee is unable to complete the case provide relevant information about the case difficulty which should impact on any rating of trainee performance. Future efforts to prospectively evaluate trainees' progress during training or to objectively assess their competency level at the end of training ought to take these factors into account.

The highly subjective assessment of endoscopic judgment also influences the overall competency rating of a fellow at the end of training. Given the risk of severe complications, it is sometimes the best medical decision even for an expert not to persist in an attempted difficult procedure if the indication is limited. For example, failure to achieve deep biliary cannulation in a young female patient with non-dilated ducts and suspected Type II sphincter of Oddi dysfunction after a short period of time generally does not warrant more vigorous attempts to obtain access and certainly not pre-cut techniques. Evaluation of competency in ERCP must somehow manage to take judgment into account in addition to technical success, cognitive skills, and procedure difficulty.

Minimum training requirements to achieve competency for ERCP

Although previous guidelines had established a minimum threshold of 100 diagnostic ERCPs to achieve competency [65], one study by Jowell *et al.*

demonstrated that 180 such cases are required to cannulate the desired duct with a success rate of at least 80% [9]. In this study, proctors prospectively graded 1796 ERCPs performed by 17 fellows. Overall ERCP competence was defined as having a rating of 1 or 2 on a 6 point subjective scale for 20 consecutive procedures. The authors found that the probability of achieving an acceptable score of 1 or 2 out of 6 for technical components without assistance did not surpass 80% until 185 ERCPs. In this study, proctors were instructed to take procedure difficulty into account when assigning the subjective score. The number required to achieve deep biliary cannulation and sphincterotomy with competence did not reach 80% at 180 cases [9].

One limitation of this study is the fact that only 3 fellows performed over 180 ERCPs during the study period. Therefore, while it is difficult to infer that fellows will achieve competency at ERCP by 180 cases, this data demonstrates that previous recommendations of 100 cases grossly underestimated the experience required to master this procedure. Another study analyzed the learning curve of 21 trainees during their first 100 ERCPs and similarly found that no fellow reached sustained acceptable biliary cannulation success rates during the study [66]. Because so little data has been collected on trainees' performance as they reach higher procedure numbers, the true number of ERCPs required to achieve competency remains uncertain except that it is far greater than 100. Recently revised ASGE credentialing guidelines suggesting a minimum experience during training of 200 cases reflect this data [10].

More important than the revised minimum number of cases required during training is the increased focus on objective outcome of trainees' performance. Especially during ERCP, the length of time that a fellow gets to attempt each portion of the procedure without assistance by the preceptor may vary considerably with the clinical situation and the comfort level of the preceptor with the progress of the case. Accordingly, the number of cases that a trainee lists as having 'performed' does not always tell the whole story of his or her degree of involvement in each case. Perhaps more relevant than the standard fellow's case log would be a record of cases in which the trainee cannulated the desired duct or performed the indicated therapeutic procedure without manual assistance from the instructor.

Competency and ERCP outcome

It is unclear what happens if one begins to practice with less than 80% success rate at the onset in terms of adverse patient outcomes and in terms of eventual development of appropriate levels of competency. More data is needed to correlate data on assessments of trainees' competence with patient outcomes as they begin to perform ERCP and other procedures on their own. Schlup *et al.*

described the ERCP learning curve of one endoscopist. In this study, an innovative CUSUM method was used to graphically illustrate the gradual skill improvement for this individual during 532 cases over 8 years, after 2 years of assisting another more experienced practitioner. The rate of selective cannulation increased from 85% during the first 2 years of supervised practice to 88%, 90%, and 96% over successive 2 year blocks. A downward slope of the CUSUM curve for 95% successful cannulation rate, reflecting the lack of further incremental improvement in performance with additional case experience was achieved after 350 cases [67]. While it is hard to generalize the results of one endoscopist, this study demonstrated that competence continues to increase with practice following formal training in a fairly steady manner until far more than the recommended minimum number of cases has been performed. Davis *et al.* looked at cumulative ERCP experience and found that endoscopists with >200 total prior cases had a higher success rate at sphincterotomy 97–99% vs. 88% [68].

Indicators of competency such as procedure success rates may depend on annual procedure case volume as much as total prior experience. In 12 low volume centers in which less than 1 sphincterotomy is performed per week, Freeman *et al.* reported a failure to achieve biliary access and drainage after sphincterotomy of 5.4% compared to 1.2 % for 5 high volume centers [69]. For all ERCPs, endoscopists performing more than 2 cases per week had significantly higher cannulation rates (96.5% vs. 91.5%) [59]. Loperfido *et al.* similarly found a failed cannulation rate of 7%vs 3.9% at centers with low volume (<200 cases/year) vs. high volume of ERCPs performed [70].

As Freeman has emphasized in several publications, failed procedures result in increased health care resource utilization with its associated costs and morbidity [71,72] In a review of 10 000 sphincterotomy cases at a single center over 15 years, while complication rates did not significantly differ between the first 10 and last 5 years, the need for second attempts to complete the procedure did decrease from 8% to 4% [73].

Competency affects not only procedure success rates but also the frequency of adverse events. For this reason, complication rates serve as another marker of competency in ERCP. A number of studies have looked at high volume vs. low volume centers in terms of adverse events, although little data is available comparing endoscopists with more and less overall experience. In a seminal study, Freeman *et al.* found that high volume centers, defined as those performing ≥1 sphincterotomy per week had fewer overall complications (8.4% vs. 11.1%), fewer severe complications (1.1% vs. 2.9%), fewer hemorrhages (1.1% vs. 2.9%), but similar rates of pancreatitis [69]. Other authors have found higher overall complication rates at lower volume centers [59,70,74] or among less experienced endoscopists [75]. Rabenstein *et al.* found that higher procedure volume (>40 sphincterotomies per year) was a more important predictor of lower adverse events than was overall case volume associated with years of experience [74].

Rate of skills acquisition for ERCP

As with colonoscopy, different fellows progress at different rates in skills acquisition. This was confirmed in the study by Jowell, with 2 fellows reaching competency after 120 ERCPs [9]. Some of this may relate to the innate abilities of the particular trainee. One extrinsic factor which may factor in to the learning curve is the frequency of hands-on work. It remains to be established whether fellows at high volume centers achieve competency at fewer numbers of procedures than their counterparts at less busy institutions. There is data described above to indicate that greater frequency of performing sphincterotomy leads to better success rates and lower complication rates [69,74]. However, no study has indicated yet that trainees learn faster or better when subject to higher daily endoscopy caseloads.

Training in therapeutic ERCP techniques

Current ASGE guidelines suggest that a minimum of 40 sphincterotomies and 10 stents be performed before competency can be assessed [10]. There are no published recommendations about other procedures such as bile duct stone removal, stricture management, and pancreatic endotherapy. Eventually, the guidelines may evolve to incorporate more specific recommendations about the expected success rates which trainees should achieve at particular therapeutic techniques before independent practice and the number of such cases typically needed to achieve these standards.

It is also recommended that 50% of procedures performed during training involve therapeutic maneuvers. As the proportion of therapeutic ERCPs at teaching centers increases, this goal should not be difficult to achieve. The principle of training endoscopists who can perform necessary therapeutic maneuvers at the same setting as the diagnostic procedure is critical. This is akin to the principle described above which considers the ability to perform snare polypectomy to be a required skill for all individuals wishing to perform colonoscopy. This diverges from former community practice, in which some practitioners would attempt diagnostic ERCP with the foreknowledge that any need for therapeutic intervention would require a referral for a second procedure. With widely available expertise in therapeutic ERCP, and given the added risks and costs of delaying therapy and subjecting patients to an additional procedure, this practice is no longer justifiable. If a trainee must be competent to perform sphincterotomy if he is to undertake any ERCP, then even 180 supervised cases may be insufficient, as sphincterotomy success rates ≥80% may not be achieved with that amount of training [9].

This emphasis on exposure to therapeutic techniques may affect the style of advanced endoscopy teaching at some institutions. At some programs, the trainee is allotted a certain amount of time with the endoscope, or allowed to handle the duodenoscope only until reaching an impasse. In this way, opportunities to gain experience with a procedure later in a case, such as stent placement, might be wasted unless the endoscope is returned to the trainee after the tutor performs the cannulation and sphincterotomy.

What is the data on the rate of skills acquisition for the most common therapeutic ERCP techniques? One study looked at the learning curve of sphincterotomy as well as the outcome of sphincterotomy performed by individuals with different levels of experience [74]. In this retrospective analysis of 1335 sphincterotomies, a small subset of 3 endoscopists had data collected on the outcome of all sphincterotomies performed starting with their initial case until they had performed over 100. Complication rates dropped to below average after 40 cases for this group, leading the authors to suggest 40 as the minimum number to perform during training. While fellows in the Jowell study did not achieve competency in sphincterotomy by 180 cases, the authors did not indicate the mean number of sphincterotomy *attempts* performed by the fellows during those 180 cases, making it impossible to extract a learning curve for sphincterotomy from this paper [9].

In the Jowell study, in which fellows were allowed to place stents even if the proctor had to perform the cannulation, competency in stent insertion occurred after 60 ERCPs. Competency in stone removal occurred after 120 procedures [9].

More data is needed to support the ASGE minimum recommendations of 40 sphincterotomies and 10 stents, as well as to characterize the learning curves for other ERCP techniques such as stricture management, sphincter of Oddi manometry and pancreatic endotherapy.

In one study [76], Harewood *et al.* described their experience in 175 patients requiring drainage of pancreatic fluid collections, and demonstrated significant improvement in success rates between the first 20 procedures and the subsequent cases (45% vs. 93%; $p = 0.0002$) and a reduction in days to resolution (50 days, initial 20 procedures vs. 33.5 days, subsequent procedures; $p = 0.05$. Such data both characterize a learning curve and help set the bar for success rates possible by experts in this particular procedure. The only problem with relying on this type of study to generalize benchmarks and training requirements is the probability that other individuals with less prior experience in therapeutic endoscopy might have difficulty achieving such high success rates and might require a much greater experience to maximize their own outcomes.

Diagnostic and therapeutic EUS

The ASGE has published guidelines for training in endoscopic ultrasound [77,78]. Development of proficiency in this procedure requires a great deal of cognitive training to identify pathology accurately. In addition to performing EUS examinations under the supervision of an expert, fellows may need to utilize a variety of didactic tools in order to develop interpretive skills and understanding of the anatomy.

Defining competency in EUS

Pooled data on reported accuracy for EUS in staging of various tumors may be used as outcome benchmarks for practitioners wishing to perform EUS (Table 11.4) [77]. As diagnostic accuracy is the best measure of procedure success rate, efforts to assess competency must include attempts to correlate findings with other staging data, including other imaging modalities, pathology, and operative findings when possible. When this correlation is not possible, then direct comparison with the findings of an expert instructor must serve as a surrogate measure of proficiency. The problem of inter-observer variability in interpretation [79] underscores the importance of clinical-pathological correlation whenever possible for both the learning process and the assessment of competency. There is a clear need for the development and validation of a feasible and objective way to measure successful performance of a EUS examination.

Data on learning curve for EUS

How long does it take a trainee to become competent to perform diagnostic EUS? A study by Hoffman *et al.* found that accurate evaluation of the

Table 11.4 Reported accuracy of EUS compared to histopathology for the local staging of esophageal carcinoma, gastric cancer, pancreatic cancer, carcinoma of the papilla of vater, and rectal cancer

Indication	n	T stage	N stage
Esophageal cancer	739	85%	79%
Gastric cancer	1163	78%	73%
Pancreatic cancer	155	90%	—
Carcinoma of papilla of Vater	94	86%	72%
Rectal cancer	19	84%	84%

Data based on compilation of all studies previously reported and listed in the references. From [77].

esophageal and gastric mucosa occurred in a median of 10–15 cases. The celiac axis could be evaluated after a median of 25 cases [80]. A survey of the American Endosonography Club suggested somewhat higher numbers of procedures required to accurately evaluate the upper gastrointestinal mucosa [81].

One study of T-staging for esophageal tumors showed that subjects required 100 procedures before being able to achieve acceptable standard rates of accuracy [82]. Another study found an 89.5 % accuracy after 75 cases [83]. Expert opinion-based ASGE recommendations suggest that novices can successfully evaluate submucosal lesions after 40–50 cases [6]. Most EUS practitioners agree that trainees must perform considerably more cases to master the more complex anatomical relationships observed in examining the pancreas, with numbers ranging from 121 to 150 cases [81,84]. One abstract, however, found that fellows could correctly identify pancreatic abnormalities after a mean of 54 procedures performed (range 13 to 134) [80]. Still, there is little prospective data to characterize the learning curve for pancreatic examination with EUS. Published ASGE guidelines on credentialing and privileging for EUS recommend a minimum number of 100 supervised cases for individuals hoping to perform non-pancreaticobiliary EUS and 150 cases for those wanting to perform all procedures (including 50 FNA procedures and 75 pancreaticobiliary cases) (Table 11.5) [78].

Increasing therapeutic capabilities such as fine needle aspiration (FNA), celiac plexus block, and pseudocyst drainage require specific additional training. A brief period of formal expert instruction may dramatically affect the learning curve for therapeutic EUS. Harewood *et al.* demonstrated that 3 experienced endosonographers (>300 total cases with >100 pancreas cases) had a

Table 11.5 Minimum number of EUS procedures before competency can be assessed

Site/lesion	Number of cases required
Mucosal tumors (e.g. cancers of esophagus, stomach, rectum)	75
Submucosal abnormalities	40
Pancreaticobiliary	75
EUS-guided FNA non-pancreatic*	25
Pancreatic**	25

* Intramural lesions or lymph nodes. Must be competent to perform mucosal EUS.
** Must be competent to perform pancreaticobiliary EUS.
For competence in imaging both mucosal and submucosal abnormalities, a minimum of 125 supervised cases is recommended.
For comprehensive competence in all aspects of EUS, a minimum of 150 supervised cases, of which 75 should be pancreaticobiliary and 50 EUS guided FNA is recommended.
From ASGE guidelines on credentialing for EUS [78].

significant improvement in EUS-FNA accuracy from 33% to 91% between their first and second 8 months of FNA experience after performing 2–3 cases with an expert mentor at the end of the first 8 month block. While the total number of cases evaluated retrospectively was small (n = 20), the cellularity of specimens was increased and the mean number of needle passes required to obtain tissue was reduced in the latter cases [85]. In a similar study Mertz [86], demonstrated a steady improvement in sensitivity for pancreatic cancer diagnosis with operator experience from 50% during the first 10 cases to 80% after 30 cases. This sustained sensitivity ≥80% from cases 30–80 supports the ASGE recommendation that individuals have at least 25 supervised FNA cases during training.

It is unknown whether high volume experience will prove as efficient as this limited expert hands-on mentoring in achieving this level of proficiency in FNA. More data is also required to define the learning curves for other therapeutic EUS applications. Published guidelines stress that (1) these procedures should not be undertaken until a trainee is fully competent in diagnostic EUS and (2) that considerable extra dedicated training is required [77,78].

Opportunities for formal advanced training in EUS are limited in the USA. Programs which offer such training are listed on the web at http://www.asge.org/gui/resources/manual/eus_training_participants.asp. Twenty-eight academic institutions are listed, 21 of which offer 4th year dedicated EUS fellowships. It is conceivable that the integration of innovative training methods such as simulators into EUS training will provide sufficient benefit to allow more academic centers to train some of their fellows to the level of competency than is currently possible.

While many gastroenterologists are attending short courses and attempting to teach themselves diagnostic EUS, a satisfactory curriculum and standard means for practicing gastroenterologists to train in EUS has not been established. If the need for endosonographers outstrips the availability of individuals who have obtained sufficient specific training in EUS as fellows, then alternative pathways for skills acquisition will need to be more clearly developed and expanded.

Complementary methods for instruction in GI endoscopy

Advances in didactic methods

Self-instruction

A variety of didactic materials may be used to complement the supervised mentoring of endoscopic procedures. Standard textbooks and atlases are useful for beginners. Procedure technique videotapes, such as the collection sponsored by the ASGE and available to ASGE members on the web may have relevance to the experienced endoscopist as well as the beginner, depending on the content of the video. Highly edited videotape offers concentrated attention to key teaching points narrated by expert endoscopists, although the editing can make the conditions appear less realistic than raw live footage. Such items may be incorporated formally into an introduction to endoscopy curriculum at a particular institution or used independently as references.

A number of new technologies offer expanded possibilities for self-tutorial. A number of CD-ROM, interactive DVD, and internet offerings are either currently available or under development. For example, several 'introduction to' CD-ROMs are available to help beginners orient to the anatomy as they learn to perform EUS. Electronic textbooks, or 'ebooks', which take advantage of hyperlink capabilities and utilize the World Wide Web for easy access, will allow trainees to explore as their own level of expertise and interests dictate. One notable example is the Visible Human Project based at the University of Colorodo. In addition to providing access to 3-D flythroughs of normal and abnormal anatomy giving CT scan and computer generated EUS images, the online *Visible Human Journal of Endoscopy* allows readers to immediately link onto the visual human anatomical database at will while reading the articles on related topics. http://www.vhjoe.com.

Self-assessment is possible through this learning modality as well. Other web-based didactic activities conducive to self-instruction include cases of the month, chat rooms, and web casts of live procedures. The developers of some of the computer simulator models discussed below hope to capitalize on web-based mentor feedback of self-instruction done on the actual simulators at remote sites. The actual importance of 'e-learning' activities in the future of endoscopy training and maintenance of skill remains to be seen, but the possibilities are considerable.

Group instruction

Review courses for gastrointestinal endoscopy come in many formats and sizes. Lectures replete with still and video illustrations are the mainstay of these offerings. The syllabus may cover a wide array of endoscopic issues and techniques or focus instead on a particular topic. These include large annual postgraduate courses serving 1000 or more registrants, smaller regional courses for a few hundred, and small workshops sponsored by local institutions for a much more limited audience. Unlike most of the self-instruction modalities, attendees have some opportunity to ask questions from instructors. Still, depending on the size of the gathering, such opportunities may be limited. Clearly, the small workshop or breakout session of larger courses featuring live commentary of edited videotape is better suited to enable interaction and active learning.

In one study by Laine *et al.*, exposure to a brief didactic teaching period to attendees at a postgraduate course significantly improved their correct characterization of stigmata of ulcer hemorrhage from 72% to 82% overall, particularly among fellows who had a 15% increase in correct answers [87]. Despite a dearth of similar data demonstrating direct benefit of short didactic presentations, this modality of instruction clearly has an important role as a complement to supervised endoscopic hands-on experience.

Laboratory demonstrations

Live endoscopy demonstrations are extremely popular with audiences. They offer a complete view of the interactions in the endoscopy unit and expose the viewers to a wide variety of situations, some unexpected. Seeing a case in real time, hearing how experts think through a problem and watching how they get out of trouble is invaluable, and not possible on most edited videotape.

Despite the excitement and educational value of this format, a number of disadvantages and limitations of live courses exist [88]. While many patients are happy to undergo procedures by expert endoscopist whom they have never met, less operator knowledge of individual patients leads to increased risk and ethical concerns. Unless live demonstrations are conducted for a small group of individuals with direct verbal access to the endoscopist, they offer limited interactive opportunities. Wide variability in the experience level of the attendees makes it difficult to tailor the cases and the discussion appropriately to the learning objectives of the audience. In fact, many of the advanced techniques demonstrated may have limited relevance to average endoscopist, who may learn more about when to refer a patient to an expert than how to perform a technique himself. When visiting faculty members perform live procedures, there are inherent risks due to unfamiliarity with the particular unit and staff. There are also potential problems stemming from pressures for faculty to showboat talents and succeed in the procedures at all costs, even when it might be better from the patient perspective to stop. The variability in pathology may present logistical difficulties, but this problem can usually be overcome at high volume centers. Down time is another potential issue, which can be minimized if more than one room can be used simultaneously for transmission. Still, the realistic complete view offered at live courses may come at the expense of efficiency of instruction. These courses are both expensive and labor intensive to organize and run.

Given the popularity of live courses, a few of these will likely continue. Local smaller live workshops performed by local endoscopists with expert visiting commentators overcome many of the above mentioned concerns. Such offerings are also likely to prosper in the future but with limited accessibility due to audience size [88–90].

One variation on a theme is the possibility of broadcasting 'live' procedures performed on animal or ex-vivo models to illustrate the key teaching points with zero risk and even allow the demonstration of how *not* to perform a technique.

Endoscopy simulators

The following section will be organized according to the basic categories of simulators that have been utilized, with particular attention to those currently commercially available for use in training. An overview of capabilities and limitations will be presented along with the most relevant validation data. A review focusing on the optimal new teaching modalities for particular procedures and for trainees at different levels of experience was recently published [91].

Static models

The concept of using static models to teach basic hand-eye coordination, use of endoscope dials, and even basic pathology recognition is well established. Schindler described using a model stomach for practice in orientation [92]. A number of static models were developed in the 1970s, including the Heinkel hemispheric anatomical model [93], Classen's upper GI plastic dummy [94], and Christopher Williams' St Marks colonoscopy plastic tubing simulator [95]. More recently, Leung and Chung described use of static model to teach ERCP [96]. A very simple rectangular box 'phantom' is available from Olympus USA, Corp which consists of a gel with embedded hypoechoic structures to simulate lymph nodes for basic instruction in EUS FNA technique. One other innovative and low tech static EUS simulator has been described. This model consists of a modified barium enema bag filled with agar and suspended with vegetables, macaroni, and water-filled latex spheres to simulate solid and cystic lesions. Intravenous tubing connected to a pump pierces the enema bag and circulates fluid through the model to simulate blood flow. In one pilot study, this apparatus was constructed for less than $50 and was used to simulate approximately 200 fine needle aspirations over a four month period [97].

The main drawback of all of these models has been their limited ability to recreate realistic conditions. For the most part, these learning devices, designed to introduce trainees to the mechanical manipulation of the endoscope within the lumen, offer limited exposure to varying pathology.

In perhaps the most comprehensive use of static models, Lucero *et al.* conducted a series of courses in which he incorporated a static model with superimposed painted pictures to represent various commonly encountered abnormalities. These courses combined didactic lessons, slides, videotape, supervised hands-on training on models, a progressive lesson plan with increasingly challenging manual and cognitive tasks, and objective skills assessments of trainees by mentors [98]. The principle psychomotor training program designed by this group is called the SimPrac-EDF y VEE (Simulator for the Practice of Fiberoptic Digestive Endoscopy and Electronic Video Endoscopy). Several types of models apart from the one developed by these authors were employed. For example a specific Bilroth II model was created to introduce trainees to this anatomy. The Classen and Heinkel models were also used to teach specific skills. The authors delineating a series of learning modules and teaching objectives and created a lesson plan employing diverse modalities to reach those objectives. During these courses, trainees had a mean duration of hands-on practice of 28 hours, with 8–25 individuals included in each particular workshop. Unfortunately, the published report of this wide experience in over 22 such courses involving 422 trainees fails to delineate many details of the observed benefit of such training. The report indicates merely that 95% of trainees demonstrated an acceptable level of skills by the end of the training [98].

Still, this concept of intensive multi-modality workshops with expert instructors, a pre-set lesson plan, integration of manual training with cognitive skills, and immediate feedback and evaluation serves as a model for future efforts employing the more realistic and sophisticated simulators which have since been developed. Each of these new simulators has features which make it most useful in teaching a particular set of skills and best suited for a particular stage of the learning process. Some suggestions for how best to integrate simulators into the typical fellowship program are included in Table 11.6.

Lucero's courses appear to be hugely labor-intensive and difficult logistically to conduct. Discovering which simulators are the most effective means of instruction for different techniques is a current area of active investigation. However, as future efforts are made to improve endoscopy training using simulators, innovators must bear in mind that any revamping of endoscopy education will require that issues of feasibility, manpower, and cost need to be addressed.

Ex-vivo artificial tissue models

The 'Phantom' Tübingen Model. The next generation of sophisticated static models was developed by Grund *et al.* at the University of Tübingen in Germany [99]. Rather than integrated painted images to represent pathology, this 'Interphant model' or 'Phantom' employs artificial electrically conductive tissue called Artitex to craft pathological lesions such as polyps and tumor strictures

Table 11.6 Comparison of available methods of endoscopic instruction

Training method	Advantages	Disadvantages	Best suited	Availability	Logistic problems	Cost
Didactic text & video	Enhance cognitive aspects of training	Interactive video & web based technologies underutilized	All stages of training	Widespread	Time allocation during busy fellowship	Low post-production costs
Supervised endoscopy training	Gold standard one-on-one feedback. Other methods cannot substitute	Limited by available expertise and infrequent pathology and patient care related issues	All stages of training	Standard for GI fellows; limited post-fellowship opportunity	Extra time needed for teaching difficult in busy units	N/A
Static models *Colon Sigmoid EGD*	Inexpensive Reusable Allow demo and practice with basic use of instrument	Limited pathology exposure. Unrealistic for	Prior to real case experience	Uncommon	Minimal upfront cost and storage issues	Low
Computer virtual reality simulators *Colon: Biopsy Polyps EGD GI bleeding ERCP: Therapuetics and fluoroscopy Flexible sigmoidoscopy*	Best exposure of different pathology in hands-on model Excellent introduction & practice for scope control & tactile feel. Unlimited reuse Self-training & assessment possible	Therapeutic techniques still not too realistic—but rapidly improving. Best used with introduction to various skills	First few months of endoscopy training ERCP/bleeding/polyp modules in year 2	Low	Lack of portability and high purchase cost are limiting factors. Very easy upkeep.	High $30–50K

Continued p. 324

Table 11.6 (cont'd)

Training method	Advantages	Disadvantages	Best suited	Availability	Logistic problems	Cost
Artificial tissue model 'Phantom'	Best static colon 'feel'	Presently requires staffing and preparation from University of Tubingen. Impractical for local hospital routine use at present	First year fellows for colon, though cheaper static models exist.	Low. Versions in the US exist but not the pre-prepared artificial tissue is not readily replaced for additional use without the team from Tubingen	Labor intensive workshops Not possible to prepare models, esp. the ERCP model without the team from Tubingen.	N/A Currently Hand-made
EGD	Best model of polypectomy.		Second year fellows:			
APC	Excellent ERCP therapeutics		Polyps APC, and strictures			
PEG	Bleeding simulation possible		Advanced trainees for ERCP & therapy			
Colon Polyp	Reusable model allows multiple trainees					
Colon Tumor						
Dilation						
Ablation						
Stenting						
ERCP (CBD+PD)						

Ex-vivo EASIE model *EGD:* *GI Bleeding* *Banding* *Injection* *Clipping* *Cautery* *APC* *ERCP (CBD)* *EMR* *Foreign body removal* *PEG*	Allows repetative practice and relaxed feedback for infrequently encountered high risk tasks. Best GI bleeding and EGD. Excellent needle knife, EMR, clipping, Biliary setup-CBD only possible Excellent for skills evaluation	Multiple instructors required. Extensive prepartion of the stomachs required. Certain skills require repeat sessions. No PD cannulation possible. Simpler models suffice for basic skills instruction	Best suited for second and third year fellows to refine basic skills and get intensive bleeding instruction Also ideal for more advanced people learning or refreshing specific skills	Low	Labor intensive workshops Compact EASIE kits are portable. Few are trained to prepare stomachs	Medium $5K per kit. Faculty/facilities may be costly to arrange
Live animal short courses "Ethicon" *ERCP* *EUS*	Realistic including motility & complications Best EUS model	High relative resource allocation. Ethical concerns	EUS	very Low	Facility dependent Very limited # of spots & workshops	High >$1K per registrant
Live courses	Live decision making by experts Entertaining with variable applicability to average endoscopist	Limited opportunity for questions and interaction Variable uncontrolled content	Limited benefit as adjunct to advanced training and experience	Several such courses held annually	Difficult to conduct Gathering faculty and patients	Moderate registration fees

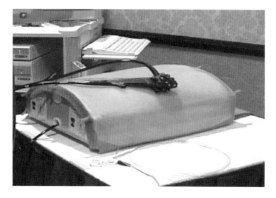

Fig. 11.6 Artificial tissue colonoscopy 'phantom' simulator, U of Tübingen.

which are sewn directly into the three-dimensional latex anatomical model (Fig. 11.6). These models still lack the realism of real bowel wall compliance and motility. However, the integrated pathology is not only realistic appearing, but also allows for the application of electrosurgical interventions. The colon model fixed structure employs a semi-flexible series of coils similar to prior static colon simulators, which gives the trainee a degree of resistance to endoscope passage to mimic the feel of an actual procedure. To allow for an even wider possibility of techniques which may be performed, Grund *et al.* have incorporated real animal tissue into the framework of their model. In particular, they craft an ampulla of Vater using a chicken heart, replete with separate pancreatic and biliary orifices, and insert this into their upper endoscopy simulator (Fig. 11.7).

When used at a training course, several polyp laden colons and chicken heart papillae can be prepared in advance and quickly inserted into the chassis of the model after the initially prepared material has been depleted. For this reason, many trainees can work on the same simulator in succession during a

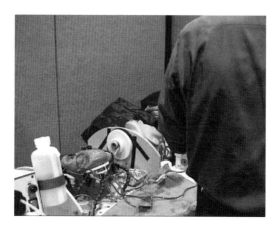

Fig. 11.7 Combine artificial tissue 'phantom' upper GI simulator with integrated chicken heart tissue papilla for ERCP simulation.

training course. Of the existing simulators, this one stands out for its realistic polypectomy, argon plasma coagulation simulation, and ERCP simulation. While fluoroscopy is not integrated, the orientation of this man-made papilla more closely resembles that of humans than the porcine papilla found in the Erlangen models described below. Pancreatic cannulation and endotherapy is also possible, in contrast to the porcine tissue models in which the pancreatic orifice is not readily accessible. Procedures that require submucosal injection are not feasible.

The major drawback to this type of simulator is that currently they are not mass produced and the pathology remains hand-prepared. For this reason, the 'Phantoms' are not widely available and can only be incorporated into training courses at considerable expense with the Tübingen team in attendance. Efforts to incorporate this simulator along with the Erlangen models into wider endoscopy curriculum innovation within Germany is underway.

The Leung ERCP simulator. A more recent innovation using the principle of artificial conductive tissue embedded into a static model has been devised by Leung for training in ERCP.

[100,101] This model uses a camera within the bile duct turned on using a foot pedal to mimic fluoroscopy and allows for sphincterotomy instruction. Rapid turnover of the artificial papilla and easy setup obviating the need for animal tissue are key advantages. Not yet commercially available, this simulator has been utilized thus far to train fellows and nurse assistants and validation work is ongoing (Fig. 11.8).

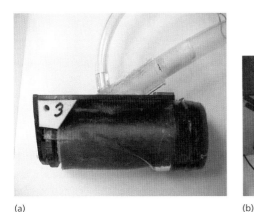
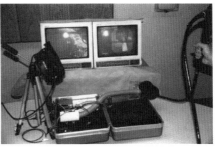

(a)   (b)

Fig. 11.8 (a) Close view artificial tissue papilla with biliary and pancreatic ducts simulated using clear tubing. (b) Leung ERCP simulator in travel kit, dual monitors, external camera, and endoscope shown inserted into plastic tubing.

Ex-vivo animal tissue simulators

Perhaps the biggest change in endoscopy education over the past 5–10 years has resulted from the development and increasing availability of ex-vivo animal tissue models. These have predominantly been used in the teaching of therapeutic upper endoscopy and ERCP as will be described below. Efforts to utilize real colon tissue in simulators and to devise EUS simulators in which porcine tissue is embedded in a gel along with objects to obtain FNA are under development, but not currently commercially available [91,102–103].

EASIE and Erlangen EndoTrainer models

In 1996, Hochberger and Neuman developed an innovative simulator using pig organs obtained from a slaughterhouse and fastened to a plastic platform [104,105]. To this model, Hochberger created a highly realistic simulation of pulsatile arterial bleeding by perforating the stomachs and inserting real arteries attached to a roller pump capable of pulsatile perfusion with cherry colored saline solution. Subsequently, other pathologies have been easily recreated using this model, including the creation of polyps, varices, and strictures [106,107].

Two types of models based on these principles now exist. In the original Erlangen EndoTrainer model, the pig organs are inserted into a dummy mannequin. This model may also be used to simulate various laparoscopic surgical procedures [108]. A smaller portable, lightweight version, the compact-EASIE retains the basic tabletop platform to which only the organs needed for endoscopy simulation are pinned. This may include just the esophagus to duodenal bulb, or may accommodate the liver and hepatobiliary tree to allow ERCP simulation involving fluoroscopy. Organ tissue packages can be supplied for use in these models either by local procurement from butchers or by special order from companies with expertise in tissue harvesting and preparation such as Endoverein Erlangen (Erlangen-Baiersdorf, Germany) in Europe or Hammerhead Design (Mt. Pleasant, SC) in the USA. Specimens may be frozen and shipped ready to be inserted into the models after thawing.

Following the development of this table-top concept by Hochberger, other similar portable model chassis have been produced and are now commercially available. The Hammerhead Design (Mt. Pleasant, SC) developed a simple plastic mould similarly to the CompactEASIE® simulator, with a somewhat shorter length of esophagus and a simplified manner of fastening the tissue for quicker turnover of specimens. The ASGE developed a simulator mould called the Endotrainer X. Both this model and the Hammerhead platform use a flexible net that is suspended over the specimen to keep the stomach in position on the mould instead of screw pins and suture used to fasten tissue into the the CompactEASIE®. In many instances, in order to simplify the preparation, the simulated blood may either be dripped in via an IV fluid apparatus or manually squirted in via a syringe, in lieu of the more realistic infusion pump. Even less realistic is the occasional use of sutured red beads to represent bleeding vessels as targets for clip application in lieu of using real vessels [102].

On all of these animal tissue-based simulators, numerous therapeutic procedures may be demonstrated, taught, and evaluated. Basic skills instruction and hand-eye coordination practice is possible, though this may not be the most efficient use of this versatile model. In one comparative study of the Erlanger EndoTrainer model vs. the compact EASIE model questionnaires completed by trainees of eleven workshops using either one or the other models showed no differences [109]; no head to head trial with objective assessments of trainees and evaluation of differences in cost and logistical factors has been conducted.

Perhaps the most well known application of these simulators is in hemostasis training [110]. The results of the randomized controlled pilot validation study of the efficacy of three serial EASIE workshops was discussed previously [36]. A similar non-randomized study was also conducted in France with similar results from a one day intensive course [111]. The Hochberger group has conducted a number of training courses using the EASIE model in other areas, including endoscopic mucosal resection (EMR), stricture management, vital staining, polypectomy, and ERCP [107,112–115]. The techniques can vary from basic biliary cannulation, wire exchanges, stone extraction, and plastic stent insertion, to choledochoscopy, laser lithotripsy, and placement of bilateral hilar metal stents. Despite its use in many ERCP workshops worldwide, there has been no published validation study to date of any model-based ERCP instruction.

The Neopapilla ERCP model

Matthes and Cohen have recently adapted the table-top ex-vivo animal model to incorporate an artifical papilla constructed from chicken heart and porcine artery tissue which is fastened to a standard stomach and duodenum package to more closely approximate the human anatomy than the native porcine anatomy [101,116]. Multiple simulated sphincterotomies are possible without exchanging the papilla and the native porcine papilla may be used as well, with or without fluoroscopy. Like the Leung model, this enables instruction in a setting where flurosocopy is not available. Another advantage over the native porcine duodenum with liver setup is the presence of a both a bile and pancreatic duct to allow training in selective cannulation and pancreatic therapeutics. As with the ex-vivo ERCP packages, conditions can be manipulated externally to simulate post-sphincterotomy bleeding, strictures and stones for therapeutic training. This model has been favorably received by a number of expert endosocpy teachers, though formal validation of benefit has not yet occurred (Fig. 11.9).

Colonoscopy ex-vivo models

An ex-vivo colon simulator has now been developed by Maiss, Hochberger and Matthes, the so called "coloEASIE" model (**colon**oscopy **E**rlangen **A**ctive **S**imulator for **I**nterventional **E**ndoscopy) [117]. The simulator serves for the training of basic and interventional colonoscopy, sigmoidoscopy and recto-proctoscopy (Fig. 11.10).

The model has a blue base and a metal spiral of stainless spring steel to which is fastened a segment of about 1 m of isolated pig colon. The pig colon is fixed with single threads at a distance of about 20 cm to the metal spiral. Multiple drillings in the base plate in combination with plugs attached to the metal spring allow different variations of the course of the colon as well as the formation of loops by changing the configuration of the metal spiral on the platform. Strictures for balloon dilation or colonic stent insertion are created by compression externally using play gum, foam plastic etc. as in the upper GI model. Polyps are created by turning first the specimen from inside to outside, lifting the mucosa with anatomical forceps and ligating a 'pseudopolyp' with a thread. The anus is fixed within a 50 mm plastic ring by sutures. At its cranial end, the colonic specimen is closed blindly. Various loops in the sigmoid and transverse colon can be created with different levels of difficulty. Therapeutic techniques such as EMR and stricture management can be taught using the coloEASIE simulator; in addition, this model allows rigid proctoscopy training including the treatment of haemorrhoids by ligation and sclerotherapy. Due to the use of biological tissue a realistic tactile feedback and anatomical surrounding is achieved. All standard endoscopes, accessories and electrosurgical devices can be used for training. The simulator can be set up in a supine, a left lateral or right lateral position by means of T-brackets and screw-attachments. To date, the coloEASIE simulator has been used in training courses for basic as well as for interventional colonoscopy and recto-proctoscopy. Initial overall feedback from participants in seven hands-on workshops was very positive and is currently the subject of a separate analysis [117].

Sedlack and colleagues have just reported an initial validation study of a bovine colon model which they have constructed. This model demonstrated good construct validity with experts outperforming fellows and fellows outperforming novices. There is scant evidence in any of the simulator literature of correlation between performance on a model and performance on real patient parameters. Given this fact, their finding that cecal intubation times on the

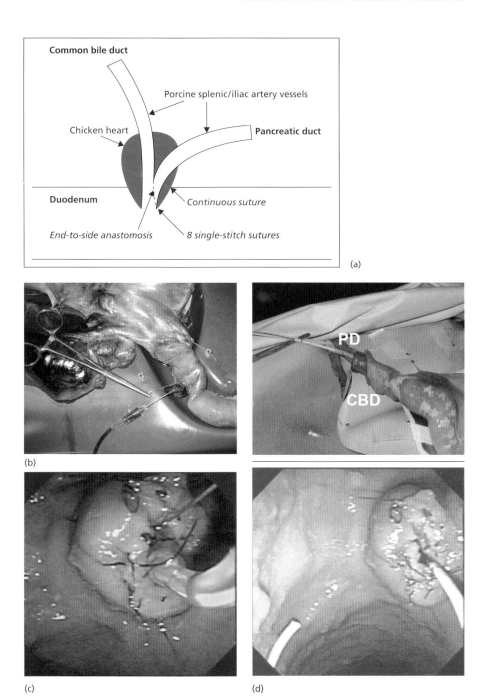

Fig. 11.9 (a) Cartoon of NeoPapilla™ model. (b) NeoPapilla™ attached to the compactEasie simulator. (c) Endoscopic view of sphincterotomy of the NeoPapilla™ with simulated bleeding. (d) Pancreatic stenting using NeoPapilla™ model.

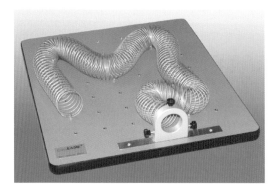

Fig. 11.10 Chassis of the 'coloEASIE' model.

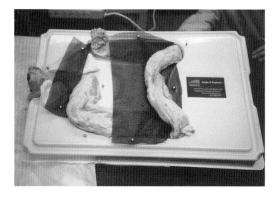

Fig. 11.11 Bovine colon ex-vivo model. Courtesy of Robert Sedlack, MD.

simulation model had a very high correlation to their respective patient-based times (r = 0.764) is most impressive. This model therefore has potential to be not only a useful means of training fellows but also an effective tool for assessment of colonoscopic competence [118] (Fig. 11.11).

Ex-vivo EUS simulation

Matsuda presented a modified Erlangen model in 2002 at the International EUS Symposium in New York. This model consisted of an esophagus and stomach package embedded in a tub filled with gelatin and surrounded by grapes to mimic mediastinal lymph nodes and plastic tubing that allowed a motor pump to pass fluid through it to create simulate the aorta [119].

Ex-vivo model based training: availability and logistical concerns

The setup and preparation needed for workshops using the ex-vivo technology is extensive. While the compact EASIE promises to facilitate dissemination of simulator training to local sites, widespread training of trainers to prepare the

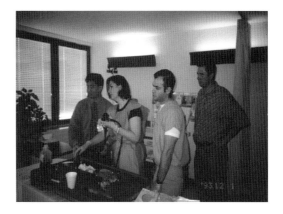

Fig. 11.12 Labor intensive hands-on simulator hemostasis training using EASIE model with 1:1 faculty to fellow ratio.

stomachs and run independent training workshops has yet to occur. Similar to the experience of Lucero *et al.* described above, training sessions using the Erlanger or EASIE models are labor intensive, with high faculty to trainee ratios (Fig. 11.12).

One key advantage of this model is the ability for trainees to perform multiple repetitions of the same technique. The use of real tissue and the capability of performing advanced therapeutic procedures make this the current simulator of choice for practitioners hoping to learn new techniques and for 2nd and 3rd year fellows hoping to get some non-pressured experience performing interventions to complement their unpredictable supervised exposure to real therapeutic endoscopy. Limited availability and logistic concerns remain obstacles to more widespread use of this important new method of endoscopy training. However, great strides have been made in recent years to incorporate ex-vivo animal tissue model work into standard fellowship training and to provide practicing gastroenterologists opportunities to learn new techniques as well.

What began as novel and entertaining demonstrations at regional courses has developed in the past 5–10 years as an increasingly integral component of endoscopic training. The New York Society for Gastrointestinal Endoscopy (NYSGE) has spearheaded with efforts to conduct intensive hands-on workshops in hemostasis for fellows using ex-vivo models and similar workshops involving various therapeutic techniques for practitioners at its annual course since 2001. In 2003, the ASGE began a major initiative to standardize and enhance Endoscopy education in the US with the development of the Interactive Technology and Training (ITT) center in Oak Brooke, Il. With major industry funding, and efforts by its training committee to create a comprehensive hands-on simulator based curriculum, the ASGE is now providing an intensive introduction to endoscopy weekend course to approximately 250 US first year GI fellows annually at the ITT.

Additionally, the ASGE has begun offering advanced hands on workshops for practicing gastroenterologists in specific areas such as double balloon endoscopy and in more general therapeutic endosocopy at which multiple techniques are taught. All of the ASGE ITT offerings blend some didactic material, interactive video case based discussion, along with the main focus on hand-on instruction and practice with expert faculty supervision. A program for advanced fellow training has not yet been established but is certainly under consideration. Many logistical hurtles, primarily funding, remain, but the interest is there, the number of faculty trained to train using the models is growing, and to some extent, data is emerging to demonstrate benefit on the models [102,110,120, 121]. Improvements in ERCP and EUS simulator training should make workshops in these areas possible without the need for live animal work.

Apart from the ASGE initiative described above, the wider availability of ready to use rentable models and pre-prepared tissue packages through companies such as Hammerhead, Inc. (Charleston, SC), and the role of industry in sponsoring local workshops and even in conducting their own ex-vivo laboratories to promote familiarity with using their accessories has dramatically increased the opportunities for hands-on simulator experience both for fellows and practitioners. Finally, hands-on sessions are now conducted at the learning center at DDW each year, at the NYSGE annual December course, and at multiple regional and local workshops and courses.

Live animal courses

Endoscopy performed on live anesthetized pigs and dogs have been performed for both research and training courses [122–124]. Such experience provides the best possible tactile 'feel' of real tissue and endoscope movements with conditions most closely resembling real endoscopy. This includes the presence of luminal fluid, motility and the ability to cause real bleeding and perforation. Live animal courses have been conducted to teach therapeutic techniques, most notably ERCP and EUS [125]. It is the only means of non-human simulation of sphincter of Oddi manometry [126].

Despite these advantages, there are several reasons why such live animal courses are likely to have only a limited role in the future of endoscopy training. Animals are very expensive to maintain and there are serious ethical considerations in using animals for training, especially when alternatives exist for teaching most techniques which do not require sacrificing animals. Such courses can only be held in specialized animal facilities. Only a limited number of attendees can participate in any given workshop. Once certain procedures such as sphincterotomy are performed, it is difficult for others to practice the same techniques on the same animal. The high costs require registration fees over $1000 per session. For these reasons, training on live animals, while potentially more realistic than inanimate simulators, is neither an efficient nor a cost-effective means of education. When such courses are held, it is important that the skills taught are limited to those techniques not well taught on other inanimate models and that attendees be at the appropriate level of training to derive the maximum benefit from the experience. It is not justifiable to sacrifice animals to provide novices with an opportunity to try out advanced techniques which they are unlikely to ever perform in their clinical practice.

The porcine anatomy leads to a few particular considerations which affect the training. First, the long stomachs often require 2 days of fasting to clear, and poor visualization due to undigested food can be problematic. The biliary papilla is located only a few cm beyond the pylorus making it difficult to achieve cannulation in the standard 'short scope' position. The pancreatic papilla is located separately distal in the duodenum, making pancreatic work difficult in the live pig model. One advantage to the porcine anatomy is the presence of a firm polypoid protrusion at the pylorus, the 'torus pylorus' which provides a nice target for practice using a needle knife [107].

In the future, live animal courses will be limited to advanced procedures such as EUS and manometry for which no comparable inanimate models exist. Live animal endoscopy labs remain well-suited for clinical investigation. Testing of new accessories and development of new techniques on live animals will continue, but a lot of the early work will be more efficiently carried out on inanimate simulators.

Computer simulation

The field of computer simulation of endoscopic procedures is rapidly developing. A number of investigators have pioneered efforts to produce models which could allow realistic experience handling the endoscope and incorporate a broad exposure to pathologic images [95,127–137]. In theory, this modality has several advantages for the trainee over some of the other educational methods discussed above. As numerous educators have recognized, computer simulation offers the best opportunity to expose trainees to a wide range of pathology. After the initial purchase cost, using computer simulators requires no setup, and learning can take place either independently or as part of larger training courses. Progressive tutorials of increasing difficulty can be constructed. Progress during training can be recorded and opportunities for feedback exist. Unlimited repetition and drilling in specific infrequently encountered procedures is possible.

Like the static models, computer simulators utilize an endoscope passed into a dummy mannequin. Recent advances in tactile feedback capability have greatly enhanced the realism of endoscopy simulators. Sensors on the endoscope tip generate the sense of tactile feedback. The incorporation of real video images

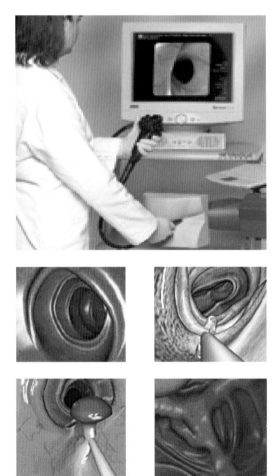

Fig. 11.13 Immersion AccuTouch®
colonoscopy simulator.

serves to further enhance the experience. It is possible to reproduce insufflation, suction, and bowel wall motility. An ASGE technology assessment statement on simulators describes in detail the innovative technological developments in this field [127]. The images on the display can be derived from interactive video stored on laser disk, computer generated images, or a combination of both.

At present two commercially available simulators have reached the market. The AccuTouch® Endoscopy Simulator (Immersion Medical) system simulator (Fig. 11.13) (http://www.immersion.com/products/medical/endoscopy.shtml) allows training in a number of procedures, including bronchoscopy, flexible sigmoidoscopy, and colonoscopy. It is possible to practice mucosal biopsy on this model. Direct performance feedback is provided by the simulator to the trainee. The development and capability of the AccuTouch® Endoscopy Simulator is presented in detail in a recent review [138].

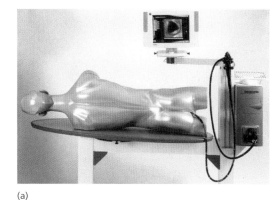

(a)

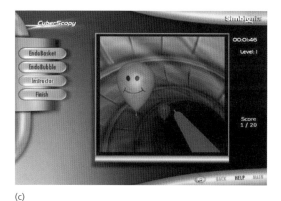

(b)

Fig. 11.14 (a) GI Mentor Simbionix colonoscopy virtual reality simulator. (b) Multiple simulated cases allow individualized training program to be set for trainee and multiple pathologies, anatomical variations, and varying degree of difficulty. (c) Special Hand-eye coordination exercises can be incorporated along with simulated procedures. In this game, the trainee must puncture all bubbles which appear with the needle without touching the wall. (*Contd. p. 338*)

(c)

The GI Mentor II (Simbionix) (http://www.simbionix.com/GI_Mentor.html) (Fig. 11.14) offers several diagnostic and therapeutic modules [133,139]. Upper and lower Endoscopy, EUS, and ERCP are all performed on the same mannequin using a special endoscope for each procedure type. An accessory channel allows the endoscopist to perform a variety of therapeutic techniques including

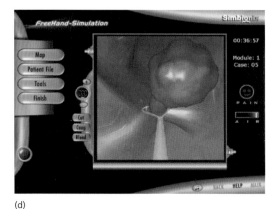

(d)

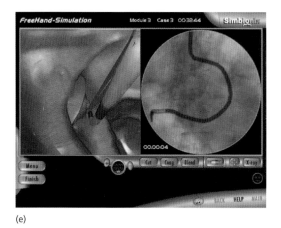

(e)

Fig. 11.14 (*cont'd*) (d) Therapeutic applications built in to the GI Mentor colonoscopy module. Tactile feel within the accessory is still under development. (e) ERCP module on GI mentor.

biopsy, polypectomy, sclerotherapy, and electrocoagulation to control active bleeding, ERCP cannulation and sphincterotomy. This simulator also includes some manual dexterity training exercises ideal for beginners to develop skills controlling the endoscope dials and using torque.

The logical descendents of the Lucero model and progressive training program, these two computer simulators incorporate a series of cases of varying pathology and technical difficulty. Specific training programs may be delineated by instructors. Trainees can get immediate feedback during and after completing each simulated procedure. In fact, the computer will even generate an expression of pain for over-insufflation or excessive looping of the instrument. Performance is recorded, including numbers and types of errors made. The instructor can review the progress of each trainee and the written procedure reports to determine whether abnormalities were correctly detected and identified; feedback messages may be sent back to the trainee. There continues to be much effort underway in the field of computer simulator development in many areas of medicine. In gastroenterology, Christopher Williams has in development a highly realistic, mathematics based colonoscopy simulator [140]. In addition, a number of computer based EUS simulators have been presented but are not yet available commercially [103].

The Simbionix computer simulator has been incorporated into a number of European endoscopy courses, most notably in Scandanavia [141–143]. Respondents to questionnaires have expressed great satisfaction with limited experience on the Simibionix simulator. However, more objective validation data is needed to justify the purchase of these models. This has been the subject of much effort over the past several years.

Validation studies of computer simulators for EGD and colonoscopy

A number of validation studies have been conducted using the Immersion and Simbionix simulators for different endoscopic procedures, and these are well summarized in a recent review by Gerson [144].

EGD validation studies

EGD computer simulation validation studies have only been conducted to date on the Simbionix GI Mentor. In one study, 22 beginners were randomized to 10 hours on the upper GI Mentor model vs. no training and compared on their performance of their first 19 or 20 real EGDs. The simulator group performed more complete procedures (87.8% vs. 70.0%; $p < 0.0001$), required less assistance (41.3% vs. 97.9%; $p < 0.0001$), and the instructor assessed performance as 'positive' more often for this group (86.8% vs. 56.7%; $p < 0.0001$) than the untrained group [145]. Two other small studies were conducted looking at novices and experts in their performance on the simulator, both showing improved performance level for experts [146,147]. In one of these studies, after training 2 hours a day for 3 weeks on the GI Mentor, the novice group improved over baseline, albeit only as demonstrated on the simulator itself, to equal the performance scores of the experts on the model [146].

These validation studies demonstrate that the endoscopic simulator appeared to be able to distinguish novices from experts who were performing upper endoscopy. Still, it should be noted that demonstration of the ability to differentiate between beginner and expert does not imply that a reproducible level of performance on this or any other simulator based test has yet been shown to be predictive of subsequent, consistent competent performance on real endoscopic procedures. It also appears that simulator training enhances the early phase of learning, although only one study has shown such a benefit in real procedure performance.

Flexible sigmoidoscopy validation studies

A small study by Tuggy compared 5 family practice residents who underwent training using the Gastro-Sim® (Interact Medical, no longer commercially available) flexible sigmoidoscopy simulator to 5 others without training as they all performed real sigmoidoscopies on the same two patients; after 6–10 hours on the simulator, residents had significantly improved insertion times and hand-eye skills measures (directional errors, percent of lumen visualized compared to those without simulator training [148]. Gerson and Van Dam compared the performance on 5 actual sigmoidoscopies of 7 internal medicine residents who received standard instruction on 10 patients to that of 9 residents who received only unlimited training time on the AccuTouch® Simulator. Superior results were achieved by trainees in the standard teaching arm in non-blinded assessments on real sigmoidoscopies. The implication is that this amount of simulator training cannot replace training on actual patients. However, the mean training time on the simulator was only 138 minutes (range 66–287 minutes) and it remains possible that either more extensive simulator work or a combination of simulator with real case experience will provide improvement over standard training methods [149].

If computer simulators are to have a role in credentialing in addition to training, they must be able to distinguish between a novice and an accomplished endoscopist. Three studies have been conducted to test for construct validity on the Immersion simulator.

Datta *et al.* showed significant differences in skill measured on the simulator between 15 novices, those with an experience of a mean of 30 sigmoidoscopies performed, and fully trained individuals with a mean of 747 prior examinations, though most of these differences were not observed when the intermediate and highly trained groups were compared alone [150].

In another validation study experts performed better than the a combination of clerical workers and residents with under 15 prior sigmoidoscopies performed, though there were no statistically significant differences in performance parameters between the expert group and the inexperienced residents alone, perhaps due to small sample size or ease of performing the simulated cases [151].

Only one small study (published only as an abstract) looked at the Simbionix simulator for sigmoidoscopy training. In the trial 13 novices demonstrated significantly lower skill on their initial testing on the simulator than a group of 11 experts. The novice group was then split and those receiving 2 hours a day instruction for 3 weeks showed significant improvement in both performance variable and manual dexterity tests over those without this experience. While this suggests that more time on the model produces better results, the small size and absence of clinical outcome correlation limit this conclusion [152].

Finally, in a prospective study from the Mayo Clinic 38 second-year internal medicine residents were randomized to either three hours of Immersion simulator-based training supervised by a senior gastroenterology fellow followed by bedside training for 9 hours, or bedside training for 12 hours. Patient satisfaction was evaluated in 1222 patients undergoing sigmoidoscopy. The median patient-reported discomfort scores were significantly lower for the simulator-trained residents compared to the residents trained by bedside teaching (p < 0.01), but all of the scores were lower than the scores from the staff-performed procedures (p < 0.01). No statistical differences were seen between the two resident groups for any of the performance parameters including ability to perform endoscopy independently, identification of pathology and/or land-marks, adequate visualization of the mucosa, or ability to perform biopsies. The authors concluded that while 3 hours of training on the simulator resulted in less patient discomfort, trainees did not perform any better on the sigmoido-scopies [153].

Therefore, while the flexible sigmoidoscopy simulator appears able to dis-tinguish novices from expert endoscopists, clinical trials have not yet shown a benefit for endoscopic training in terms of performance measures. The reasons for this lack of benefit could include inadequate sample size, insufficient amount of training time on the endoscopic simulator, or lack of appropriate clinical difficulty with the current simulator software. However, the evidence from one trial suggests that usage of a sigmoidoscopy simulator may be associ-ated with less discomfort for patients during the examination.

Colonoscopy simulator validation studies

Construct validity has been shown consistently for the colonoscopy simulators. Sedlack and Kolars evaluated the performance on two colonoscopies on the Immersion simulator for 10 faculty experts, six gastroenterology fellows at the end of their first year of colonoscopy training, and six medicine residents with-out prior endoscopic experience. There were significant differences for the total procedure time, insertion time, and time in red-out between the experts and the other test groups combined , but the faculty described the cases as easier than actual colonoscopy [154].

Similar results were obtained in a Danish study using the Simbionix GI Mentor, finding faculty to perform better in terms of percent mucosa visualized, time with looping, and pain than a group of residents undergoing training and medical students, but again no differences between the trainees and the students [155]. Two other construct validity studies have reached similar findings [156,157].

Does virtual reality computer training benefit fellows learning to perform colonoscopy? The evidence supports that sufficient simulator work does, indeed, have a positive impact, though mainly in the initial phase of learning. The best evidence for this was a large multicenter randomized controlled trial published in 2006 [49]. In this study, 45 first year GI fellows from 16 centers were randomized to either 10 versus 0 hours on the GI Mentor during the initial 8 weeks of fellowship prior to performing real colonoscopies. The subsequent 200 real examinations were then scored by proctors blinded as to the simulator experience of the trainees according to objective criteria of both technical and cognitive performance. The group of fellows who underwent the course of simulator training had significantly greater objective measures of success throughout the learning curve, although the simulator training did not influence the median number of procedures within which fellows reached 90% objective competency. In fact, corrected for the number of evaluation forms collected, the median number of 184 cases performed bears a remarkable similarity to the number observed by Cass *et al.* in their prospective evaluation of 135 fellows [O. Cass, personal communication]. This trial suggests that some of the negative efficacy results from prior sigmoidosocpy may be explained by lesser amount of time spent on the models. Importantly, the greatest differences between the two groups were found within the first 80 cases performed.

Two other studies using the GI Mentor showed some improvement in various performance parameters as measured on the simulator itself over time [158,159]. Such data, however, is less compelling than objective improvement assessed on real procedures.

In a small prospective study to determine the efficacy of training on the Immersion simulator, 8 fellows were randomized to either six hours of work on the simulator vs. no simulator training. The simulator group perfomed significantly better overall than their traditionally trained counterparts in the intial phase of performing real colonoscopies. The simulator group demonstrated improved depth of insertion, independent completion, and ability to identify landmarks out to 30 colonoscopies, though after this number of cases performed, there was no longer any difference between groups [160]. This study corroborates the findings of the Simbionix validation randomized trail described above.

Many questions still remain regarding the optimal role and the magnitude of benefit of computer simulators in sigmoidoscopy and colonoscopy training. Defining the optimal amount and frequency of simulator training prior to beginning real supervised cases will be essential. The data presented above suggest that at least 6–10 unsupervised hours are a minimum requirement at the onset of training. Does ongoing simulator work during standard endoscopy training enhance the benefit of this modality of training? Do GI fellows, by virtue of their increased case volume during actual training with both upper and lower Endoscopy, learn faster, and does simulator training have different benefits for different kinds of trainees? Even if the benefit is less pronounced for non-gastroenterologists, the fact that specialties which have fewer actual training cases to offer their trainees have the biggest incentive to invest in any technology which might accelerate the learning curve. Another open question is whether simulator training will affect only the initial phase of endoscopy learning. Even if initial benefit is limited to the first 30–80 real procedures for upper or lower endoscopy, the impact of prior simulator experience on patient satisfaction during the initial stages of training will also need to be further explored. Does instructor feedback make a difference in the effectiveness of simulator training? This question has not been adequately addressed. One study in which 26 individuals with varying experience were evaluated over the course of 5 procedures on the Immersion simulator without any feedback showed no progress on the model [161]. However, this does not rule out that they might have progressed with the much larger number of cases performed in other validation trials. With future optimizing of the 'simulator-based' curriculum, it is possible that the learning curve might be shifted sufficiently to the left to reduce the time required to train to competency in colonoscopy and reduce the added costs associated with training. One caveat is that if subsequent study indicates that computer simulators, like the ex-vivo models, are best utilized with the instructor present, then this will undermine one of the theoretical advantages of computer work: the potential for independent study and reduced manpower devoted to teaching. The answers to all of these questions will determine whether the impact of the virtual reality computer simulators on training will justify the significant cost involved.

Assessment of computer simulators for therapeutic endoscopy, ERCP and EUS

At present the therapeutic modules for the Simbionix simulator are best suited mainly for *introductory* orientation to polypectomy, hemostasis, and ERCP. In one advanced ERCP training course for practitioners, attendees and faculty were asked to compare their impressions of the relative utility of 20–30 minutes spent using the live pig model, the Erlangen ex-vivo model and the Simbionix GI Mentor ERCP module, and the computer model rated lowest in both realism and usefulness [162]. For ERCP and therapeutic techniques, present computer technology offers the potential to incorporate didactic lessons, specific questions for the endoscopist concerning accessory set-up and generator settings, and opportunities for self-assessment quizzes to complement the hands-on technical experience. It might be a more efficient use of limited resources for trainees to spend time on computer simulators in this manner at the onset of therapeutic training and then proceed to ex-vivo workshops once they have had some experience familiarizing themselves with the equipment and procedures.

The Simbionix EUS module, and other EUS simulators in development but not presently commercially available, carry particular promise but await validation of efficacy.

Computer simulator overview

At present, computer simulators appear to have a lot to offer trainees in terms of showing diverse pathology and teaching beginners hands-eye coordination and scope handling. Unique aspects of this type of training are the simulation of contractions, feedback on comfort, opportunity for self-instruction without constant expert supervision, quantification of skills, and offsite skills assessment by instructors. Current available models appear less useful for more experienced endoscopists, although capabilities are expanding rapidly.

The major obstacle to expanded use of these simulators remains the cost and logistics of making them accessible to trainees. At costs ranging from $40 000 to $100 000 most individual departments cannot afford to purchase computer simulators. Potential solutions to the feasibility problem currently limiting dissemination of this technology include regional shared facilities, use of internet based servers to transmit simulator modules to remote sites via broadband access, and the addition of simulator modules for other specialties so that hospitals could purchase one unit for use in various departments. Recent reviews have explored these future logistical considerations in more detail [120,121].

Much thought has been applied to the question of how to best devote limited financial and manpower resources to the use of various simulators and models for various groups of trainees. Gerson has provided an excellent evidence based review and the summarized results are shown with permission in Table 11.7. A possible algorithm for the incorporation of the various learning modalities available to complement supervised procedures in the process of endoscopy education is shown in Fig. 11.15.

Credentialing and granting of privileges

The process of privileging and credentialing endoscopists is designed to maximize patient safety and outcomes by insuring that individuals performing procedures are sufficiently competent to perform them at the time the privileges are being requested. Decisions by institutions about whom to privilege for which procedures and about whom to grant renewal of privileges depend on both the credentials of an applicant and documentation of current ability

Table 11.7a Studies using simulation for upper endoscopy, hemostasis, and ERCP

Author (year & reference)	Study type & evidence	Subjects & simulator	Outcomes	Findings
Upper endoscopy				
Fertilsch, 2002 [7]	Validation Evidence – [B]	13 novices 11 experts	Virtual endoscopies and skill tests	Experts significantly better; simulator-trained group reached expert level
Moorthy, 2004 [8]	Validation [B]	11 novice 11 fellows 10 experts	Performance after 2 cases on simulator	Able to distinguish novice from expert
Hemostasis				
Hochberger 2004 [27]	Comparison of Endotrainer (4 courses) to compact-EASIE (7 courses) [B]	291 trainees	Questionnaire Modules for variceal bleed or injection for peptic ulcer	No difference in preferences between models
Maiss, 2005 [28]	Training Course compact-EASIE simulator [B]	32 GI Fellows	Panel of experts evaluated manual skills, injection, hemoclipping	All fellows improved. Fellows with more experience at baseline showed greater improvement
Hochberger, 2005 [29]	Randomized Controlled Trial—EASIE simulator [A]	28 GI Fellows bedside training versus bedside training & 3 courses on EASIE over 7 months	Grading by mentors and blinded experts	Fellows in simulator arm showed improvement for all skills; bedside-trained only improved in variceal ligation
ERCP				
Neumann, 2000 [34]	Validation [D]	Senior endoscopist	Ability to simulate ERCP	Successful simulation of stone extraction and stent placement
Sedlack, 2003 [35])	Comparison trial [B]	10 novices 10 faculty	Rating of each model for realism, utility in training	Erlangen model most realistic and useful for ERCP training

Table 11.7b Usage of endoscopic simulators for flexible sigmoidoscopy

Author (year & reference)	Study type & evidence	Subjects & simulator	Outcomes	Findings
Tuggy, 1998 [9]	Clinical trial [B]	5 control 5 simulator-trained Gastro-Sim (Interact Medical)	Hand-eye skills	Simulator group significantly faster insertion times and shorter duration
Datta, 2002 [10]	Validation [B]	15 Novice 15 Intermediate 15 Expert Immersion medical	Incremental and significant improvement in all parameters according to experience	Simulator able to distinguish experience level
MacDonald, 2003 [11]	Validation [B]	10 clerical workers 19 residents 5 experts Immersion medical	Performance on simulated cases	Experts performed better but had higher perforation rates
Gerson, 2003 [12]	Randomized Clinical Trial [A]	Internal medicine residents 9 simulator-trained 7 bedside trained Immersion medical	Ability to reach splenic flexure, perform retroflexion, patient satisfaction & Discomfort	Bedside training superior in all outcomes No difference in patient discomfort
Sedlack, 2004 [13]	Randomized Clinical Trial [A]	Internal medicine residents 19 simulator-trained 19 bedside trained Immersion medical	Ability to reach flexure, perform biopsy, patient discomfort	Less patient discomfort in simulator group. No difference in procedural skills

Table 11.7c Published studies using medical simulation for colonoscopy

Author (year & reference)	Study type & evidence	Subjects & simulator	Outcomes	Findings
Sedlack, 2002 [16]	Validation [B]	10 experts 5 partially trained 2 novices Immersion medical	Determine optimal usage for simulator	Simulator most effective early in training
Sedlack, 2003 [17]	Validation [B]	10 experts 6 fellows 6 residents Immersion medical	Performance on 2 virtual exams and rating of simulator	Procedure time, insertion time, and time in red out better for experts
Mahmood, 2003 [19]	Validation [B]	10 novice 7 Intermediate 5 Expert Immersion medical	Performance on simulator	Experts superior compared to other 2 groups for all parameters
Eversbusch, 2004 [21]	Validation [B]	8 experts 10 residents 10 medical students Simbionix	Performance on 10 consecutive trials on simulator	Experts best performance; learning curve plateau on 2nd repetition for experts, 5th for residents, and 7th for students
Mahmood, 2004 [23]	Validation [B]	26 postdoctoral fellows without endoscopic experience Immersion medical	Repeated same random module 5 times either with or without feedback	No improvement in skills without feedback

Continued p. 348

Table 11.7c (*cont'd*)

Author (year & reference)	Study type & evidence	Subjects & simulator	Outcomes	Findings
Sedlack, 2004 [24]	Clinical trial [B]	8 novice fellows; 4 simulator-trained for 6 hours Immersion medical	Performance during 15 actual colonoscopies	Simulator-trained fellows outperformed bedside trained up to 30 procedures except for time of insertion (p < 0.05)
Grancharov, 2005 [18]	Validation [B]	8 experts 10 residents 10 medical students Simbionix	Performance on simulator	Experts superior performance; no difference between residents and students
Felsher, 2005 [20]	Validation [B]	75 faculty, fellows, and residents Simbionix	Performance on 2 virtual exams	Experts superior for all parameters
Clark, 2005 [22]	Clinical trial [B]	5 PGY-1 and 8 senior surgical residents with monthly simulator training Simbionix	Simulator performance over 2 years	Junior residents improved efficiency by 59%, seniors by 88%
Cohen, 2006 [25]	Clinical trial [A]	45 first year gastroenterology fellows, 23 randomized to simulator training for 10 hours and 22 randomized to no simulator training	Objective and subjective competency during 200 colonoscopies	Simulator-trained group showed higher objective competency during the first 80 cases. No difference in patient discomfort

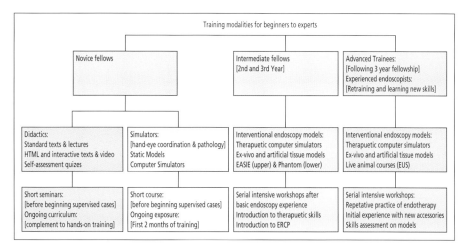

Fig. 11.15 Algorithm for complementary training modalities to standard supervised endoscopy.

to perform the requested procedures at a pre-determined acceptable level of success.

Credentialing

Credentialing is the review of evidence that a prospective endoscopist has proper licensure, education, adequate training to qualify them for privileges at an institution. Training directors are asked to attest to the competence level of trainees after completing the training program. This certification refers to both technical and cognitive skill level attained by the trainee. Trainees' procedure logs also provide documentation of the number and type of procedures performed.

Such information is used by institutions to help determine whether to grant privileges to individuals. Information regarding the number of procedures a fellow actually performed without assistance, the difficulty level of cases done, and the success rates achieved is not generally available for either the training directors or for subsequent review by credentialing committees.

Other relevant data provided to institutional credentialing committees may include licensing information, specialty board certification, and documentation of attendance at post-graduate courses and other CME programs. Statements written by endoscopy teachers may also serve to support a trainee's application for privileges at a particular institution.

As far as subspecialty board certification in gastroenterology, endoscopic interpretation of findings, indications and management decisions are certainly covered on standardized tests. However, no practical demonstration of endo-scopic skill is incorporated into credentialing examinations.

Privileging

Similar to assessment of competency discussed above, review of credentials and determination of privileging requests should follow a few basic principles. These are specified in guidelines for credentialing and granting privileges published by the ASGE [10,78]. First, each procedure should be considered separately. Second, besides flexible sigmoidoscopy, individuals seeking privileges for diagnostic endoscopy should have the ability and should seek the privileges to perform those common therapeutic manoeuvres which are typically encountered.

As discussed above, one should not grant colonoscopy privileges to some-one who cannot perform and provide the credentials to support that they can perform polypectomy. Applicants must be able to document completion of appropriate forms of training and attainment of sufficient levels of both techni-cal and cognitive competence. As with guidelines about competence, privileges guidelines stress the fact that minimum numbers of procedures performed does not ensure competency.

Proctoring

Most information available to privileging boards is either indirect evidence of technical ability or written indication of cognitive skill. No separate standard-ized endoscopy certification examination or practical demonstration of skill on patients or simulators is presently practiced. The feasibility, acceptance, and demand for such certification are all open questions at this time. Direct demon-stration of technical proficiency is possible at local institutions. It has been advocated that proctoring be conducted for all endoscopic procedures [163–166]. However, formal proctoring of individuals applying for privileges is not yet widely practiced.

The ASGE has published specific guidelines for hospitals intending to establish proctoring programs [167]. Proctoring protocols may be established for first-time applicants, for practicing gastroenterologists wishing to perform new tech-niques, for routine re-credentialing purposes, and even for quality assurance purposes when potential problems are identified in a hospital unit. Proctors themselves serve on behalf of the institution and must themselves be experi-enced endoscopists with expertise in the procedures they are asked to evaluate.

Ideally, the institution will invite outside experts to serve as proctors when no one already at the institution is qualified to do so for a particular procedure.

While the guidelines state that proctors should be free of conflict of interest, this may be difficult to achieve in practice. Policies regarding proctoring and the implications of a failure to demonstrate acceptable levels of competency during proctored examinations need to be clearly delineated and written into hospital bylaws. For this process to work, the governing board in charge of privileging must determine an appropriate number of cases for each procedure type to be observed over a specified time period.

Standard evaluation forms for each major procedure should be submitted along with confidential written assessments to the governing body for decisions regarding privileging. Appeal mechanisms for applicants must be specified. The guidelines emphasize that proctors are not supposed to have any role in the actual procedures in terms of either patient contact or advice given to the applicant. Proctors should only intervene in the event of observed substandard care with potential immediate harm to patients. Complete documentation of proctoring activities is essential to minimize liability. Patients do need to be informed of the proctors' presence and role and this also needs to be recorded [167,168].

Renewal of privileges and privileging in new procedures

The ASGE has published guidelines on the process of privilege renewal [169] (http://www.asge.org/gui/resources/manual/pc maintaining.asp). Re-credentialing of practitioners by hospitals is required at least every two years, as stipulated in the Joint Commission (JCAHO) Comprehensive Accreditation Manual for Hospitals [170]. Renewal of privileges depends on documentation of the following:
- Case volume sufficient to maintain skills.
- Objective data on procedure success rates and complications.
- Participation in relevant continuing educational activities.

Data on the number of cases performed is perhaps the most easily obtained for the purpose of privilege renewal. As discussed above, there is some evidence that higher procedure volume leads to better patient outcomes and fewer complications. Individuals with very little experience in certain procedures may elect not to seek renewal for one or more technique. Just how many cases per year an endoscopist must perform to maintain acceptable quality of care is poorly characterized for most procedures [38].

In the absence of such data, those required to grant privilege renewals are left to make their own determinations as to whether documented procedure volume is adequate to maintain skills. If an endoscopist has not performed enough cases to maintain skills, a privileging board can recommend that the practitioner seek some additional training. The gold standard in privilege renewal process really is procedure outcome data. This sort of objective information should become more readily available to privileging boards as they gain improved access to it under the auspices of quality assurance efforts. The effort to define quality measures and get practicing endoscopist and trainees to collect data on their own performance record has not yet had the benefit of sufficient pressure to drive the process [171]. Certainly, more stringent requirements to do so by credentialing and re-credentialing bodies will provide a strong impetus; however, to date, hospitals and departments have been slow to adopt even existing ASGE recommendations into their requirements. Ultimately, with some technical support to make the data collection automatic using the electronic report generators and additional external pressure from insurers or from patients, more of this hard outcome data will become available and should become the primary basis for getting and maintaining privileges.

CME activity is also expected of individuals applying for privilege renewal. But, how effective are refresher courses or even intensive hands-on simulator tutorials in skills maintenance? If these are effective tools in this regard, how often should an endoscopist participate in such activities? The answer would clearly vary with an individual's actual case volume and total prior experience. At present there is little objective data to address these important questions.

New procedures

New procedures present an interesting problem for credentialing committees. For these techniques, requesting physicians are unlikely to have received much formal mentored training and little is known about the learning curve for the procedure [172]. There may be great variance in the overall endoscopic expertise and experience of the individual seeking privileges. For these reasons, some objective criteria of competency and some formal process of proctoring are particularly important in the process of granting privileges in new techniques [78,173].

An important distinction must be made between major new procedures such as EUS requiring formal preceptorship and minor new techniques which might be adequately learned from didactic materials and attendance at short courses. An example of a minor new skill deemed as an extension of normal practice would be the use of a new accessory.

Privileging for non-gastroenterologists and non-physician providers

Increasing demands for endoscopic procedures provide impetus for non-gastroenterologists and even non-physicians to perform certain endoscopic procedures. One advantage of formal, standardized institutional privileging processes which base decisions on objective documentation of competency and outcome is the common approach to prospective endoscopists regardless of specialty.

Recommendations for training vary widely among different specialties, as described above. Common privileging standards based on objective criteria would circumvent any disagreement by different specialties about minimum required training. For example, if a hospital credentialing and privileging board decides that applicants should have completed a minimum of 100 colonoscopies in training with and document at least a 90% cecal intubation rate to merit privileges in colonoscopy, these would apply to gastroenterologists, surgeons, and family practitioners alike.

Such uniformity of standards would serve to minimize bias as to which providers are allowed to perform which procedures, while maintaining quality standards for the endoscopy that is performed in an institution. Interestingly, in many instances in which paramedical personnel perform screening flexible sigmoidoscopy, the criteria used to privilege these individuals are actually more stringent than those requirements applied to physicians [40].

One interesting wrinkle to the credentialing and privileging issue is the practice of office based endoscopy. With current reimbursement forces creating large sites-of-service differentials in provider fees, the prosect of increased performance of endoscopy in the unregulated office settings poses questions pertaining to training in addition to the obvious questions regarding patient safety implications. The ASGE guidelines for privileging and credentialing are intended to cover endoscopy performed by any provider regardless of specialty and regardless of setting. While ethical and medico-legal considerations should serve to prevent unqualified individuals from performing office based endoscopic procedures, this remains a less regulated environment than the hospital. With a number of states beginning to require all facilities in which office surgery is performed to be subject to some form of accreditation, some of these concerns may be addressed.

The future of credentialing and privileging

While it is hard to predict how the process will change in the coming years, it is likely that standard guidelines will be more widely adopted. Local variation in practice may diminish with greater acceptance of these guidelines. Formal proctoring programs as described above may become more common. It is uncertain how government regulation, patient advocacy groups, and third party payers will influence the process.

Two themes which appear in most published statements on competency and granting of privileges are an increasing reliance on objective measurement of competency to establish credentials and the importance of procedure outcome data. As such data become better collected and more readily available to hospital privileging boards, it will certainly have increasing importance in the privileging process and the renewal of privileges.

The use of new technology for credentialing

The role of new technology for skills assessment has the potential to transform this process, but this remains problematic for a number of reasons. Simulators have the potential for current skills demonstration without patient risk and in a time-efficient manner [174]. However, access to simulators with proctors to evaluate skills on them is limited at present. As described above, preliminary data is currently being collected to validate the utility of various simulators as effective learning tools.

An essential question in the simulator field is the applicability of skills demonstration on simulators to performance on real endoscopy. If good correlation of performance evaluations on computer simulators and/or animal tissue models with proctored evaluations on real examination can be demonstrated, there will be a great impetus for wider dissemination of simulators.

Once reliable simulator based tests of technical and cognitive skill can be developed and validated, medical departments and hospitals may feel impelled to purchase simulators to facilitate the credentialing and privileging process. Once such a role in assessing skill for the purpose of credentialing can be established for simulators, this strong financial incentive for their purchase should greatly expand the availability of these tools for use in training.

Outstanding issues and future trends

The technology of endoscopy has been progressing rapidly, dramatically expanding the diagnostic and therapeutic potential of the procedures performed. Slowly, the training process is evolving, as it must, into a more controlled process which incorporates data concerning acquisition of competency.

Standard supervised practice on real patients will be supplemented by alternative training modalities at appropriate stages in the training process. This will begin with more didactic and interactive media presentations of technique and pathology recognition for novices along with simulators to teach hand-eye coordination and control of the instruments. Trainees will thereby begin real endoscopy with a running start, and free patients from the delays and potential discomfort of being subject to true beginners.

Hands-on training workshops for therapeutic techniques will enhance basic skills and teach specific procedures in order to provide opportunities for independent performance of techniques, repetitive practice of skills, and relaxed feedback not reliably available during the usual course of training.

Live courses and annotated video presentations will complement but by no means substitute for dedicated training in advanced procedures and skills. Short courses involving hands-on techniques may serve multiple purposes: starting off points for more concentrated supervised training, intensive comprehensive training in certain specific new techniques such as the use of a new accessory, and retraining opportunities for endoscopists. Increasingly, when fellows complete their endoscopy training and when practitioners learn a new technique, they will be required to demonstrate evidence of satisfactory procedure success rates before getting privileged to practice these techniques without supervision.

Besides transforming the credentialing and privileging process, outcome data on procedure success, complications, and patient satisfaction will be the best validation for future efforts to improve the effectiveness and efficiency of endoscopy training.

References

1 Sivak MV. The art of endoscopic instruction. *Gastrointest Endosc Clin N Am* 1995; 5: 299–310.

2 Church JN. Learning colonoscopy: the need for patience (patients). *Am J Gastroenterol* 1993; 88: 1569.

3 Katz PO. Providing feedback. *Gastrointest Endosc Clin N Am* 1995; 5: 347–55.

4 Borland JL. Retraining in endoscopy. *Gastrointest Endosc Clin N Am* 1995; 5: 363–72.

5 American Society for Gastrointestinal Endoscopy. Guidelines for clinical application. Statement on role of short courses in endoscopic training. American Society for Gastrointestinal Endoscopy. *Gastrointest Endosc* 1999; 50: 913–14.

6 American Society for Gastrointestinal Endoscopy. Principles of training in gastrointestinal endoscopy. *Gastrointest Endosc* 1999; 49: 845–50.

7 Cass OW, Freeman ML, Cohen J *et al*. Acquisition of competency in endoscopic skills (ACES) during training: a multicenter study [Abstract]. *Gastrointest Endosc* 1996; 43: 308.

8 Cass OW, Freeman ML, Peine CJ *et al*. Objective evaluation of endoscopy skills during training. *Ann Intern Med* 1993; 118: 40–44.

9 Jowell PS, Baillie J, Branch S *et al*. Quantitative assessment of procedural competence: A prospective study of training in endoscopic retrograde cholangiopancreatography. *Ann Intern Med* 1996; 125: 983–9.

10 American Society for Gastrointestinal Endoscopy. Guidelines for Credentialing and Granting Privileges for Gastrointestinal Endoscopy. *Gastrointest Endosc* 2002; 55: 780–3.

11 Bjorkman DJ, Popp Jr. JW. Measuring the quality of endoscopy. *Gastrointest Endosc* 2006; 63: S1-S2 and *Am J Gastroenterol* 2006; 101: 864–5. http://www.asge.org/nspages/practice/patientcare/sop/establishment/2006_quality.pdf

12 Faigel DO, Pike IM, Baron TH, Chak A, Cohen J *et al*. Quality indicators for gastrointestinal endoscopy procedures: an introduction. *Gastrointest Endosc* 2006; 63: S3–S9 and *Am J Gastroenterol* 2006; 101: 866–72.

13 Cohen J, Safdi MA, Deal SE, Baron TH, Chak A *et al*. Quality indicators for esophagogastroduodenoscopy. *Gastrointest Endosc* 2006; 63: S10–S15 and *Am J Gastroenterol* 2006; 101: 886–91.

14 Rex DK, Petrini JL, Baron TH, Chak A, Cohen J *et al*. Quality indicators for colonoscopy. *Gastrointest Endosc* 2006; 63: S16–S28 and *Am J Gastroenterol* 2006; 101: 873–85.

15 Baron TH, Petersen BT, Mergener K, Chak A, Cohen J *et al.* Quality indicators for endoscopic retrograde cholangiopancreatography. *Gastrointest Endosc* 2006; 63: S29–S34 and *Am J Gastroenterol* 2006; 101: 892–7.

16 Jacobson BC, Chak A, Hoffman B, Baron TH, Cohen J *et al.* Quality indicators for endoscopic ultrasonography. *Gastrointest Endosc* 2006; 63:S35–S38 and *Am J Gastroenterol* 2006; 101: 898–901.

17 Cotton PB, Hawes RH, Barkun A, Ginsberg G, Amann S *et al.* Excellence in endoscopy: toward practical metrics. *Gastrointest Endosc* 2006; 63: 286–91.

18 Coppola AG, Raufman JP, Sharma VK. Unregulated gastrointestinal endoscopy credentialing practices: a national survey (abstract). *Gastrointest Endosc* 2001; 53: AB55.

19 Freeman ML. Training and competence in gastrointestinal endoscopy. *Reviews in Gastroenterological Disorders* 2001; 1: 73–86.

20 Wigton RS, Nicolas JOA, Blank LL. Procedural skills of the general internists: a survey of 2500 physicians. *Ann Intern Med* 1989; 111: 1023–34.

21 Wigton RS, Blank LL, Nicolas JOA. Procedural skills training in internal medicine residencies. *Ann Intern Med* 1989; 111: 932–8.

22 Wigton RS, Blank LL, Monsour H, Nicolas JOA. Procedural skills of practicing gastroenterologists. A national survey of 700 members of the American College of Physicians. *Ann Intern Med* 1990: 113; 540–6.

23 American Board of Internal Medicine. Results of procedure survey of gastroenterology program directors. *Am Board Intern Med Newsletter Spring/Summer* 1990: 4–5.

24 Federation of Digestive Disease Societies. Guidelines for Training in Endoscopy. Manchester, MA: Federation of Digestive Disease Societies, 1981.

25 Society for American Gastrointestinal Surgeons. Granting Privileges for Gastrointestinal Endoscopy by Surgeons. SAGES publication no 11. Los Angeles: Society for American Gastrointestinal Surgeons; 1991.

26 Rodney WM, Hocutt JE, Coleman WH *et al.* Esophagogastroscopy by family physicians: a national multisite study of 717 procedures. *J Am Board Fam Pract* 1990; 3: 73–9.

27 European Union of Medical Specialists, European Board of Gastroenterology. Requirements for the specialty gastroenterology. In: *Charter on Training of Medical Specialists in the EU.* Brussels, Belgium: European Union of Medical Specialists, European Board of Gastroenterology 1995. Available from: URL: http://www.uems.be/gastrointestinal-e.htm.

28 Farthing MJG, Walt RP, Allan RN *et al.* A national training programme for gastroenterology and hepatology. *Gut* 1996; 38: 459–70.

29 Conjoint Committee for Recognition of Training in Gastrointestinal Endoscopy. Information for Supervisors: Changes to Endoscopic Training. Sydney: The Conjoint Committee for Recognition of Training in Gastrointestinal Endoscopy; 1997.

30 German Society of Surgery. Standards and guidelines of flexible surgical endoscopy. Recommendations of the Surgical Study Group of Endoscopy and Sonography of the German Society of Surgery and the Working Group of German Surgeons on learning and quality assurance in intraluminal endoscopy in surgery.German Society of Surgery. *Chirurg* 1999; 70: 245–6.

31 Rodney WM, Weber JR, Swedberg JA *et al.* Esophagogastroduodenoscopy by family physicians Phase II: A national multisite study of 2500 procedures. *Fam Pract Res* 1993; 13: 121–131.

32 Schauer PR, Schwesinger WH, Page CP *et al.* Complications of surgical endoscopy. *Surg Endosc* 1997; 11: 8–11.

33 Sieg A, Hachmoeller-Eisenbach U, Eisenbach T. Prospective evaluation of complications in outpatient GI endoscopy: a survey among German gastroenterologists. *Gastrointest Endosc* 2001; 53: 620–27.

34 The Gastroenterology Leadership Council. Training the Gastroenterologist of the future: The gastroenterology core curriculum. *Gastroenterology* 1996; 110:1266–1300.

35 American Society for Gastrointestinal Endoscopy. Principles of privileging and credentialing for endoscopy and colonoscopy. Granting privileges for GI endoscopy. *Gastrointest Endosc* 2002; 55: 145–8.

36 Hochberger J, Matthes K, Maiss J, Koebnick C, Hahn EG, NYSGE Study Group, Cohen J. Training with the compactEASIE biologic endoscopy simulator significantly improves hemostatic technical skill of gastroenterology fellows: A randomized controlled comparison with clinical endoscopy training alone. *Gastrointest Endosc* 2005; 61: 204–14.

37 Stevens PD, Finegold J, Garcia-Carrasquillo RJ *et al.* Effectiveness of a protocol-based team approach to gastrointestinal hemorrhage [Abstract]. *Gastrointest Endosc* 1997; 45: AB102.

38 American Society for Gastrointestinal Endoscopy. Maintaining competency in endoscopic skills. *Gastrointest Endoscopy* 1995: 42: 620–1.

39 Hawes R, Lehman GA, Hast J *et al.* Training resident physicians in fiberoptic sigmoidoscopy. How many supervised examinations are required to achieve competence? *Am J Med* 1986;80: 465–470.

40 Cash BD, Schoenfeld PS, Ransohoff DF. Licensure, use, and training of paramedical personnel to perform screening flexible sigmoidoscopy. *Gastrointest Endosc* 1999; 49: 163–9.

41 Lieberman DA, Weiss DG, Bond JH *et al.* Use of colonoscopy to screen asymptomatic adults for colorectal cancer. *N Engl J Med* 2000; 343: 162–8.

42 Rex DK, Rahmani EY, Haseman JH *et al.* Relative sensitivity of colonoscopy and barium enema for detection of colorectal cancer in clinical practice. *Gastroenterol* 1997; 112: 17–23.

43 Parry BA, Williams SM. Competency and the colonoscopists: a learning curve. *Aust N Z J Surg* 1991; 61: 419–22.

44 Marshall JB. Technical proficiency of trainees performing colonoscopy: a learning curve. *Gastrointest Endosc* 1995; 42: 287–91.

45 Chak A, Cooper GS, Blades EW *et al.* Prospective assessment of colonoscopic intubation skills in trainees. *Gastrointest Endosc* 1996; 44: 54–57.

46 Church JN. Training. In: Church JN. *Endoscopy of the Colon, Rectum and Anus*. New York: Igaku Shoin; 1995: 214–25.

47 Tassios PS, Ladus SD, Grammenos I *et al.* Acquisition of competence in colonoscopy: the learning curve of trainees. *Endoscopy* 1999; 31: 702–6.

48 Cass OW. Training to competence in gastrointestinal endoscopy: a plea for continuous measuring of objective end points. *Endoscopy* 1999; 31: 751–4.

49 Cohen J, Cohen SA, Vora KC, NYSGE Study Group, Burdick JS, Hawes RH, Xue X. Multicenter Randomized Controlled Trial of the Impact of Virtual Reality Simulator Training on the Acquisition of Competency in Colonoscopy. *Gastrointest Endosc* 2006; 64: 361–8.

50 Rodney WM, Dabov G, Cronin C. Evolving colonoscopy skills in a rural family practice: the first 293 cases. *Fam Pract Res J* 1993;1343–52.

51 Harper MB, Pope JB, Mayeaux EJ *et al.* Colonoscopy experience at a family practice residency: a comparison to gastroenterology and general surgery services. *Fam Med* 1997; 29: 575–9.

52 Hopper W, Kyker KA, Rodney WM. Colonoscopy by a family physician: a 9-year experience of 1048 procedures. *J Fam Pract* 1996; 43: 561–6.

53 Godreau CJ. Office-based colonoscopy in a family practice. *Fam Pract Res J* 1992; 12: 313–20.

54 Haseman JH, Lemmel GT, Rahmani EY, Rex DK. Failure of colonoscopy to detect colorectal cancer. *Gastrointest Endosc* 1997; 45: 451–5.

55 Wexner SD, Forde KA, Sellers G *et al.* How well can surgeons perform colonoscopy? *Surg Endosc* 1998; 12: 1410–14.

56 Bond JH, Frakes JT. Who should perform colonoscopy? How much training is needed? *Gastrointest Endosc* 1999; 49: 657–9.

57 American Society for Gastrointestinal Endoscopy. Guidelines for advanced endoscopic training. *Gastrointest Endosc* 2001; 53: 846–8.

58 Chutkan RK, Ahmad AS, Cohen J, *et al.* ERCP core curriculum. prepared by the ASGE Training Committee. *Gastrointestinal Endosc* 2006 ; 63: 361–76.

59 Freeman ML, Nelson DB, DiSario JA *et al.* Risk factors for post ERCP pancreatitis: a prospective, multicenter study [Abstract]. *Gastrointest Endosc* 1999; 49: AB72.

60 Choudari CP, Sherman S, Fogel EL *et al.* Success of ERCP at a referral center after a previously unsuccessful attempt. *Gastrointest Endosc* 2000; 52: 478–83.

61 Rollhauser C, Benjamin SB, Al-Kawas FH. Success of ERCP at an academic center after refer-ral for a failed cannulation or failure to complete therapeutic goal [Abstract]. *Gastrointest Endosc* 1997; 45: AB146.

62 Cunningham JT, Tarnasky PR, Hawes RH, Cotton PB. Repeat ERCP after prior failure can be safely performed with a high degree of diagnostic and therapeutic success [Abstract]. *Am J Gastroenterol* 1997; 92.

63 Tanner AR. ERCP: Present practice in a single region. *Eur J Gastroenterol Hepatol* 1996; 8: 145.

64 Schutz SM, Abbott RM. Grading ERCPs by degree of difficulty: a new concept to produce more meaningful outcome data. *Gastrointest Endosc* 2000; 51: 535–9.

65 Vennes JA, Ament M, Boyce HW Jr., Cotton PB, Jensen DM *et al.* Principles of training in gastrointestinal endoscopy. American Society for Gastrointestinal Endoscopy, Standard of Training Committees, 1989–1990. *Gastrointest Endosc* 1992; 38: 743–7.

66 Watkins JL, Etzkorn KP, Wiley TE, DeGuzman L, Harig JM. Assessment of technical compe-tence during ERCP training. *Gastrointest Endosc* 1996; 44: 411–15.

67 Schlup MMT, Williams SM, Barbezat GO. ERCP: a review of technical competency and workload in a small unit. *Gastrointest Endosc* 1997; 46: 48–52.

68 Davis WZ, Cotton PB, Arias R *et al.* ERCP and sphincterotomy in the context of laparoscopic cholecystectomy: academic and community practice patterns and results. *Am J Gastroenterol* 1997; 92: 597–601.

69 Freeman ML, Nelson DB, Sherman S, Haber GB, Herman ME *et al.* Complications of endo-scopic biliary sphincterotomy. *N Engl J Med* 1996; 335: 9–18.

70 Loperfido S, Angelini G, Benedetti G *et al.* Major early complications from diagnostic and therapeutic ERCP: a prospective multicenter study. *Gastrointest Endosc* 1998; 48: 1–10.

71 Freeman ML, Nelson DB, Eisen GM *et al.* Failures and complications of attempted therapeu-tic ERCP: impact on outcomes and costs [Abstract]. Gastrointest Endosc 1998; 47: AB114.

72 Freeman ML. Procedure-specific outcomes assessment for endoscopic retrograde cholan-giopancreatography. *Gastrointest Endosc Clin N Am* 1999; 9: 639–47.

73 Escourrou J, Delvaux M, Buscail L *et al.* Clinical results of endoscopic sphincterotomy: com-parison of 2 activity periods in the same endoscopy unit. *Gastrointest Endosc* 1990; 36: 205–6.

74 Rabenstein T, Schneider HT, Nicklas M, Ruppert T, Katalinic A *et al.* Impact of skill and experience of the endoscopist on the outcome of endoscopic sphincterotomy techniques. *Gastrointest Endosc* 1999; 50: 628–36.

75 Bilbao MK, Dotter CT, Lee TG *et al.* Complications of endoscopic retrograde cholangiopan-creatography (ERCP). A study of 10 000 cases. *Gastroenterol* 1976; 70: 314–20.

76 Harewood GC, Wright CA, Baron TH. Impact on patient outcomes of experience in pancre-atic fluid collection drainage. *Gastrointest Endosc* 2003; 58: 230–5.

77 American Society for Gastrointestinal Endoscopy. Guidelines for training in endoscopic ultra-sound. Guidelines for clinical application. *Gastrointest Endosc* 1999; 49: 829–33.

78 American Society for Gastrointestinal Endoscopy. Guidelines for credentialing and granting privileges for endoscopic ultrasound. *Gastrointest Endosc* 2001; 54: 811–4. http://www.asge.org/gui/resources/manual/pc_credential_ultrasound.asp

79 Catalano MF, Sivak MV, Bedford RA *et al.* Observer variation and reproducibility of endo-scopic ultrasonography. *Gastrointest Endosc* 1995; 41: 115–20.

80 Hoffman BJ, Wallace MB, Bloubeidi MA *et al.* How many supervised procedures does it take to become competent in EUS?—results of a multi-center three year study [Abstract]. *Gastrintest Endosc* 2000; 51AB: 139.

81 Hoffman BJ, Hawes RH. Endoscopic ultrasound and clinical competence. *Gastrointest Endosc Clin N Am* 1995; 5: 879–84.

82 Fockens P, Vanden Brande JH, Van Dullemen HA *et al.* Endosonographic T-staging of esophageal carcinoma: a learning curve. *Gastrointest Endosc* 1996; 44: 58–62.

83 Schlick T, Heintz A, Junginger T. The examiner's learning effect and its influence on the qual-ity of endoscopic ultrasonography in carcinoma of the esophagus and gastric cardia. *Surg Endosc* 1999; 13: 894–8.

84 Boyce HW. Training in endoscopic ultrasonography. *Gastrointest Endosc* 1996; 43: S12–5.

85 Harewood GC, Wiersema LM, Halling AC, Keeney GL, Salamao DR, Wiersema MJ. Influence of EUS training and pathology interpretation on accuracy of EUS-guided fine needle aspiration of pancreatic masses. *Gastrointest Endosc* 2002; 55: 669–73.

86 Mertz H, Gautam S. The learning curve for EUS-guided FNA of pancreatic cancer. *Gastrointest Endosc* 2004; 59: 33–37.

87 Laine L, Freeman M, Cohen H. Lack of uniformity in evaluation of endoscopic prognostic features of bleeding ulcers. *Gastrointest Endosc* 1994; 40: 411–17.

88 Cotton PB. Live endoscopy demonstrations are great, but. . . . *Gastrointest Endosc* 2000; 51: 627–9.

89 Waye JD, Axon A, Riemann JF, Chung S. Continuing education in endoscopy: live courses or video format? *Gastrointest Endosc* 2000; 52: 447–51.

90 Carr-Locke DL, Gostout CJ, Van Dam, J. A guideline for live endoscopy courses: an ASGE White Paper. *Gastrointest Endosc* 2001; 53: 685–8.

91 Sedlack RE. Simulators in Training: Defining the Optimal Role for Various Simulation Models in the Training Environment. *Gastrointestinal Endoscopy Clinics of North America* 2006; 16: 553–63.

92 Schindler R. *Gastroscopy: the Endoscopic Study of Gastric Pathology*. Chicago: University of Chicago Press, 1937: 74–75.

93 Heinkel VK, Kimmig JM. Megenphantome zur ausbiling in der gastrokamera-magenuntersuchung. *Z Gastroenterol* 1971; 9: 331.

94 Classen M, Ruppin H. Practical training using a new gastrointestinal phantom. *Endoscopy* 1974; 6: 127–31.

95 Williams CB, Saunders BP, Bladen JS. Development of Colonoscopy Teaching Simulation. *Endoscopy* 2000; 32: 901–5.

96 Leung JW, Chung RS. Training in ERCP [letter]. *Gastrointest Endosc* 1992; 38: 517.

97 Sorbi D, Vazquez-Sequeiros E, Wiersema MJ. A simple phantom for learning EUS-guided FNA. *Gastrointest Endosc* 2003; 57(4): 580–3.

98 Lucero RS, Zarate JO, Espinella F, Davolos J, Apud A *et al.* Introducing digestive endoscopy with the 'SimPrac-EDF y VEE' simulator, other organ models and mannquins: Teaching experience in 21 courses attended by 422 physicians. *Endoscopy* 1995; 27: 93–100.

99 Grund KE, Bräutigam D, Zindel C *et al.* Interventionsfähiges Tübinger Simulationsmodell INTERPHANT für die flexible Endoskopie. *Endoskopie heute* 1998; 11: 134.

100 Rojany M, Leung J, Wilson R. Mechanical simulator for ERCP training. *AJG* 2005: 100: S84–85.

101 Baillie J. Endoscopic retrograde cholangiopancreatography simulation. *Gastrointest Endosc Clin N Am* 2006; 16: 529–42.

102 Hochberger J, Maiss J. Currently available simulators: ex vivo models. *Gastrointest Endosc Clin N Am* 2006; 16: 435–49.

103 Kefalides PT, Gress F. Simulator training for endoscopic ultrasound. *Gastrointest Endosc Clin N Am* 2006; 16: 543–52.

104 Hochberger J, Neumann M, Hohenberger W, Hahn EG. Neues Bio-Trainingsmodell für die operative flexible Endoskopie. *Endoskopie heute* 1997; 1: 117–18.

105 Hochberger J, Neumann M, Hohenberger W, Hahn EG. Neuer Endoskopie-Trainer für die therapeutische flexible Endoskopie. *Z Gastroenterol* 1997; 35: 722–3.

106 Hochberger J, Maiss J, Hahn EG. The Erlangen EASIE model for a close-to reality team-training of doctors and nurses in interventional endoscopy. In: Bhutani MS, Tandon RK (Eds). *Advances in Gastrointestinal Endoscopy*. New Delhi: Jaypee Brothers Medical Publishers (P) LTD, 2001.

107 Hochberger J, Maiss J, Magdeburg B, Cohen J, Hahn EG. Training simulators and education in gastrointestinal endoscopy: Current status and perspectives in 2001. *Endoscopy* 2001; 33: 541–9.

108 Neumann M, Mayer G, Ell C, Felzmann T, Reingruber B, *et al.* The Erlangen endo-trainer: life-like simulation for diagnostic and interventional endoscopic retrograde Cholangiography. *Endoscopy* 2000; 32 (11): 906–10.

109 Hochberger J, Euler K, Naegel A, Hahn EG, Maiss J. The compact Erlangen Active Simulator for Interventional Endoscopy: a prospective comparison in structured team-training courses on 'endoscopic hemostasis' for doctors and nurses to the 'Endo-Trainer' model. *Scand J Gastroenterol.* 2004; 39: 895–902.

110 Matthes K. Simulator training in endoscopic hemostasis. *Gastrointest Endosc Clin N Am* 2006; 16: 511–27.

111 Maiss J, Wiesnet J, Proeschel A, Matthes K, Prat F *et al.* Objective benefit of a 1-day training course in endoscopic hemostasis using the 'compactEASIE' endoscopy simulator. *Endoscopy.* 2005; 37(6): 552–8.

112 Hochberger J, Maiss J, Nägel A, Tex S, Hahn EG. Polypectomy/vital endoscopic staining/ Mucosectomy—a new structured team–training in a close to reality Endoscopy Simulator (EASIE). *Endoscopy* 2000; 32(Suppl.1): E23.

113 Hochberger J, Maiss J, Neumann M, Hildebrand V, Bayer J, Hahn EG. EASIE-Team-Training in Endoscopic Hemostasis—Acceptance of a systematic training in interventional endoscopy by 134 trainees. [Abstract.] *Gastrointest Endosc* 1999; 49: AB143.

114 Hochberger J, Neumann M, Maiss J, Hohenberger W, Hahn EG. EASIE—Erlangen Active Simulator for Interventional Endoscopy—A new bio-simulation-model—first experiences gained in training workshops. [Abstract.] *Gastroitest Endosc* 1998; 47: AB116.

115 Neumann M, Mayer G, Ell C, Felzmann T, Reingruber B *et al.* The Erlangen Endo-Trainer: life-like simulation for diagnostic and interventional endoscopic retrograde cholangiography. *Endoscopy* 2000; 32: 906–10.

116 Matthes K, Cohen J. The Neo-Papilla: a new modification of procine ex vivo simulators for ERCP training. *Gastrointest Endosc* 2006; 64: 570–6.

117 Maiss J, Matthes K, Naegel A, Hahn EG, Hochberger J. Der coloEASIE-Simulator - Ein neues Trainingsmodell für die interventionelle Kolo- und Rektoskopie (The coloEASIE-Simulator - A new Training Model for Interventional Colonoscopy and Rectoscopy). *Endo heute* 2005; 18: 190–3.

118 Sedlack RE, Baron TH, Downing SM, Schwartz AJ. Validation of a colonoscopy simulation model for skills assessment. *Am J Gastroenterol* 2007; 102: 64–74.

119 Matsuda KHR. How shall we experience endoscopic ultrasound before the actual first procedure? Development of a modified erlanger active simulator for interventional endoscopy (easie) model for endoscopic ultrasound training. *Gastrointest Endosc* 2002; 56: A1.

120 Cisler JJ, Martin JA. Logistical considerations for endoscopy simulators. *Gastrointest Endosc Clin N Am* 2006; 16: 565–75.

121 Cohen J. The First International Conference on Endoscopy Simulation: Consensus Statement. *Gastrointest Endosc Clin N Am* 2006; 16: 583–91.

122 Gholson CF, Provenza JM, Silver RC, Bacon BR. Endoscopic retrograde cholaniography in the swine: a new model for endoscopic training and hepatobiliary research. *Gastrointest Endosc* 1990; 36: 600–3.

123 Falkenstein DB, Abrams RM, Kessler RE, Jones B, Johnson G, Zimmon DS. Endoscopic retrograde cholangiopancreatography in the dog: a model for training and research. *Gastrointest Endosc* 1974; 21: 25–6.

124 Noar MD. An established porcine model for animate training in diagnostic and therapeutic ERCP. *Endoscopy* 1995; 27: 77–80.

125 Bhutani MS, Hoffman BJ, Hawes RH. A swine model for teaching endoscopic ultrasound (EUS) imaging and intervention under EUS guidance. *Endoscopy* 1998; 30: 605–9.

126 Pasricha PJ, Tietjen TG, Kalloo AN. Biliary manometry in swine: a unique endoscopic model. *Endoscopy* 1995; 27: 70–2.

127 American Society for Gastrointestinal Endoscopy. Technology status evaluation report. Endoscopy simulators. *Gastrointest Endosc* 1999; 50: 935–7.

128 Williams CB, Baillie J, Gillies DF, Borislow D, Cotton PB. Teaching gastrointestinal endoscopy by computer simulation: a prototype for colonoscopy and ERCP. *Gastrointest Endosc* 1990; 36: 49–54.

129 Noar MD. Robotics interactive endoscopy simulation of ERCP/sphincterotomy and EGD. *Endoscopy* 1992 24(Suppl.2): 539–41.

130 Noar MD. The next generation of endoscopy simulation: Minimally invasive surgical skills simulation. *Endoscopy* 1995; 27: 81–85.

131 Noar MD, Soehendra N. Endoscopy simulation training devices. *Endoscopy* 1992; 24: 159–66.

132 Beer-Gabel M, Delmontte S, Muntlak L. Computer assisted training in endoscopy (CATE): from a simulator to a learning station. *Endoscopy* 1992; 24 (Suppl. 2): 534–8.

133 Bar-Meir S. A new endoscopic simulator. *Endoscopy* 2000; 32 (11): 898–900.

134 Baillie J, Jowell P. ERCP training in the 1990s. Time for new ideas. *Gastrointest Endosc Clin N Am* 1994; 4(2): 409–21.

135 Gessner CE, Jowell PS, Baillie J. Novel methods for endoscopic training. *Gastrointest Endosc Clin N Am* 1995; 5: 323–36.

136 Bar-Meir S. Endoscopy simulators: the state of the art, 2000. *Gastrointest Endosc* 2000; 52: 201–3.

137 Gerson LB, Van Dam J. The future of simulators in GI endoscopy: An unlikely possibility or a virtual reality? [Editorial.] *Gastrointest Endosc* 2002; 55: 608–11.

138 Long V, Kalloo AN. AccuTouch Endoscopy Simulator: development, applications and early experience. *Gastrointest Endosc Clin N Am* 2006; 16: 479–87.

139 Bar-Meir S. Simbionix Simulator. *Gastrointest Endosc Clin N Am* 2006; 16: 471–8.

140 Williams CB, Thomas-Gibson S. Rational colonoscopy, realistic simulation, and accelerated teaching. *Gastrointest Endosc Clin N Am* 2006; 16: 457–70.

141 Aabakken L, Osnes M, Rosseland AR, Fork FT, Liedberg G et al. Hands-on endoscopy training: an evaluation of the SADE endoscopy course. *Endoscopy* 1995; 27: 66–9.

142 Aabakken L, Adamsen S, Kruse A. Performance of a colonoscopy simulator: experience from a hands-on endoscopy course. *Endoscopy* 2000; 32: 911–13.

143 Adamsen S. Simulators and gastrointestinal endoscopy training. *Endoscopy* 2000; 32: 895–7.

144 Gerson LB. Evidence-based assessment of endoscopic simulators for training. *Gastrointest Endosc Clin N Am* 2006; 16: 489–509.

145 Di Giulio E, Fregonese D, Casetti T, Cestari R, Chilovi F et al. Training with a computer-based simulator achieves basic manual skills required for upper endoscopy: a randomized controlled trial. *Gastrointest Endosc* 2004; 60: 196–200.

146 Ferlitsch A, Glauninger P, Gupper A, Schillinger M, Haefner M et al. Evaluation of a virtual endoscopy simulator for training in gastrointestinal endoscopy. *Endoscopy.* 2002; 34: 698–702.

147 Moorthy K, Munz Y, Jiwanji M, Bann S, Chang A, Darzi A. Validity and reliability of a virtual reality upper gastrointestinal simulator and cross validation using structured assessment of individual performance with video playback. *Surg Endosc* 2004; 18: 328–33.

148 Tuggy ML. Virtual reality flexible sigmoidoscopy simulator training: Impact on resident performance. *J Am Board Fam Pract* 1998; 11: 426–33.

149 Gerson LB, Van Dam J. A prospective randomized trial comparing a virtual reality simulator to bedside teaching for training in sigmoidoscopy. *Endoscopy.* 2003; 35: 569–75.

150 Datta V, Mandalia M, Mackay S, Darzi A. The PreOp flexible sigmoidoscopy trainer. Validation and early evaluation of a virtual reality based system. *Surg Endosc* 2002; 16: 1459–63.

151 MacDonald J, Ketchum J, Williams RG, Rogers LQ. A lay person versus a trained endoscopist: can the preop endoscopy simulator detect a difference? *Surg Endosc* 2003; 17: 896–8.

152 Ferlitsch A, Glauninger P, Gupper A, Schillinger M, Heafner AG et al. Virtual endoscopy simulation for training of gastrointestinal endoscopy. [Abstract.] *Gastrointest Endosc* 2001; 53: AB78.

153 Sedlack RE, Kolars JC, Alexander JA. Computer simulation training enhances patient comfort during endoscopy. *Clin Gastroenterol Hepatol* 2004; 2: 348–52.

154 Sedlack RE, Kolars JC. Validation of a computer-based colonoscopy simulator. *Gastrointest Endosc* 2003; 57: 214–8.

155 Grantcharov TP, Carstensen L, Schulze S. Objective assessment of gastrointestinal endoscopy skills using a virtual reality simulator. *JSLS* 2005; 9: 130–3.

156 Mahmood T, Darzi A. A study to validate the colonoscopy simulator. *Surg Endosc* 2003; 17: 1583–9.

157 Felsher JJ, Olesevich M, Farres H, Rosen M, Fanning A *et al*. Validation of a flexible endoscopy simulator. *Am J Surg* 2005; 189: 497–500.

158 Eversbusch A, Grantcharov TP. Learning curves and impact of psychomotor training on performance in simulated colonoscopy: a randomized trial using a virtual reality endoscopy trainer. *Surg Endosc* 2004; 18: 1514–8.

159 Clark JA, Volchok JA, Hazey JW, Sadighi PJ, Fanelli RD. Initial experience using an endoscopic simulator to train surgical residents in flexible endoscopy in a community medical center residency program. *Curr Surg* 2005; 62: 59–63.

160 Sedlack RE, Kolars JC. Computer simulator training enhances the competency of gastroenterology fellows at colonoscopy: results of a pilot study. *Am J Gastroenterol* 2004; 99: 33–7.

161 Mahmood T, Darzi A. The learning curve for a colonoscopy simulator in the absence of any feedback: no feedback, no learning. *Surg Endosc* 2004; 18: 1224–30.

162 Sedlack R, Petersen B, Binmoeller K, Kolars J. A direct comparison of ERCP teaching models. *Gastrointest Endosc* 2003; 57: 886–90.

163 Health and Public Policy Committee. American College of Physicians. Clinical competence in the use of flexible sigmoidoscopy for screening purposes. *Ann Intern Med* 1987; 107: 589–91.

164 Health and Public Policy Committee American College of Physicians. Clinical competence in diagnostic esophagogastroduodenoscopy. *Ann Intern Med* 1987; 107: 937–9.

165 Health and Public Policy Committee American College of Physicians. Clinical competence in colonoscopy. *Ann Intern Med* 1987; 107: 772–4.

166 Health and Public Policy Committee American College of Physicians. Clinical competence in diagnostic ERCP. *Ann Intern Med* 1988; 108: 142–4.

167 American Society for Gastrointestinal Endoscopy. Proctoring and Hospital Endoscopy Privileges: guidelines for clinical application. *Gastrointest Endosc* 1999; 50: 901–5.

168 Sundermeyer M. Prevention of hospital liability for granting privileges to unqualified physicians. *Gastrointest Endosc Clin N Am* 1995; 5: 433–5.

169 American Society for Gastrointestinal Endoscopy. Renewal of endoscopic privileges: guidelines for clinical application. *Gastrointest Endosc* 1999; 49: 823–5.

170 Joint Commission Comprehensive Accreditation Manual for Hospitals 1997.

171 Cotton PB. Simulators in competence assessment and credentialing: prospects and problems. *Gastrointest Endosc Clin N Am* 2006; 16: 577–81.

172 Fleischer DE. Advanced training in endoscopy. *Gastrointest Endosc Clin N Am* 1995; 5: 311–22.

173 American Society for Gastrointestinal Endoscopy. Guidelines for clinical application. Methods of privileging for new technology in gastrointestinal endoscopy. American Society for Gastrointestinal Endoscopy. *Gastrointest Endosc* 1999; 50: 899–900.

174 Rodney WM. Will virtual reality simulators end the credentialing arms race in gastrointestinal endoscopy or the need for family physician faculty with endoscopic skills? *J Am Board Fam Pract* 1998; 11: 492.

CHAPTER 12

Towards excellence and accountability

PETER B. COTTON AND ROLAND VALORI

Synopsis

Documenting and improving quality has become a hot topic in the world of endoscopy. Key issues are what to measure, how to collect the data, and how to encourage/enforce compliance.

Introduction

No one—practitioner, payer, patient (or plaintiff)—can doubt the importance of ensuring that interventional procedures are performed well. Professional organizations representing endoscopy around the world have published numerous recommendations and guidelines on various aspects of this quality agenda [1,2]. These include methods for training, evaluation of competence, principles for the granting of privileges to perform procedures, and methods for recredentialing (revalidation). The mirror of excellence is accountability. There is increasing interest in defining the metrics and mechanisms for documenting levels of endoscopic performance, which will allow appropriate comparisons (benchmarking), and refinement of standards.

The proliferation of thoughtful publications on this subject has had relatively little effect so far in the complex and diffuse world of endoscopic practice. Guidelines are not mandatory, and peer pressure has limited influence. Training program directors have little objective data with which to judge the competence of their graduates, and credentialing bodies have even less. In addition, there is (as yet) no consensus on what level of performance is really acceptable. In the United States, many of the routine procedures are performed by doctors (general internists and surgeons) who have not undergone formal gastroenterology training. These endoscopists may see the recommendations of the gastroenterology and endoscopy societies as being too stringent, and also self-serving. Finally, most routine procedures (in the USA) are performed in offices and freestanding endoscopy centers and therefore are not subject to the (albeit flawed) credentialing process that apply to endoscopy in hospital environments.

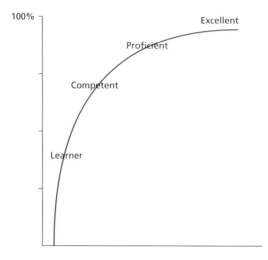

Fig. 12.1 The learning curve for endoscopy expertise.

Achieving competence—the goal of training

Endoscopists can be categorized broadly into four levels of performance—from beginner/learner through states of competence, proficiency, to excellence (Fig. 12.1). Competence defines the level of performance at which independent practice is justified, i.e. the completion of initial training. The key issues are:

1 What needs to be learned to become competent?
2 What level of performance is needed for 'competence'?
3 Who makes that determination?
4 How is competence assessed and documented?

The appropriate application of endoscopy requires cognitive knowledge, technical skills, and some humanity. Until recently, it was assumed that a standard period of gastroenterology training (e.g. GI Fellowship in the USA, or a Specialist Registrar position in the UK) would get trainee endoscopists to a reasonable level of competence. However, this is clearly not always the case, even for standard procedures such as colonoscopy. The situation for advanced procedures (e.g. ERCP and EUS) is even more unsatisfactory.

What experience is necessary in training? the fallacy of numbers

In the late 1980s, professional societies began to recommend minimum numbers of cases during training. Initially, the American Society for Gastrointestinal Endoscopy (ASGE) suggested that endoscopists might be competent after approximately 100 upper endoscopies, 100 colonoscopies, and 100 ERCPs (provided that these included the relevant common therapeutic applications) [1]. However, these numbers were not based on data, and there was never a clear definition of what should 'count' as a case; how much of the procedure must the trainee do? The reliance on numbers was softened somewhat by the inclusion of the word 'threshold' in later ASGE recommendations. This was intended to indicate that trainees could ask their Training Program Directors whether they were indeed competent only after they reached that threshold number of cases. However, this subtlety was widely ignored. More important, several studies showed clearly that these numbers were too low. This was brought into bright focus by the seminal study at Duke University which showed that ERCP trainees were only barely reaching 80% competence after participating in 180–200 procedures [3]. This study and others led to an escalation of the numbers recommended by the ASGE (EGD 130, colon 140, ERCP 200), and by other professional organizations [1]. The Australian Gastroenterology Society proposed the most rigorous test for ERCP, indicating that trainees need to have completed 200 ERCP procedures, unassisted. The fact that professional societies representing surgeons and internists initially recommended much lower numbers [1] was confusing and contentious.

Some of these issues of competence and numbers are amplified in Chapter 11.

It is now obvious that mere numbers are poor markers for expertise. Would we submit ourselves to a procedure by one of our graduates if the sole determinant of competence was the number of procedures that he or she had experienced (or just observed)? We need meaningful objective outcome data.

Beyond numbers: tools to measure competence

In order to measure endoscopic performance, it is necessary to dissect out the essential elements of the procedures, and then to develop a list of the essential 'competencies', covering the domains of knowledge, technical skill, and attitude. Some competencies can be assessed by standard written tests, others by documenting the achievement of technical milestones. Computer simulation may well become an important part of the assessment process. Evaluating attitudes, appropriate application of knowledge (judgement), and technical skills require proctoring of real cases, so-called DOPS (direct observation of procedural skills). The Joint Advisory Group (JAG) in Britain, which represents all parties interested in endoscopy, has recently defined processes for assessing competence of trainees [4]. This group is now applying a competence test for colonoscopy, for established endoscopists who have not been through a competency test as a trainee. This accreditation test was stimulated by the introduction of a national bowel cancer screening program. All colonoscopies performed in the program are undertaken by accredited colonoscopists. This has lead to concern about a two-tier system developing but the intention is that this new standard should eventually become the norm.

What level of competence is good enough? how is it recognized?

When we have the tools to measure performance, we then will have to decide on the 'pass mark' for competence, and to agree who is in a position to make that determination. Should it be the professional organizations (who may be seen as self-serving, and often fail to find a consensus), the payers (who come in many guises), or the consumers? All have different agendas.

Another issue is how endoscopic competence should be certified. An endoscopy diploma (procedure specific) would seem to be the obvious answer, but there is no move towards that concept in the USA. The JAG issues certificates of competence in Britain that are recognized by physicians and nurses. The surgical colleges in Britain have now accepted the principle of JAG certification, but less willingly because of the implications for all surgical procedures.

Endoscopic performance beyond training

Once a trainee is deemed 'competent', a process is required to ensure that acceptable performance is maintained. Hopefully, skills will increase progressively in practice. Competent endoscopists should become proficient, and some will become true experts (Fig. 12.1). Performance is influenced by the extent and quality of prior training, by case volume, by the availability of mentoring by senior colleagues, and by continuing education activities. An important but unanswered question is how many procedures need to be done on an annual basis to ensure continuing adequate performance (let alone to enhance it). Numbers in this context are important not only to maintain expertise but also to provide sample sizes sufficient to detect areas of concern within a reasonable time frame. For example, adverse endoscopic event rates are so low that it could take many years for variance to be recognized and remedial action taken.

Making individual endoscopists aware of their skill levels compared to their colleagues is a strong stimulus to improve performance [5]. This 'benchmarking' can be done only if there is a continuous and reliable measurement process in place, and a central system for analysis and feedback.

Issues in measuring endoscopic performance

Most published data on the outcomes of endoscopy come from expert centers, or from motivated collaborative groups [1,2,6], and concentrate on technical 'success rates' and complications. For colonoscopy, attention has been focused mainly on cecal intubation rates. Studies from experts and major multicenter research studies suggest that completion rates often exceed 95% [7,8]. However, the non-experts rarely publish their data, so that it is difficult to know much about overall standards in the community. A database audit of almost 20 000 colonoscopies from seven hospitals in the USA showed that only 54% of 108 endoscopists reached the cecum in more than 90% of cases [9], and even lower rates have been reported [10]. However, it is obvious that the goal of colonoscopy is not merely to reach the cecum, but rather to examine the whole mucosa and to detect/manage all lesions with acceptable levels of comfort and safety. A good example of more meaningful quality data comes from a community study which correlated polyp detection rates with withdrawal durations [11]. Recent comparative studies with CT colonography have shown that colonoscopy is not 'as good as gold' [12]. However, polyp detection rates themselves are just a surrogate marker of careful inspection; missed cancers are arguably much more important. A Canadian population based study showed signification variation in miss rates for cancer [13]. The same group have subsequently explored factors that predict incomplete colonoscopy: age, female sex and having the procedure in a private office [14]. These studies re-enforce the view that careful colonoscopy does make a difference to patients.

There are very few data on the complications of colonoscopy in community practice, and even fewer of patient acceptability. Two British studies, one of unselected practice and the other of a screening pilot, showed wide variation in perforation rates of from 1 : 769 to 1 : 4000 [5,15]. Several more widespread audits are underway in Britain (www.healthcarecommission.org.uk).

These general surveys are of interest, but we need to embrace a new paradigm—the collection of performance data for and by individual endoscopists.

The report card agenda

The American Society for Gastrointestinal Endoscopy (ASGE) recommended in 2000 that all endoscopists should keep track of their practice, but there is little evidence that many have done so. A key issue is what parameters to measure. The most comprehensive review of endoscopy performance metrics was produced by a joint working party of the ASGE and ACG [16]. An attempt to provide slightly simpler metrics was published recently [17], and other working parties are in progress. Some data points are obvious (e.g. annual procedure numbers, case mix, certain technical endpoints), and can be incorporated easily into a report card. These should be available to any interested parties, whether payers, credentialing bodies, patients, and even lawyers [18].

Sceptics of this approach put forward several arguments. They are concerned about the quality of the data, which may not be verifiable independently, and that the need to report outcomes may stimulate interventionists to avoid the most difficult and risky cases. Perhaps the most powerful point is that there is little evidence that their use in other fields (for example in cardiac surgery) has yet influenced the choices of patients or indeed payers. The final problem is that this exercise will be time consuming and expensive. Some of these concerns will fade as all endoscopy reporting becomes electronic. The performance data can be generated automatically at the time of the procedure, and easily uploaded into systems for benchmarking. Furthermore, such systems allow adjustment for case mix.

The argument for collecting and sharing data remains strong. If we do not collect the data, others will do it for us, and we will have little control over its relevance or quality. Secondly, documentation of our experience will provide some legal protection to individual endoscopists, and indeed, to those who credential them. Perhaps the most persuasive argument is that endoscopists with report cards will have a practice advantage in the future. Patients (and payers) will increasingly ask their providers for objective data on their expertise, and may well go elsewhere if it is not forthcoming or reassuring. Furthermore, there is a strong tide running in the USA for 'pay for performance', in other words tying reimbursement to outcomes. It really is time for action to supersede discussion. Professionals proud of their practice should set an example and start documenting their practice and outcomes. We should wear our data as badges of quality.

Benchmarking

If enough endoscopists collect their data, and agree to share them (albeit anonymously) in a voluntary 'quality network', it will be possible to compare practice and outcomes, and to develop benchmarks of performance. When such data are fed back to participants, they act as a powerful incentive for self-improvement [5]. Benchmarks can help to define and to raise standards. An important question is who will pay for the necessary infrastructure.

The quality of endoscopy units

The quality of an endoscopy experience depends on the environment in which it is performed, as well as on the individual practitioner, in the same way that the experience in a restaurant depends on more than the individual chef (or server). Thus it is logical to extend the concept of report cards to document the structure and function of endoscopy units. This concept has been embraced in the United Kingdom with the development of a 'global rating scale (GRS)' for endoscopy units (www.grs.nhs.uk). Initially this was simply a self-administered questionnaire on aspects of practice and process. It is now a web-based reporting tool backed up with specific measures of processes, data, and performance. The GRS has been accepted as the service standard for accreditation of endoscopy units participating in the national bowel cancer screening programme (www.bcsp.nhs.uk) and for those wishing to be accredited to train endoscopists (www.thejag.org.uk). The GRS is now being adopted by providers outside the state system with more widespread use has the potential to be used as a commissioning tool. Furthermore, the GRS has been underpinned with a knowledge management system to support quality improvement.

Conclusion

Everyone is (or should be) interested in improving the performance of endoscopy, and its documentation. We are convinced that this agenda can be advanced effectively and easily by the widespread acceptance of ongoing collection and sharing of quality data, for example, the use of report cards for endoscopists, and for endoscopy units. In most environments this will be a voluntary exercise initially, but there will be increasing peer pressure to participate. Aggregation of the data in a voluntary 'quality network' will allow benchmarking, and stimulate improvement. It is the right thing to do.

Outstanding issues and future trends

Numerous professional bodies and groups in several countries are now addressing the key issues of endoscopy performance measurement and enhancement. Soon there will be a consensus on the basic metrics, and methods for collecting and sharing the data, a process which will be greatly facilitated by electronic reporting. The resistance to 'report cards' will be overcome as their practice advantages are better appreciated, and as our patients learn to ask for the data. It remains to be seen who will provide the infrastructure needed to support this agenda, and how exactly the data will impact the quality of endoscopy in different practice environments.

References

1 Cohen J. (2004). Endoscopic training and credentialing. In: *Advanced endoscopy, e-book/annual* (ed. Cotton PB), www.gastrohep.com
2 Freeman ML. Training and competence in gastrointestinal endoscopy. *Rev Gastroenterol Disord* 2001; 1: 73–86.
3 Jowell PS, Baillie J, Branch MS, Affronti MD, Browning CL, Bute BP. Quantitative assessment of procedural competence: a prospective study of training in endoscopic retrograde cholangiopancreatography. *Ann Intern Med* 1996; 125: 983–8.
4 www.thejag.org.uk

5 Ball JE, Osbourne J, Jowett S, Pellen M, Welfare MR. Quality improvement program to achieve acceptable colonoscopy completion rates: prospective before and after study. *BMJ* 2004; 329: 665–7.

6 Cotton PB, Leung JWC (2005). *Advanced digestive endoscopy: ERCP.* Blackwell Publishing, Oxford.

7 Rex DK, Bond JH, Winawer S, Levin TR, Burt RW, Johnson DA *et al.* Quality in the technical performance of colonoscopy and the continuous quality improvement process for colonoscopy: recommendations of the U.S. Multi-Society Task Force on Colorectal Cancer. *Am J Gastroenterol* 2002; 97: 1296–305.

8 Cotton PB, Durkalski VL, Pineau BC, Palesch Y, Mauldin PD, Hoffman B *et al.* Computer tomographic colonography (virtual colonoscopy): a multicenter comparison with standard colonoscopy for detection of colorectal neoplasia lesions. *JAMA* 2004; 291: 1713–19.

9 Cotton PB, Connor P, McGee D, Jowell P, Nickl N, Schutz S *et al.* Colonoscopy: practice variation among 69 hospital-based endoscopists. *Gastrointest Endosc* 2003; 57: 352–7.

10 Bowles CJ, Leicester R, Romaya C, Swarbrick E, Williams CB, Epstein O. A prospective study of colonoscopy practice in the UK today: are we adequately prepared for national colorectal cancer screening tomorrow? *Gut* 2004; 53: 277–83.

11 Barclay RI, Vicari JJ, Doughty AS, Johanson JF, Greenlaw RI. Variation in adenoma detection rates and colonoscopic withdrawal times during screening colonoscopy. N Engl J Med. 2006; 355: 2533-41

12 Lieberman D. Colonoscopy: as good as gold? *Ann Int Med* 2004; 141: 401–3.

13 Bressler B, Paszat LF, Vinden C, Li C, He J, Rabeneck L. Colonoscopic miss rates for right-sided colon cancer: a population-based analysis. *Gastroenterology* 2004; 127: 452–4.

14 Shah HA, Paszat LF, Saskin R, Stukel TA, Rabeneck L. Factors associated with incomplete colonoscopy: a population-based study. *Gastroenterology* 2007; 132: 2297–2303.

15 UK Colorectal Cancer Screening Pilot Group. Results of the first round of a demonstration pilot of screening for colorectal cancer in the United Kingdom. *BMJ* 2004; 329: 133.

16 Faigel DO, Pike IM, Baron TH *et al.* Quality indicators for gastrointestinal endoscopy. *Gastrointest Endosc.* 2006; 63 (4 suppl): S3–9.

17 Cotton PB, Hawes RH, Barkun A, Ginsberg GG, Amman S, Cohen J *et al.* Excellence in endoscopy: toward practical metrics. *Gastrointest Endosc* 2006; 63: 286–91.

18 Cotton PB. How many times have you done this procedure, doctor? 2002; 97: 522–3.

Index

Page numbers in *italics* represent figures, those in **bold** represent tables.